Curriculum Development
and
Evaluation in Nursing

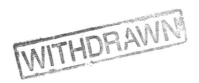

Curriculum Development and Evaluation in Nursing

Sarah B. Keating, EdD, RN, FAAN

Visiting Professor, Orvis School of Nursing
University of Nevada, Reno
Reno, Nevada

Professor Emerita and Former Dean
Samuel Merritt and Saint Mary's Colleges
Oakland and Moraga, California

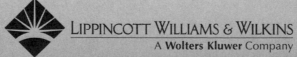

LIPPINCOTT WILLIAMS & WILKINS
A **Wolters Kluwer** Company

Philadelphia • Baltimore • New York • London
Buenos Aires • Hong Kong • Sydney • Tokyo

Senior Acquisitions Editor: Quincy McDonald
Managing Editor: Joseph Morita
Editorial Assistant: Marie Rim
Project Manager: Cynthia Rudy
Senior Production Manager: Helen Ewan
Senior Managing Editor / Production: Erika Kors
Art Director: Brett MacNaughton
Interior Designer: BJ Crim
Cover Designer: Melissa Walter
Senior Manufacturing Manager: William Alberti
Production Services / Compositor: TechBooks
Printer: R. R. Donnelley–Crawfordsville

9   8   7   6   5   4

Library of Congress Cataloging-in-Publication Data

Keating, Sarah B.
   Curriculum development and evaluation in nursing / Sarah B. Keating.
      p. cm.
   Includes bibliographical references and index.
      ISBN 13: 978-0-7817-4770-7
      ISBN 10: 0-7817-4770-8 (alk. paper)
      1. Nursing—Study and teaching. 2. Curriculum planning. 3. Curriculum evaluation. I. Title.
   RT71.K43 2006
   610.73′071′1—dc22

                                                                        2004025159

Care has been taken to confirm the accuracy of the information presented and to describe generally accepted practices. However, the authors, editors, and publisher are not responsible for errors or omissions or for any consequences from application of the information in this book and make no warranty, express or implied, with respect to the content of the publication.

The author, editors, and publisher have exerted every effort to ensure that drug selection and dosage set forth in this text are in accordance with the current recommendations and practice at the time of publication. However, in view of ongoing research, changes in government regulations, and the constant flow of information relating to drug therapy and drug reactions, the reader is urged to check the package insert for each drug for any change in indications and dosage and for added warnings and precautions. This is particularly important when the recommended agent is a new or infrequently employed drug.

Some drugs and medical devices presented in this publication have Food and Drug Administration (FDA) clearance for limited use in restricted research settings. It is the responsibility of the health care provider to ascertain the FDA status of each drug or device planned for use in his or her clinical practice.

LWW.com

For Susan and Stacen

CONTRIBUTORS

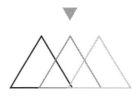

Diana L. Biordi, PhD, RN, FAAN
Professor and Assistant Dean
Research and Graduate Affairs
Kent State University College of Nursing
Kent, Ohio
(Chapter 9)

Therese A. Black, MS, RN, CNS
Nursing Faculty
Western Nevada Community College
Carson City, Nevada
(Chapter 4)

Marilyn E. Flood, PhD, RN
Associate Dean, Emeritus
School of Nursing
University of California San Francisco
San Francisco, California
(Chapter 1)

Mary Ann Haw, PhD, RN
Professor, San Francisco State University
    School of Nursing
Project Director, St. Mary's Center
    Community Nursing Project
San Francisco and Oakland, California
(Chapters 3 and 13)

Abby M. Heydman, PhD, RN
Professor, Saint Mary's College of California
Professor Emeritus, Samuel Merritt College
Oakland and Moraga, California
(Chapter 12)

Kathleen Huttlinger, PhD, RN
Professor and Director, Center for Nursing Research
Kent State University College of Nursing
Kent, Ohio
(Chapter 9)

Julie E. Johnson, PhD, RN, FAAN
Dean and Professor
Kent State College of Nursing
Kent, Ohio
(Chapter 2)

Sarah B. Keating, EdD, RN, FAAN
Visiting Professor, Orvis School of Nursing
University of Nevada, Reno
Reno, NV
Professor Emerita and Former Dean
Samuel Merritt and Saint Mary's Colleges
Oakland and Moraga, California
(Chapters 5, 6, 7, 10, 13, 14, and 15)

Ellen M. Lewis, MSN, RN, FAAN
Program Administrator Nursing & Allied Health
Clinical Professor, OB/GYN
University of California, Irvine
Irvine, California
(Chapter 11)

Robyn Marchal Nelson, DNSc, RN
Chair and Professor, Division of Nursing
California State University, Sacramento
Sacramento, California
(Chapter 8)

Arlene A. Sargent, EdD, MSN, RN
Director of Education and Research
Kaiser Permanente
Oakland, California
(Chapter 11)

Diane D. Welch, MSN, RN
Director of Nursing Programs
Sacramento City College
Sacramento, California
(Chapter 8)

REVIEWERS

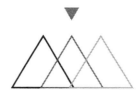

Margaret M. Anderson, EdD, RN, CNAA
Professor and Chair
Department of Nursing and Health
Northern Kentucky University
Highland Heights, Kentucky

Wanda Bonnel, PhD, RN
Associate Professor
University of Kansas School of Nursing
Kansas City, Kansas

William K. Cody, PhD, RN
Professor and Chair
Family and Community Nursing Department
UNC Charlotte School of Nursing
Charlotte, North Carolina

Ann M. Gothler, PhD, RN
Professor of Nursing
The Sage Colleges
Clifton Park, New York

Lisa-Anne Hagerman, EdD, MBA, BScN, RN
Assistant Professor
Trent University
Peterborough, Ontario, Canada

Lisa M. Lewis, PhD, RN
Instructor of Nursing Education
Teachers College, Columbia University
New York, New York

Elizabeth Mathewson, BScN, RN, MPH, COHN, CRSP
Professor of Nursing
Sir Sandford Fleming College
Peterborough, Ontario, Canada

Marylou K. McHugh, EdD, RN
Adjunct Associate Professor
Drexel University College of Nursing and
    Health Professions
Philadelphia, Pennsylvania

Lauren E. O'Hare, EdD, RN
Assistant Professor of Nursing
Wagner College
Staten Island, New York

Carole Orchard, MD, EdD, BSN
Director and Associate Professor
Memorial University School of Nursing
St. John's, Newfoundland, Canada

Linda A. Streit, RN, DSN, CCRN
Professor and Assistant Dean, Graduate Program
Georgia Baptist College of Nursing of Mercer
    University
Alpharetta, Georgia

Laura Talbot, PhD, EdD, RN, CS
Assistant Professor
Johns Hopkins University
Baltimore, Maryland

PREFACE

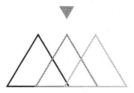

In the early 21st century, nursing shortages continue and are expected to last until at least 2020. Compounding the problem is an especially dire shortage of nursing faculty owing to too few graduate-prepared teachers and increasing numbers of older faculty retiring. The workforce shortage problem has received nationwide attention, and as a result, there has been an increase in applicants to schools of nursing; yet there are inadequate numbers of faculty members to serve the incoming students. Though the numbers of doctoral programs in nursing are rising dramatically, and there are increasing numbers of programs offered online, not all of these programs include formal courses and experiences in the art of teaching. Many of the new graduates of master's and doctorate programs are superb clinicians and researchers, but they lack curriculum development and teaching and learning knowledge and skills. In response to these issues, many schools of nursing are offering post-graduate certificates in education and degree programs with a major or minor in education at the master's and doctoral levels.

Having taught curriculum development and evaluation in nursing at the graduate level, I discovered the need for a current text on the topic. In 1982, Em Bevis published the first edition of her text, *Curriculum Building in Nursing: A Process,* which served for several decades as the leading textbook on curriculum development. In 1989, she joined with Jean Watson in publishing *Toward a Caring Curriculum: A New Pedagogy for Nursing.* This text moved away from the behaviorist theories of teaching and learning that were prevalent in nursing education and toward an emphasis on the learner and on caring. Both texts continue to serve in the development of nursing curricula; however, there is a need to build upon these precepts and add the 21st century's emphasis on transformative and constructivist learning theories, the delivery of curricula through technology, accountability in education, and the measurement of program outcomes through total quality management.

This text is meant as an introduction to curriculum development and evaluation and is intended for students in graduate programs preparing for the role of faculty members, new teachers in nursing who do not have formal education or experience in curriculum building, preceptors and mentors for students, and nurse educators in the practice setting. While the majority of nursing faculty for diploma and associate degree programs hold master's degrees and the doctorate is the preferred degree for baccalaureate and higher degree programs, this text is intended to introduce both levels to the art and science of curriculum building. Thus, it is a recipe of sorts that serves as a template for curriculum development and evaluation activities. Many of the theories and concepts used throughout this text can be adapted to staff development and health education; however, Chapter 13 devotes itself to the topic and provides specific information for nurse educators functioning in the health care setting.

It seems appropriate at this point to present the definition of curriculum as developed by this author: *A curriculum is the formal plan of study that provides the philosophical underpinnings, goals, and guidelines for the delivery of a specific educational program.* The text uses this definition of the formal curriculum throughout while recognizing the existence of the "informal" curriculum. The informal curriculum consists of activities that students, staff, or consumers experience outside of the formal, planned curriculum. Examples of the informal curriculum are interpersonal relationships, athletic/recreational activities, study groups, student, staff, and community organization activities, and special events. Although the text focuses on the planned curriculum, nurse educators should keep the informal curriculum in mind for its influences on the formal curriculum and its use in reinforcing learning activities derived from the planned curriculum.

Throughout the text, citations from the literature are referenced and represent the most recent theories at the time of publication or classic theories in nursing and education. Readers are urged to supplement these references as nursing education and other related disciplines continue to build a body of knowledge in education that is evidence-based—that is, teaching and learning activities that are based on research and generate and validate theories, concepts, and models in education and related sciences. The text begins with an introduction to curriculum through a view of the history of nursing education and its influence. As an overview, the second chapter presents the role of faculty in curriculum development and evaluation and makes the important point that faculty has the responsibility for curriculum. Without a view of the curriculum as a whole, teaching becomes parochial and of little benefit to the learners and the instructors.

The text touches briefly on instructional design through a review of learning theories, educational taxonomies, and the development of critical thinking. These concepts and theories are integral to the curriculum. Knowledge from them and preference for selected theories and taxonomies eventually provide the guidelines for the implementation of curriculum (instructional design). The text is not meant to introduce instructional design theories and guidelines, because there are already many excellent nursing texts that apply to teaching. Instead, the text is a detailed elucidation on curriculum development and evaluation.

To validate the relevance and demand for a new educational program or for those programs undergoing revision, a needs assessment is necessary. This text uses a model of the assessment of the external and internal frame factors that influence the program for gathering the data for a needs assessment and making curricular decisions based on the findings. To illustrate the application of a needs assessment, a case study is introduced and appears again in ensuing chapters that discuss the development of a curriculum with all of its components and its application through a distance education program. It should be noted that the case study is a fictionalized version of an actual feasibility study for an outreach program that subsequently proved to be quite successful.

Several chapters present a discussion of current undergraduate and graduate curricula and raise issues facing nurse educators for the future. The pivotal role of evaluation is discussed through a review of master planning and its relationship to strategic planning. Program evaluation models are discussed in light of their application to nursing curricula, and an overview of the important role of accreditation in nursing education gives advice on preparing reports and participating in site visits. While one section of the text focuses on evaluation, its concepts are interspersed throughout other chapters because it influences needs assessments and curriculum development.

The rapid changes that distance education programs and technology have had on nursing education are a major issue. The text traces the history of distance education and reviews its types and their advantages and disadvantages. Current issues and a look to the future end the text, with several proposed curricula that are meant to provoke controversy and discussion. Though the proposed curricula are not new, the progress on their implementation is painfully slow. The author pleads for speeding up the process to bring nursing education into the 21st century and to bring it in line with other health care disciplines.

The text is meant as a practical guide for developing and evaluating curricula. At the same time, it is hoped that the last chapter, with its issues and proposed curricula for entry into nursing at the doctoral level, will instigate debate and result in action that retains valuable knowledge from the past and applies newer, innovative techniques to the delivery of nursing education programs. These programs must be developed to meet the needs of society, the health care system, and the profession.

Sarah B. Keating, EdD, RN, FAAN

CONTENTS

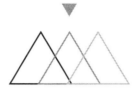

Introduction to the History of Curriculum Development and Faculty Role

▼

Sarah B. Keating, EdD, RN, FAAN

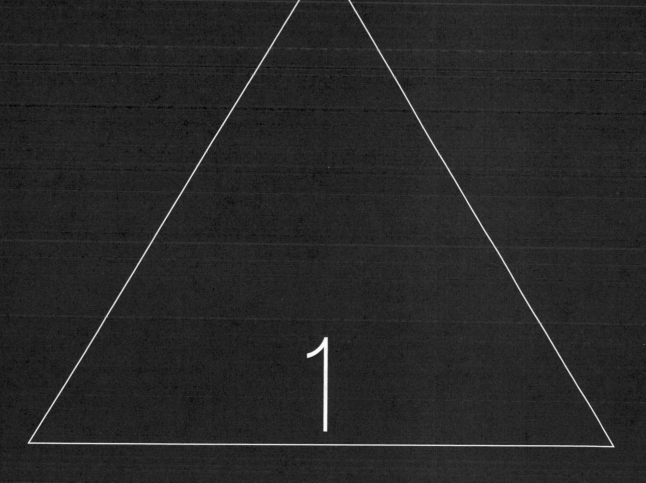

1

▲ OVERVIEW OF CURRICULUM DEVELOPMENT AND EVALUATION IN NURSING

This text devotes itself to the processes of curriculum development and evaluation. To initiate the discourse, a definition of curriculum is in order. For the purposes of the textbook, the definition is as follows: *a curriculum is the formal plan of study that provides the philosophical underpinnings, goals, and guidelines for the delivery of a specific educational program.* The text uses this formal definition throughout while recognizing the existence of the "informal" curriculum. The informal curriculum consists of activities that students, staff, or consumers experience outside of the formal, planned curriculum. Examples of the informal curriculum are interpersonal relationships; athletic/recreational activities; study groups; student, staff, and community organization activities; special events; and so forth. Although the remainder of the text will focus on the formal curriculum, nurse educators should keep the informal curriculum in mind for its influence and use it to reinforce learning activities derived from the planned curriculum.

To place curriculum development and evaluation in perspective, it is wise to examine the history of nursing education in North America and the lessons it can provide for today's curriculum developers and those in the future. Section 1 sets the stage for the process through an examination of nursing education's place in the history of higher education and the role of faculty and administrators in developing and evaluating curricula. Nursing curricula are currently undergoing transformation. Today's emphasis on continuous quality management, accountability, benchmarking, and learning organizations places yet another perspective on curriculum development and evaluation. Nursing faculty must consider all of these factors when examining the curriculum and considering change. Today and tomorrow's curricula call for an integration of processes that are learner and transactional focused and at the same time, ensure excellence in education by building in outcome measures to determine quality of the program.

▲ NURSING CURRICULA: HISTORY AND EVOLUTION

Chapter 1 traces the history of American nursing education from the time of the first Nightingale schools of nursing to the present. The trends in professional education and society's needs impacted nursing programs that started from apprentice-type schools to a majority of the programs now in institutions of higher learning. Lest those in the profession forget, liberal arts plays a major role in nursing education and sets the foundation for the development of critical thinking, cultural awareness, and a strong science background so necessary to the nursing process. Chapter 1 discusses historical events in society and the world that influenced nursing practice and education as well as major changes in the health care system. The major world wars increased the demand for nurses and the nursing education system responded by preparing a workforce ready to meet the increased demand. The emergence of nursing education that took place in community colleges in the mid-20th century initiated continuing debate about entry into practice. All of these trends and the events that brought them about and the issues they raise for the future are also discussed in Chapter 1.

Faculty Role in Curriculum Development and Evaluation

Curriculum development and evaluation are the processes by which faculty in education programs continually assess curricula and their outcomes. Based on the results of the assessment, educators refine existing curricula through minor or major revisions. In some instances, new programs are needed and the same processes that support assessment and revision produce the justification for and establishment of new programs.

It is a cardinal rule in academics that the curriculum "belongs to the faculty." In higher education, faculty members are deemed as the experts in their specific discipline or in the case of nursing, clinical specialties; therefore, they are the people who determine the content that must be transferred to and assimilated by the learner. At the same time, they should be expert teachers in the delivery of information—that is, the pedagogy, or in the case of adult learners, the oft-used term andragogy. Curriculum planning and the art of teaching are learned skills, and nursing faculty members have a responsibility to include them in their repertoire of expertise as well as being content specialists.

Nursing faculty must periodically review a program to maintain a vibrant curriculum that responds to changes in society, health care needs of the population, the health care system, and learners' needs. It is important to measure the curriculum's success in preparing nurses for the current environment as well as for the future. Currency of practice as well as that of the future must be built into the curriculum, because it will be several years before students graduate. There is an inherent requirement of the curriculum to produce caring, competent, and confident practitioners or clinicians. At the same time, the curriculum must meet professional and accreditation standards. While it is unpopular to think that curricula build upon accreditation criteria, in truth, integrating these standards into curriculum development helps faculty to prepare for program approval or review and accreditation.

Chapter 2 discusses the role and responsibilities that faculty assumes in undertaking curriculum development and evaluation. Among the responsibilities are agreement on the curriculum's mission/vision, philosophy/values, and selected organizational framework, and setting overall objectives. Additionally, faculty continually monitors the curriculum for its relevance to the health care system and needs of society and makes recommendations for changes if they are indicated. Faculty retains academic freedom in implementing the curriculum and choosing individual methods of instruction; however, individuals cannot change the pre-set goals and objectives of the program that the faculty-as-a-whole developed.

The governance of colleges and universities usually includes curriculum committees or their equivalent composed of elected faculty members. These committees are at the program level and college-wide or university-wide levels. Curriculum committees in schools of nursing receive recommendations from faculty for curriculum changes and periodically review the curriculum for its currency, authenticity, and diligence in realizing the mission, philosophy, and goals.

In addition to the day-to-day activities of curriculum development, faculty is responsible for evaluating its outcomes. Faculty members discover the need for revisions in the process of delivering the curriculum and develop formative evaluation strategies such as student examinations and course evaluations. Outcomes from the total program are measured through summative evaluation methods such as follow-up surveys of graduates and their employers and NCLEX results. Faculty plays an important role in developing the measures and responding to the feedback from graduates, employers, and other consumers of the program. To bring the curriculum into reality and out of the "Ivory Tower," faculty must include students, alumni, employers, and the people whom their graduates serve in the curriculum-building process. Partnerships among government agencies, industry, consumers, and educators are demanded from cost-effective and quality viewpoints.

Chapter 2 discusses the philosophical underpinnings of the faculty role in curriculum planning. It describes the classic hierarchy of curriculum approval processes in institutions of higher learning and the importance of nursing faculty participation within the governance of the institution. Trends in the nursing faculty role in curriculum development and evaluation are identified, and issues for the future are raised.

Best-Laid Plans:
A Century of Nursing Curricula

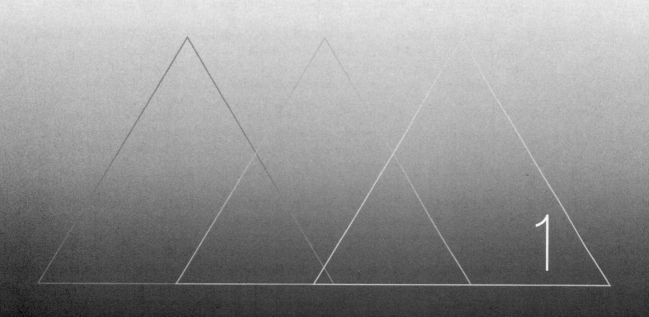

Marilyn E. Flood, PhD, RN

OBJECTIVES

Upon completion of Chapter 1, the student will be able to:

1. Compare the nursing curricular events of the 1890s with those of the 1950s.
2. Identify at least two reasons why the 1965 Position Paper occasioned so much controversy.
3. Describe significant milestones identified in the development of one program type, i.e., diploma, baccalaureate, associate degree, master's, or doctoral.
4. Provide a rationale for identifying the decade most pivotal to the development of doctoral education and provide reasons.
5. Explain the sense in which the Cadet Nurse Corps phenomenon and period was transitional—i.e., continued characteristics of preceding decades but shifted into a direction that was foundational to the next period.
6. Evaluate the impact of the history of nursing education on current and future curriculum development and evaluation activities.

▲ OVERVIEW

The roots of current curricular arrangements are entwined with the development of nursing as a distinct occupation focused on providing health-related care to strangers. Nursing developed to improve existing institutions, and then made new hospitals workable. As a consequence, hospital characteristics, from the social class of patients to the architecture of buildings, influenced nursing's roots. Medicine gradually became a dominant influence in hospitals. Nursing curricula had to take medicine's developing science and technology into account, reflect the changing boundary with medicine, and clarify the nature of nursing within medicine's hegemony.

Although postsecondary education had increasingly centered in collegiate institutions before and after World War I, nursing education remained substantially enmeshed in hospital service through the 1950s. However, both baccalaureate and associate degree programs were noticeably visible by the end of that decade. Baccalaureate preparation in nursing, which in the 1920s had been envisioned as a goal for the leaders of the profession, gradually transmuted into a basic foundational expectation for nurses. Associate degree programs, coming on the scene as junior or community colleges multiplied after World War II, married the advantages of decentralized, locally based preparation with the advantages of higher education funding, the ethos of an educational environment, and shorter elapsed time from enrollment to graduation as compared to diploma programs.

Master's curricula evolved in this same period, folding into their offerings some of the formerly freestanding postbasic specialist courses in teaching, administration, and public health. They gradually became truly postbaccalaureate curricula, and subsequently came to be oriented primarily around specialized nursing content in clinical areas. As nursing's central disciplinary identity became distinct and differentiated, the need for the capacity to train nurse researchers became pressing. Doctoral curricula were born of this need.

The 1940s, including the activity fomented in connection with the Cadet Nurse Corps, and the optimistic post–World War II planning, was a transitional decade. Certainly, forces promoting the postwar changes began their influence before 1940, and change came gradually in the following decades, but the 1940s were pivotal.

The triangulation of subject, setting, and student characteristics served to frame curriculum planning for several decades (Bevis, 1989; Bevis and Watson, 1989; Schubert, 1986) and is an equally useful framework for seeking the "why" and "whither" of nursing curriculum evolution over time. For example, conceptions about the subject of nursing changed substantially over time. Both health care and educational settings, to say nothing of the larger social order around them, changed from era to era. Additionally, students brought substantially different qualifications, expectations, and characteristics to interact with the curricula. Almost nothing happened just because "nursing decided it," but it is equally true that organized nursing, and grassroots nurses, played a significant part in shaping ideas that came to be reflected in curricula.

▲ IN THE BEGINNING

The U.S. Civil War was a catalyst for the eventual development of nursing as a paid occupation. During the war, women gave life-saving care under trying circumstances. Other women gained experience and visibility in their home cities by organizing war support efforts related to the health and welfare of soldiers. After the war, these organizing skills were brought to bear on the state of hospitals (Smith-Rosenberg, 1985). Although there were earlier training efforts of various kinds, the "standard story" usually begins with the founding in 1873 of three training schools (in New Haven, New York, and Boston), which were modeled on the Nightingale School in London (Goodnow, 1934). By 1880, there were 15 schools, and by 1890, there were 35. Most of these schools, and the 2,000 more that would be founded in the next 30 years, consisted primarily of on-the-job training mixed with regimented living and working. This "curriculum" was intended to develop proper character traits and habits (Tomes, 1984). The "pupils" were the nursing service for the hospital, which offered its imprimatur, in the form of diplomas and pins, for enduring this training for the stipulated time. The programs grew from 1 year, to 2 years, and then to 3 years by the mid-1890s. The hours of work were like those of women in households, i.e. from arising in the morning to retiring to sleep at night. Students came one by one as they were available and their services were needed. The patients were mostly poor, without families and/or homes to provide care. From the institution's standpoint, graduates were a byproduct rather than a purpose for the training school. "Trained nurses" generally gave private care in wealthy homes, administered/trained pupils in a training school, or cared for the poor in their homes after graduation (Reverby, 1984).

Despite the existence of the training schools and some public awareness of the abilities of the "trained nurse," the domestic roots of nursing were still very much in evidence. Every woman expected to nurse family members. Older women, who had extensive family experience and needed to earn a living, would care for neighbors or contacts by word-of-mouth-referrals (Reverby, 1987). In some places, short courses in nursing were offered and advertised to women who wanted to learn better in-family care and to those who were preparing to take care of strangers in a hospital (D'Antonio, 1987, 1993). The title of the Clara Weeks-Shaw's *A Text-Book for Nursing: For the Use of Training Schools, Families, and Private Students,* first published in 1885, clearly reflects the breadth of the nursing audience in that era. Inside its pages, however, the hospital context has considerable attention, and the third edition in 1902 identifies the primary audience as "professional" nurses rather than "amateurs." It assumed that students had an elementary acquaintance with anatomy and physiology, "which is now a fundamental part of training."

Physician-authored texts about nursing and for nurses were commonplace, while nurse-authorship was pioneered in Britain. Clara Weeks (later Weeks-Shaw), a graduate of the New York Hospital in 1880 and founding superintendent of the Paterson General Hospital School from 1883 to1888, wrote the first widely disseminated text in the United States (Obituary, 1940). The possession of such a text decreased the dependence of graduates on their course notes and supplied information that otherwise would have been missed because of cancelled lectures or note-taking student exhaustion. The text reinforced the idea that nursing required more than fine character and exerted a subtle standardizing effect on training school expectations. Such a text today, with its reference to managing the fire in the fireplace during the night and to candles as light sources, jars readers into considering differences of setting. The approximately 100 names in the comprehensive list of medicines, including ether, oxygen, topical agents, and multiple names for the same substance, subverted efforts to keep nurses ignorant of the names of medicines they were administering. Although the topics of venesection and transfusion are listed, venesection was by cut-down at the elbow and transfusion referred to administration of a quart of normal saline over a half hour by a glass canula placed in the vein (Weeks-Shaw, 1902).

The 1890s

The International Congress of Charities, Correction and Philanthropy met in Chicago as part of the Columbian Exposition of 1893. Isabel Hampton, the founding principal of the training school and superintendent of nurses at Johns Hopkins Hospital, played a leading role in planning the nursing sessions for the congress. At a plenary session she presented a paper, "Educational Standards for Nurses," which overtly argued for the responsibility of hospitals to provide actual education for students and the urgent need for superintendents to work together to establish standards (James, 2002). The paper included her proposal to extend the training period to 3 years to allow the shortening of the "practical training" to 8 hours per day, and to make it possible to admit pupils into classes with "stated times for entrance into the school, and the teaching year...divided according to the academic terms usually adopted in our public schools and colleges" (Robb, 1907). During the week of the congress, Hampton instigated an informal meeting of nursing superintendents that laid the groundwork for the formation of the American Society of Superintendents of Training Schools in the United States and Canada (ASSTS), which later, in 1911, was renamed the National League of Nursing Education (NLNE). Certainly a landmark event within nursing, this was the first association of a professional nature organized and controlled by women (Bullough & Bullough, 1978).

The year 1893 also marked the publication of Hampton's *Nursing: Its Principles and Practice for Hospital and Private Use.* The first 25 pages are devoted to a description of a training school, including physical facilities, contents of a reference library, a 2-year curriculum plan—for both didactic content and planned, regular clinical rotations from service to service—and examinations. Hampton notably omitted reference to the pupil nurse residence as a character-training instrument in the training school system, though she noted in other contexts the importance of the residence for the health and social development of students (Dodd, 2001). Clearly, she was pushing for a progressive professional education and a professional identity for nursing.

In this century, professionhood seems an obvious direction for the efforts of Hampton and others such as Lillian Wald and Lavinia Dock, who have been canonized as early leaders. But throughout the first 75 years of nursing's history as an intentional occupation, many nurses would have deeply disagreed with this as a goal. Barbara Melosh (1982) aptly describes the image many held of nursing as "not merely a profession," but a calling, or an expression of true womanhood. Coexisting with these ideals, she acknowledges, were nurses who intended to give good care but who primarily just needed a means of livelihood. A part of Hampton's genius was her ability to embody the womanly service ideals and to talk in the language of calling, while focusing her efforts toward professionalization and arguing for the health and welfare of nurses. For her these were not divergent goals, but aspects of an integrated whole.

Hampton's Johns Hopkins was absolutely atypical of training schools and was sometimes spoken of as a normal school for nursing. It offered a model of what might have been done had other training schools been as well resourced socially, educationally, and financially (Baldwin, 2002). Although an organizational mechanism (the ASSTS/NLNE) had been initiated to set standards and provide a network of like-minded superintendents with high educational aspirations, the momentum for hospital founding with corequisite training schools drove the demand for pupils and their 12-hour days or nights of work on the wards. Many schools gave just enough on-the-job training to adequately meet their own hospital's needs. In 1890, there were 35 training schools. By 1900, there were 432, and by 1905, 862. The number of training schools peaked at 2,155 in 1926, and then a long contraction began. Hampton's proposal for a 3-year program length was rapidly adopted by hospitals large and small, but without the 8-hour day.

Retrospective From 1940

From the vantage point of administrator-educators in 1940, the 1890s were a world away. They had just lived through a decade of the Depression that resisted governmental fixes. The immediate circumstances of the prior decade demanded innovation to meet new problems. Patients who formerly hired private nurses to care for them in the hospital instead came to the wards composed of four- to 10-bedrooms rather than 30-bed halls, where the student service provided care. Students came as members of a nursing class, and attrition was hard to predict; therefore, the ballooning census on the wards made it necessary to hire graduate nurses temporarily that were often unemployed private duty nurses. The most notable change since 1890 was that people who had homes and families came to hospitals for care rather than receiving care at home (Vogel, 1980). In scattered local areas, systems of health insurance were now available, making this a factor for the care of covered patients and for hospitals. Except in remote places, surgery and its after-care were now hospital events. Nurses still did private duty nursing in homes, but increasingly they cared for their individual patients in the hospital context. Public health nursing attracted graduates who wanted more autonomy and engagement with broader health concerns. Several factors (e.g., hospital architecture, physician expectations, nursing efforts, and general culture change) contributed to increased expectations for cognitive learning by students. With markedly increased numbers of applicants during the Depression, many more schools were able to select capable students and to grant diplomas that signified both cognitive learning and character.

National Reports and Standards 1911–1937

The Grading Committee worked from 1926 to 1934 to produce educational programs' "gradings" based on answers to survey forms. Each school received individualized feedback about its own characteristics in comparison to all other participating schools (Committee on the Grading of Nursing Schools, 1931). The NLNE's 1927 *A Curriculum for Schools of Nursing* (see next page) provided the implicit framework for the surveys and reports. Although the original hope was that the committee would rank schools into A, B, and C categories, the committee pointed out that the work and cost of visiting 2,205 schools made this impossible.

Even without this actual "grading," the gradings provided more data than nursing ever had about its schools. For example, it found that the average U.S. nursing school had 10 faculty members: the superintendent of the hospital, the superintendent of nurses, the night supervisor, the day supervisor, two heads of special departments (usually operating room and delivery room), one assistant in a special department, two other head nurses, and one instructor. This median varied by region from four to 17 faculty members. Forty-two percent of the faculty had not completed high school. Forty-five percent of superintendents of nursing came to their positions more recently than the senior students' admission dates.

Hospital schools in the period between World Wars I and II presented a highly variable picture. Some still offered only apprenticeship learning. However, without "master craftswoman" nurses and with a social milieu more consonant with turn-of-the-century culture, they gave nursing a backward, rigid quality that was susceptible to caricature. Others were pushing their limits to provide stimulating learning and an environment more akin to other educational institutions (Egenes, 1998).

The Grading Committee's reports joined a series of reports dating back to 1910, when the American Hospital Association formed a committee to make recommendations regarding the length of the nurse training course, a model curriculum, and the training of nurse helpers. The resulting model curriculum for large general hospitals and small hospitals, which could affiliate with larger, was a graded 3-year curriculum. It contained different subjects to be taught in each of the 3 years and was intended for students who had at least 1 year of high school. It included a plan for a 3-month preliminary period that was primarily educational with a secondary emphasis on practice. Notably, it took the position that specialty hospitals should not have training schools (with the exception of psychiatric hospital schools, which could affiliate with general hospitals), and it completely ignored the charge to deal with the subject of nurse helpers or assistants. This report included a topical listing of curriculum content with broad ranges of possible hours per topic (Aikens, 1911).

In 1917, 1927, and 1937, the NLNE published a series of curriculum recommendations in book form. The reaction to the title of the first, *Standard Curriculum...*, led to naming the second *A Curriculum...* and the third *A Curriculum Guide....* The first was developed by a relatively small group, but the second and third involved a long process with broad input, which, even apart from the product, served an important function. The published curricula were intended to set the pace, i.e., to reflect a generalization about what the better schools were doing or aimed to do. As such, they give a picture of change over the 20-year period but cannot be regarded as providing a snapshot of a typical school. Each volume represents substantial change from the previous, and where the same course topical area exists in all three, the level of detail and specificity increased with each decade. Indeed, the markedly increased length and wordy style of the 1937 volume appropriately carries in the title the word "guide."

Each *Curriculum* book increased the number of classroom hours and decreased the recommended hours of patient care, in effect making the nursing service more expensive. Each *Curriculum* also increased the prerequisite educational level: 4 years of high school, but temporary tolerance of 2 years in 1917; 4 years of high school in 1927; and 1 to 2 years of college or normal school in addition to high school by 1937 (National League of Nursing Education, 1917, 1927, 1937). This was a selective standard, which was more easily met by students from urban homes. In 1920, only 16.8% of the age cohort graduated from high school; in 1930, 20%; and in 1940, 50.8% (Tyack, 1974). It was not until the 1930s, with the depressed labor market and enforcement of child labor and mandatory attendance laws, that one-third of the age cohort nationally attended high school. With the beginnings of a nursing school accreditation mechanism before World War II, and the postwar National Nursing Accrediting Service, the functions that the *Curriculum* books were intended to serve were now incarnated by consultants and supplanted by concise written standards (Committee of the Six National Nursing Organizations on Unification of Accrediting Services, 1949).

NURSING AND HIGHER EDUCATION

Starting in the early 1900s, universities began to enfold such nontraditional fields as education, business administration, and engineering. These had originally been taught in freestanding, single-purpose institutions (Veysey, 1965). In the period between World Wars I and II, the university became the dominant institution in the postsecondary landscape (Graham, 1978). From 1920 to 1940, the percentage of women attending college from the 18-to-21-year-old cohort rose from 7.6% to 12.2%. Men's college-going rates rose faster, and thus the percentage of women in the student body dropped from 43% in 1920 to 40.2% in 1940 (Eisenmann, 2000; Solomon, 1985).

Nursing made overtures to a few colleges and universities prior to World War I. In 1899, the American Society of Superintendents of Training Schools developed the Hospital Economics program for nurses who had potential as superintendents of hospitals and training schools. The program involved 8 months of study using many courses existing in the Domestic Science department, but with a custom-designed course on teaching and a Hospital Economics course that would be taught by nurses. It was expected that the nurse-students could earn sufficient money doing 3 to 4 months of private duty before or after the 8 months to cover the $400 cost of the course (Robb, 1907). This relationship with Teachers College grew and was cemented by the endowment in 1910 of a Chair in Nursing, occupied for many years by M. Adelaide Nutting. The nursing faculty at Teachers College continued to be unusually influential in nursing education through the 1950s, when other centers began to share influence.

In the first decade of the 1900s, technical institutes such as Drexel in Philadelphia, Pratt in Brooklyn, and Mechanics in Rochester, as well as Simmons College in Boston and Northwestern University in Chicago, offered coursework to nursing students in the preliminary period (Robb, 1907). The designers of the 1917 *Standard Curriculum* gave some thought to the relationship of nursing education to the collegiate system. In an appendix, they provided their calculations that led them to suggest that the theoretical work in a nursing school was equivalent to 36 units, or about 1 year of college, and the clinical work another 51 units. Also in 1917–1918, with popular patriotism running high and nursing the only entrée for women to direct involvement in World War I, more than 400 college graduates who attended a 12-week preliminary course on the Vassar campus in 1918 subsequently attended schools of nursing across the country. Participating schools committed to a program of just 2 additional years of study. Student motivation waned with the early armistice and the rigid atmosphere in some of the schools, so only 42% of the original group graduated from schools of nursing (Armeny, 1983; Gage, 1918; Roberts, 1954).

Over time, a number of ideas were put forward for changing the organization and sponsorship of nursing instruction, among them the idea of aligning nursing within institutions of higher education. However, few voices actively campaigned for this idea even as late as the 1930s, despite the recommendation of the Rockefeller-funded Goldmark report *Nursing and Nursing Education in the United States* in the early 1920s (1923). Initially such a program was envisioned solely for the leaders of training schools.

Educators who wanted a university context for nursing, and thereby concentration on educational goals and emancipation from dependence on the hospitals' student work-study schemes, looked hopefully at the Yale University School of Nursing, funded by the Rockefeller Foundation starting in 1924 and headed by the determined and respected Annie W. Goodrich. Similarly encouraging was the program at Western Reserve University, endowed by Francis

Payne Bolton in 1923 following considerable prior work within the Cleveland civic community. Vanderbilt was endowed by a combination of Rockefeller, Carnegie, and Commonwealth Funds in 1930. University of Chicago established a school of nursing in 1925 which benefitted from an endowment from the distinguished but discontinued Illinois Training School (Hanson, 1991). Dillard University established a school in 1942 with substantial foundation support and governmental war-related funds. Mary Tennant, nursing adviser in the Rockefeller Foundation, pronounced the Dillard Division of Nursing "one of the most interesting developments in nursing education in the country, irrespective of race" (Hine, 1989). Although these were milestone events, endowments did not cure all that was ailing in nursing education. Neither did they lead immediately to programs that would be accreditable by the standards of later decades (Faddis, 1973; Kalisch & Kalisch, 1978; Sheahan, 1980).

According to the *Journal of the American Medical Association*, 25 universities granted bachelor's degrees to nurses by 1926 (JAMA, 1927). By the end of the 1930s a bewildering array of "collegiate" programs existed, partly because baccalaureate programs were being invented by trial and error within the combinations of opportunities and constraints presented in each local hospital and university pair (Petry, 1937).

▲ THE CADET NURSE CORPS

World War II, with its demands for all able-bodied young men for military service, mobilized available women for employment or volunteer service. Indeed every resident was engaged in the effort by the mandates of food, clothing, and gasoline rationing, and by persuasion toward everything from tending victory gardens to buying savings bonds. From mid-1941 to mid-1943, with the help of federal aid, nursing schools increased their enrollments by 13,000 over the baseline year, and 4,000 postdiploma nurses completed postbasic course work to enable them to fill the places of nurses who had enlisted, and some inactive nurses returned to practice (Roberts, 1954). Despite the effort necessary to bring about this increase, hospitals were floundering and more nurses were needed for the military services.

Congress passed the Bolton Act, which authorized the complex of activities known as the Cadet Nurse Corps (CNC) in June 1943. It was conceived as a mechanism to avoid civilian hospital collapse (in the absence of the one-fourth of all active nurses who went to war), to provide nursing to the military, and to ensure an adequate education for student nurse cadets. The goal was to recruit 65,000 high school graduates into nursing schools in the first year (1943–1944) and 60,000 the next year. This represented 10% of girls graduating from high school and the whole percentage of those who would expect to go to college! The program exceeded the goals for both years (Kalisch & Kalisch, 1978).

Hospitals sponsoring training schools recognized that CNC schools would out-recruit noncadet schools, thereby almost certainly guaranteeing their closure or radical shrinkage. Thus they signed on, despite the fact that hospitals had to establish a separate accounting system for school costs, literally meet the requirements of their state boards of nurse examiners to the satisfaction of the CNC consultants, and allow their students to leave for federal service during the last 6 months of their programs, when they would otherwise be most valuable to their home schools. Schools received partial funding from a separate appropriation for modifications necessary to build classrooms and library space and to secure additional student housing. Visiting consultants looked at faculty numbers and qualifications, clinical facilities available for learning, curricula, hours of student clinical and class work, the school's ability to accelerate course work to fit in 30 months, and the optimal number of students the school could accommodate (Robinson & Perry, 2001). Only high school graduates could qualify to become cadets (Petry, 1943). Schools were pressed to increase the size of their classes and number of classes admitted per year, to use local colleges for basic sciences to conserve nurse instructor time, and to make affiliations with psychiatric hospitals, both for educational reasons and secondarily to free up dormitory space for more students to be admitted. Consultants could give 3-, 6-, or 12-month conditional approval while deficiencies were corrected (Robinson & Perry, 2001). Given the pressure to keep CNC-approved status, schools made painful changes.

Students, who were estimated to be providing 80% of care in civilian hospitals, experienced a changed practice context. They now had to decide what they could safely delegate to Red Cross volunteers and any paid aides available. Extra responsibility for nursing arose from the shortage of physicians. With grossly short staffing, nurses had to set priorities carefully. All of these circumstances altered student learning, whether or not they were codified in course content or lesson plans. The intense work of the consultants, who provided interpretation and linkage between the United States Public Health Service (USPHS) in Washington and each school, and their strategy of simultaneously naming deficiencies and identifying improvement goals was a critical factor in the success of the program and in the improvement in nursing education. Without the financial resources of the federal government to defray student costs, to assist with certain costs to schools, and to provide the consultation, auditing, and public relations/recruitment functions, the goals could not have been met. Lucile Petry, the director of the Division of Nursing Education in the USPHS, combined a sense of the social significance of nursing with first-hand experience in nursing education and a humility that equipped her to work with all kinds of people and generously give credit to everyone involved in the massive undertaking. Opinions differed on such questions as the cut-off point for irredeemably weak schools, but overall the effort was pronounced a substantial success for nursing (Roberts, 1954).

After the end of the war in 1945, much of the remainder of the decade was devoted to reversing the changes occasioned by mobilization and absorbing the new postwar reality. Among the benefits for returning military—including nurses—was funding for higher education. This gave unexpected access to colleges and universities and expanded the public's aspirations for higher education.

▲1950–2000

Nursing curricula were transformed in the years from 1950 to 2000. Change in the intervening years was at least as great as from 1890 to 1940. Consider, for example, the gradual sorting out of the wildly idiosyncratic arrangements that were forged between hospital schools and colleges in the preceding decades and the bewildering array of postbasic courses for nurses offered by various units of colleges and universities. Even degree-granting programs, both bachelor's and master's, were variable in sequencing, unit value and scheduling, and terminal expectations in the 1950s. Experiments to sponsor nurse programs in junior or community colleges were underway in the 1950s. Even the hospital-sponsored diploma programs, which dramatically decreased in number during these years, were substantially transformed into educationally focused efforts. By the early 1970s, the rich but disorderly profusion of the 1950s was regularized, most immediately through the influence of accreditation processes. By the late 1960s, master's programs were beginning to prepare clinical nurse specialists and the literature described nurse practitioner roles. Coronary care and intensive care units were requiring staff nurses to exercise judgment and take action in a far wider range of clinical situations than formerly acknowledged within nursing's scope of practice, and educators were trying to sort out the implications of this for both graduate and undergraduate programs. These developments in practice, together with educators' decisions to focus graduate preparation on nursing rather than on teaching and administration, transformed master's programs. Research capacity grew and research training in doctoral programs developed.

The relentless drumbeat of talk about "the hospital nursing shortage" continued through much of these 50 years, with a hiatus only in the early 1990s. Given the expansion in bed capacity fueled by Hill-Burton legislation and subsequent similar funding, expanded private insurance coverage, the advent of Medicare and Medicaid, and the development of technology to treat a wider range of patients intensively, the increased demand for nurses was not surprising. Supply-side solutions could not keep up with demand, even though nurses gradually increased their workforce participation rates to a very high level. Nurse wages, however, did not rise sufficiently to give hospitals incentives to treat nurses as a scarce resource and thus bring supply and demand into equilibrium (Lynaugh & Brush, 1996).

Accreditation

From the standpoint of the ordinary nursing school, the possibility of actual accreditation became a reality in the 1950s. The National League for Nursing Education (NLNE) developed standards for accreditation and made pilot visits from 1934 to 1938. By 1939, schools could list themselves to be visited so that they could qualify to be on the first list published by NLNE. Despite the greatly increased work, turnover, and general disruption created by the war, 100 schools mustered both the courage and energy required to prepare for accreditation evaluation and were judged creditable by 1945. The substantial number of schools that qualified for provisional accreditation, however, was due for revisiting by the end of the war. The Association of Collegiate Schools of Nursing (ACSN), formed in 1932, exercised a kind of "accreditation" via its requirements for full and associate membership, but its standards primarily influenced schools that aspired to be part of this group or that attended conferences it cosponsored. Only 26 schools were accredited by ACSN in 1949. The National Organization for Public Health Nursing (NOPHN) had accredited postbasic programs in public health since 1920, but more recently had considered specialty programs at both baccalaureate and master's levels and the public health content in generalist baccalaureate programs (Harms, 1954). By 1948, these organizations, along with the Council of Nursing Education of Catholic Hospitals, ceded their accrediting role to the National Nursing Accrediting Service (NNAS), which published its first combined list of accredited programs just 1 month before the survey-based interim classification of schools was published by the National Committee for the Improvement of Nursing Services (NCINS) in 1949 (Petry, 1949). The classification put schools in either Group I, the top 25% of schools, or Group II, the middle 50%, leaving other schools unlisted and unclassified.

The NNAS, much like the Cadet Nurse program before it, elected a strategy designed to entice schools with at least minimal strengths to improve. It published the first list of temporarily accredited schools in 1952, giving these schools 5 years to make improvements and qualify for full accreditation. During the intervening time, it provided many special meetings, self-evaluation guides, and consultant visits to the schools. By 1957, the number of fully accredited schools increased by 72.4% (Kalisch & Kalisch, 1978). Changes in hospital school programs were catalyzed and channeled by accreditation norms (Committee of the Six National Nursing Organizations on Unification of Accrediting Services, 1949). Ultimately, the forces that drove change were primarily external, ranging from public expectations of postsecondary education mediated through hospital trustees and physicians to competition among programs for potential students, who now had access to information about accreditation and who were recruited heavily by schools that still had substantial responsibility for nursing service. By 1950, all states participated in the State Board Test Pool examination, another measuring rod that induced improvement or closure of weaker schools.

Despite the influential Carnegie- and Sage-funded *Nursing for the Future* in 1948, which recommended a broad-based move of nursing education into general higher education, nursing's earliest centralized accreditation mechanism concentrated considerable energy on improving diploma schools, as had the Grading Committee before it (Brown, 1948, Roberts, 1954). Why this seeming mismatch between aspirations and effort? Partly it sprang from realism: Students were in hospital schools, whether ideal or not, so they needed the best possible preparation because nursing services would reflect this quality. (Postgraduation learning via staff development or socialization into the traditions of a service was not considered a significant factor.) Further, the quality of many of the baccalaureate programs left a great deal to be desired and their capacity for more students was limited, so these could not be promoted as an immediate or ideal substitute for diploma programs. Although by 1957 there were 18 associate degree programs (Kalisch & Kalisch, 1978), no one foresaw the speed of their multiplication in the next decade. Finally, nursing's collective sense of social responsibility burdened it with finding ways to continue to provide essential services, both within the hospital and elsewhere, as its educational house moved from the base of the hospital to the foundation of higher education (Lynaugh, 2002).

Baccalaureate Education

The diverse baccalaureate curricula of the 1930s multiplied by the 1950s. As one educator wrote in 1954:

> Baccalaureate programs still seem to be in the experimental stage. They vary in purpose, structure, subject matter content, admission requirements, matriculation requirements, and degrees granted upon their completion. Some schools offering baccalaureate programs still aim to prepare nurses for specialized positions. Others, advancing from this traditional concept, seek to prepare graduates for generalized nursing in beginning positions (Harms, 1954).

Although a few programs threaded general education and foundational science courses through 5 years of study, the majority structured their programs with 2 years of college courses before or after the 3 years of nursing preparation, or book-ended the nursing years with the split 2 years of college work (Bridgman, 1949). Margaret Bridgman, an educator from Skidmore College who consulted with a large number of nursing schools, made favorable reference to the "upper division nursing major" in her volume directed toward both college and nursing educators (Bridgman, 1953). The paramount issues, she said, were whether or not (1) the academic institution and academic goals had meaningful involvement and influence in the program as a whole, and (2) degree-goal and diploma-goal students were comingled in nursing courses. Programs, which failed the first test criterion, were termed the "affiliated" type. In 1950, 129 of 195 schools offering a basic (prelicensure) program were of the affiliated type. In 1953, 104 of the 199 schools still offered both degree and diploma programs (Harms, 1954), and given the pragmatics of programs, probably comingled the two types of students in courses. To further complicate the situation, only 9,000 of the 21,000 baccalaureate students in 1950 were prelicensure students. The remaining 12,000 postdiploma baccalaureate students were not evenly distributed among schools, thus some programs found themselves with a sprinkling of prelicensure students among a class of experienced diploma graduates.

Bridgman recommended that postdiploma students be evaluated individually and provisionally with a tentative grant of credit based on prior learning, including nursing schoolwork, and successful completion of a term of academic work. The student's program would be made up of "deficiencies" in general education and prerequisite courses, and then courses in the major itself. Credit-granting practices varied considerably from place to place; thus, a nurse could easily spend 1½ to 3 years earning the baccalaureate (Bridgman, 1953). National nursing organizations elected not to update the curriculum guide in the late 1940s, perhaps because the 1937 guide still presented challenges, but Bridgman provided "suggestions for content" using the categories of:

1. knowledge from the physical and biologic sciences,
2. communication skills,
3. the major in nursing,
4. knowledge from social science (sociology, social anthropology, and psychology), and
5. general education, all of which she thought should ideally be interrelated throughout the program.

Of the 199 colleges and universities offering programs leading to bachelor's degrees in 1953, the National Nursing Accrediting Service accredited 51 basic programs.

Given the constant expansion of knowledge relevant to nursing, it was doubly difficult for programs with a history of a 5-year curriculum to shrink to 4 academic years in the 1960s and early 1970s. The expanded assessment skills expected of coronary and critical care nurses, together with the master's-level emphasis in clinical nurse specialist and certificate nurse practitioner programs, stimulated the inclusion of more sophisticated skills in baccalaureate programs in the early to mid-1970s. In response to nursing service agitation to narrow the gap between new graduate organizing skills and initial employment expectations, and much talk about "reality shock," baccalaureate programs structured curricula to allow a final experience in which students were immersed in clinical care and focused on skills of organization and integration, stimulated by a multi-patient assignment.

Associate degree–prepared nurses of the early 1980s found expectations and mechanisms for matriculating into baccalaureate programs much more clearly defined than described by Bridgman; indeed, some baccalaureate programs were designed specifically for associate degree graduates. The ever-expanding body of nursing knowledge forced repeated decisions about which content was most essential and what clinical settings would bring about best learning. By the 1990s, as hospital censuses plummeted and sick patients shuttled back and forth between home and ambulatory settings, programs were forced to consider increasing community-based clinical experience with its attendant challenges to find placements and provide geographically dispersed instruction.

Associate Degree Programs

Programs of the 1950s in senior colleges had to cope with the entrenched traditions of both hospitals and universities as they struggled to make changes. By contrast, associate degree nursing programs began with a clean slate. They were initially welcomed by community colleges. The lure of having an additional supply of nurses promoted at least grudging cooperation from clinical agencies, although hospital nursing staff and administrators in many places had misgivings about the curricular arrangements and limited clinical experience of students.

At the height of the government-supported access to college for veterans after World War II, the President's Commission on Higher Education projected that a much higher proportion of young Americans had the ability to do postsecondary work than before the war. The commission envisioned low-cost-to-student education at both the community colleges and the former normal schools that were increasingly redesignated as colleges (the President's Commission on Higher Education, 1947). Junior colleges had existed for some time and California developed many public junior colleges, which had dual classification as grades 13 and 14 of secondary education and years 1 and 2 of college (Lavine, 1986). Emphasis formerly had been on preparing students to qualify for junior year standing in senior colleges. The postwar conversation in educational circles focused on transforming the "junior" college into a "community" college, which would provide preparation for fields and required only 2 years of postsecondary study, while continuing to fulfill the transfer function. In this period, the excitement and the new thinking in junior college circles was on development of terminal programs to serve the needs of local students and local employers (Haase, 1990).

In early 1950, representatives of NLNE approached their counterparts at the American Association of Junior Colleges (AAJC) suggesting that they form a joint committee, including the Association of Collegiate Schools of Nursing, to study nursing education. The focus was to be the "Brown report", that is, *Nursing for the Future* authored by Esther Lucille Brown, a social anthropologist with the Russell Sage Foundation (Brown, 1948). The immediate context for the committee, from the nursing side, was significant: In 1947, the board of NLNE adopted the policy goal that nursing education should be located in the higher education system. Also in 1947, the faculty at Teachers College Columbia launched a planning process that involved Eli Ginzberg, a young economist, who thought that nursing could be thought of as a whole set of functions and roles rather than a single role or type of worker. He posited that nursing needed at least two types of practitioners, one professional and one technical (Haase, 1990).

Starting in the fall of 1947, Brown began her conferences with nursing leaders and visits to more than 50 schools, completing her report so that it could be disseminated in September 1948. In one section of the report, she compared nursing to engineering, with its highly valued technical workers. She believed that perhaps a "graduate bedside nurse" needed more preparation than a practical nurse, but less than a full-fledged professional nurse. In early

1949, NLNE sought funding for the joint work with community colleges, and found Russell Sage and W.K. Kellogg Foundations responsive with substantial support (Haase, 1990).

By May of 1950, nurse members of the AAJE-NLNE-ACSN Joint Committee reported to the NLNE board that two possibilities were under consideration: (1) a 2-year program in nursing with transfer at the end of the 2 years to a senior university and (2) a 3-year program to end in an Associate in Arts or Associate in Science degree and qualification to take the state board licensing examination. Later in the year the Joint Committee indicated its interest in (1) education of practical nurses, (2) providing associate degree study that would form the base for baccalaureate study, and (3) in-service training for hospital staffs. Concurrently in 1950, Mildred Montag, a doctoral student at Teachers College, Columbia, used her dissertation to work out the philosophy and plan for a new kind of nursing program, and designed a plan for testing the viability of such a program. She was subsequently appointed to the Joint Committee in 1951 and became the project director for the anonymously funded Cooperative Research Project (CRP) in Junior and Community College Education for Nursing in early 1952 (Haase, 1990).

The CRP pilot programs were 2 years long or 2 years plus a summer. Initially they were one-third general education and two-thirds nursing, but they moved toward equal proportions of each by the end of the project. The curricula, although controlled by faculty in each school, tended to focus on variations in health in their first year, and then deviations from normal, i.e., physical and mental illness, in the second year. These "broad fields" were accompanied by campus nursing laboratory learning and by clinical learning experiences in a wide variety of client- or patient-care settings, but with a major hospital component. Students in the pilot programs were somewhat older than diploma or baccalaureate students and some were married (a nonstarter in diploma programs) and had children. Men were a small percentage of the students, but tripled the representation in diploma programs. State board examination pass rates for graduates of the pilot group were comparable to those of other programs.

From the mid-1950s to mid-1970s, when the associate degree program growth rate peaked, the number of programs doubled about every 4 years. By 1975 there were 618 associate degree programs in nursing, comprising 45% of basic nursing programs and graduating a comparable percentage of new graduates each year. Diploma programs comprised 31% of basic programs, though given the recency of associate degree program development, the vast majority of nurses in practice still had come originally from diploma programs (Haase, 1990; Rines, 1977). By 1959, W.K. Kellogg Foundation assistance to the expansion of associate degree nursing education totaled more than $3 million. The Nurse Training Act of 1964 and subsequent federal legislation funding nursing also contributed to program growth (Scott, 1972).

Over the ensuing years, elapsed time from enrollment to graduation lengthened, due in part to the expanding knowledge base needed to be "a bedside nurse," but also, pressures from elsewhere on campuses to expand general education, sequencing requirements of the nursing faculty, the level of preparation and ability that students brought, and/or student choice. Much time was devoted to communicating with hospital nursing service representatives to identify students' competencies at graduation so that new graduate orientations and staff development plans articulated with them. Curricular offerings were fine-tuned to ensure that these baseline competencies were met. When "the bedside" was no longer in the hospital, questions about preparation for practice in the home-care context arose temporarily, but the familiar condition of hospital "nursing shortage" laid these to rest.

Nursing Education Civil War

The cultural upheaval that characterized the mid-1960s through the 1970s had its counterpart in nursing. Within nursing, a rift grew between those who believed an incremental approach would eventually get nursing education situated optimally, undefined though it was, and those who believed that the eventual goal should be clearly specified far in advance so that changes could take the goal into account. Nurses involved in day-to-day patient care and many diploma nurse educators tended to cluster in the first group, and those, particularly educators, who were in national or regional leadership positions were in the second group. The latter group was focused on the professional end of the nursing continuum, working to achieve the fullest possible academic and professional recognition for nursing so that its advocacy and action would have broad credibility and influence.

From this perspective, the American Nurses Association 1965 position paper, "Educational Preparation for Nurse Practitioners and Assistants to Nurses," seemed like the next logical step (ANA, 1965). After all, for more than 15 years the NLNE, reconstituted and combined with the NOPHN, ACSN, and National Association of Industrial Nurses (NAIN) in 1952 to be the National League for Nursing (NLN), had been saying that education for nursing belonged in institutions of higher education. The idea that nursing was a continuum, comprised of vocational, technical, and professional segments, had been talked about intermittently in those same circles during that entire period.

Unfortunately, the Position Paper dropped like a bomb on people who had never heard these conversations. It was said to ignore diploma schools and nurses altogether, classify associate degree–prepared nurses as technical nurses, and downgrade vocational/practical nurse preparation. Fundamental questions, such as the "fit" of the three-part typology with the range of nursing work, the location and nature of the boundaries between the segments of the continuum, and the regulatory and licensure implications of such a plan, could hardly be debated because of the emotionality that surrounded the specter of the loss of access to the "RN" title for associate and diploma nurses and what appeared to be the hijacking of the term "professional."

Regardless of nursing program background, the term "professional" had been applied to all that was good. General usage, likewise, cast "professional" in positive terms. A person who did a project or handled a situation "professionally" knew it was well done. A student who "looked professional" knew she had met certain standards (however little clean shoelaces may have to do with actual professionalism). A student who studied to be a "professional nurse" would qualify to take the state board examination and in the years just before the position paper, thought she would give comprehensive, individualized care to patients. "Technical" just did not have the same ring to it: "Technical" sounded limited and mechanical; "technical" sounded "less than." However knowledgeable, talented, and essential technical workers were in the discourse of educational macroplanners and economists, the word translated poorly to the world of nursing. Immense amounts of creative and emotional energy were diverted into this conflict.

The crisis was gradually defused, partly by action on the recommendations of the next committee to study nursing, "The National Commission for the Study of Nursing and Nursing Education" (1970), commonly known as the Lysaught Commission, which reported in 1970.

Among the recommendations in *Abstract for action* were (1) statewide planning for the number and distribution of nursing education programs, (2) career mobility for individual nurses, and (3) cooperation of nursing service and education in working to improve patient care. As the world around community colleges changed so that more and more people, particularly women, resumed formal education after a hiatus and senior colleges had good experience with community college graduates who sought baccalaureates, the concepts of "career mobility" and "articulation" came into nursing discourse. By 1972, the NLN prepared a collection titled, "The Associate Degree Program—A Step to the Baccalaureate Degree in Nursing." However, according to Patricia Haase, a historian of associate degree programs, it was also true that "(i)t was assumed by some in baccalaureate education that the curricula of the two nursing programs were not related, that they occupied two separate universes" (Haase, 1990). Rapprochement was gradually achieved, but sensitivities, which have their roots in this conflict, exist to this day.

Master's Programs

Master's programs differentiated from undergraduate programs and developed a distinctive focus in the 30 years from 1950 to 1980. Initially, the dire need for faculty in all three types of prelicensure programs prompted the impulse to establish first-level graduate programs. Federal funding for traineeships and program development, starting in 1957, provided resources for expansion. The outlines of advanced clinical knowledge and practice gradually emerged, first in the discussion and preparation for the clinical nurse specialist role in the acute care practice context. Almost concurrent with this, though using a continuing education approach, nursing and medical educators were designing programs for preparation of nurse practitioners for outpatient care.

Master's programs were few and relatively small in the 1950s. The 1951 report of the National Nursing Accrediting Service (NNAS) Postgraduate Board of Review noted that in some instances the same set of courses led to a master's degree for students who held a baccalaureate and to a baccalaureate degree for students who had no prior degree. Some of the clearly differentiated master's programs had so many prerequisites that few students qualified for admission without clearing multiple "deficiencies" by taking additional course work. The report opined that few programs focused on nursing "in its broadest sense," as contrasted with teaching and administration. And even this narrower focus seemed to be designed for the 2,000 hospitals that had schools of nursing rather than the 4,500 hospitals that didn't have them (NNAS Postgraduate Board of Review, 1953).

A Work Conference on Graduate Nurse Education, sponsored by the NLN Division of Nursing Education in the fall of 1952, concluded that master's graduates needed competencies in interpersonal relations, communication skills, their selected functional area (e.g., teaching or administration), promotion of community welfare, and "sufficient familiarity with the principles and methods of research to conduct and/or participate in systematic investigation of nursing problems and evaluate and use research findings" (Harms, 1954). But a 1954 study comparing six leading schools' master's curricula identified wide variability in actual practice. Program lengths were nominally 1 year for students without deficiencies, but this actually ranged from 24 to 38 semester credits. Although research was an agreed-upon master's focus, only one of the six schools had one course that by title could be identified as addressing this area. And names of degrees varied widely (Harms, 1954).

Given the relatively few students seeking admission and the small size of programs, regional planning became important, particularly in the South and West. In regional activity that was the precursor to the formation of the Southern Council on Collegiate Education for Nursing (SCCEN), it was agreed in 1952 that six universities—Universities of Alabama, Maryland, North Carolina, and Texas, and Vanderbilt and Emory Universities—would come together to plan five new master's programs to serve the South. This Regional Project in Graduate Education in Nursing garnered funding from both W.K. Kellogg and Commonwealth Foundations. By 1955, all six programs were admitting students (Reitt, 1987).

In the West, the Western Conference of Nursing Education was convened in early 1956 by the Western Interstate Commission for Higher Education (WICHE). Nursing educators, nurse leaders in various other positions, and nonnurse representatives from higher education from the western states gathered to advise WICHE on the development of nursing education programs in the area. A 2-month study of nursing education in the West, conducted by Helen Nahm, laid the groundwork for the meeting. This report provided the group with the essence of hundreds of interviews conducted with educators in nursing and related fields in the eight states, as well as nurse manpower data by state for 1954. Respondents reportedly believed that graduate programs in nursing should contain more work in social science fields, advanced preparation in physical and biologic science fields, strong foundations in education, courses basic to research, courses in philosophy, research in some area of nursing, and "graduate courses in a clinical nursing area which are truly of graduate caliber" (WICHE, 1956). Subsequently, the Western Interstate Council for Higher Education in Nursing (WICHEN) sponsored joint work that developed early master's-level clinical content and terminal competencies in the early and mid-1960s (WICHEN, 1967; Brown, 1978).

Enrollment in master's programs almost doubled between 1951 and 1962, growing from 1,290 to 2,472 (Harms, 1954; Kalisch & Kalisch, 1978). During the 1960s, clinical area emphases replaced functional specializations as the organizing frames for curricula. This shift in focus to nursing itself not only clarified and enriched baccalaureate curricula in later decades (Lynaugh & Brush, 1996), but it also freed doctoral-level training to focus directly on nursing knowledge development.

The clinical specialist role, idealized by educators, combined advanced clinical area knowledge with sophisticated care giving, care integration, and care improvement skills. The concept of such a master's-level role was discussed as early as 1949, and the first program embodying the concept was developed in 1954 (Smoyak, 1976). A number of papers on the subject came into the literature in the 1960s. The NLN Council of Baccalaureate and Higher Degree Programs devoted its third annual meeting in 1968 to the topic of clinical nurse specialist (CNS) preparation. Plenary papers, reflecting the flux of the period, blurred the concepts of clinically expert knowledge and the CNS role, and described preparation for the role variously as master's and doctoral work. The published *Proceedings* of the meeting, however, closed with a summary role description that bears striking resemblance to the current general outlines of the role (National League for Nursing Council of Baccalaureate and Higher Degree Programs, 1969). Although this idealized role description existed, the circumstances of each employing agency differed; therefore, the mix and emphasis of responsibilities varied from place to place, and various agencies combined clinical specialist functions with others, such as supervision or staff development, in actual practice.

Political pressure for access to care, interacting with the shortage and misdistribution of physicians and recognition that nurses could competently do a subset of physician work, led to federal support for the spread of nurse practitioner (NP) programs (National Commission for the Study of Nursing and Nursing Education, 1971; Bullough, 1976). Until the mid-1970s, most nurse practitioner preparation was designed and offered as non–degree-related continuing education. The first national conference on family nurse practitioner curricula convened in January 1976. At that point, programs ranged from 4-month certificate level offerings to specialties set within master's programs, with divergent characteristics depending on rural or urban settings. Certificate programs accounted for 71% of NP program grants funded by the Division of Nursing of the U.S. Public Health Service that year. Just 9 years later, in 1985, 81% of NP program grants went to master's level programs without any change in the authorizing law and presumably the award criteria (Geolot, 1987). Multiple factors drove or accommodated this change: Practice settings had higher expectations, fears of nurse educators about preserving the essence of nursing subsided, sufficient numbers of potential students saw value in a graduate degree, and the faculty members who reconceptualized the curricula were persuasive. Not insignificantly, federal funds were available to assist with the costs of transition. Curricular trends over the 20-year period included a proportionate decrease in time spent on health assessment and medical management; the movement of pharmacology from a free-standing course to integration in medical management courses, and back again to free-standing; increased emphasis on health promotion and chronic illness management; and development of common clinical core courses in schools where multiple nurse practitioner specialty tracks existed (Geolot, 1987).

Although graduate education in the 1960s and 1970s appears inventive and creative in retrospect, educators at the time found the simultaneous and sometimes conflicting changes difficult to reconcile. Clinical specialists were easiest to see as a development of the familiar base of nursing. But wariness, if not suspicion, greeted nurse practitioners, who seemed tainted by too-close associations with medicine and the work of medicine. Outside of academia, critical care nurses, an example of practice-born specialists, formed their own specialty association, raising questions about the fragmentation of nursing. Regional medical programs spearheaded continuing education efforts for both nurses and physicians that furthered nurse competence, but outside of standard nursing education channels. And then, from within nursing, came the idea of primary nursing. The recurrent question "What is nursing?" sometimes shaded into a pessimistic "nursing will soon disappear" lament in this period (Gunter, 1967). Clinical specialization, whether at the advanced-practice or staff nurse level, signaled a fundamental shift within nursing, occasioning uneasiness or frank antagonism because of the deeply held valuing of "sameness" in nursing. This sameness was equated to "equity", which was at odds with "expertness". For some, to be "special[ized]" implied that others were not (Smoyak, 1976).

Most large master's programs had multiple specialties by the mid-1980s, but these only weakly correlated with the major specialty organizations and with certification mechanisms (Styles, 1989). The clinical expertise and interest of nursing faculty, links to local resources, community needs for a particular specialty, and federal/state/local voluntary organization financial initiatives to address specific health problems all drove the pattern of specialty development (Burns et al., 1993). Nursing specialty organizations, reflecting current practice perspectives, exerted a substantial shaping influence on specialty curricular content in their respective areas. The rapid expansion—27%— in the number of master's programs in the last half of the 1980s (Burns et. al, 1993) may also have spurred creative naming of specialties for purposes of student recruitment. Efforts to rationalize the relationships of the specialties to one another, and where possible to achieve common use of resources, were the natural response to this proliferation.

By the 1990s, permutations of what had been considered clinical specialist content were being combined with nurse practitioner approaches. And advanced-practice nurses of both types were beginning to question whether the two roles were, after all, so different from each other (Elder & Bullough, 1990). Changes in health care financing and delivery were prompting clinical nurse specialist programs to include content to prepare graduates to deal with cost and reimbursement dimensions of care for populations (Wolf, 1990), and were pressuring practitioner programs to prepare graduates to care for patients with less stable conditions.

The *Essentials of College and University Education for Professional Nursing* (AACN, 1986), with its ambitious goals for a substantial liberal arts background, served as a springboard for the development of programs at the master's level for nonnurse college graduates. Students completed prelicensure generalist preparation before focusing in a specialty area, leading to the master's as the first professional degree (Wu & Connelly, 1992). Very few such programs had existed in the prior 2 decades (Diers, 1976; Plummer & Phelan, 1976), but external conditions favored their development in the 1990s. The *Essentials of Master's Education for Advanced Practice Nursing* codified the broad areas of agreement about master's preparation among educators (AACN, 1996) and this, together with accreditation mechanisms and a shared external environment, nudged programs toward common curricular characteristics.

Doctoral Programs

Educators began to focus on the hope of developing doctoral work in nursing in the midst of the chaotic educational diversity of the 1950s. The need for doctorally prepared faculty to teach master's students, who it was hoped would graduate and teach in the multiplying baccalaureate programs, fueled part of the interest in this topic. But for leaders already involved in higher education, it was painfully clear that nursing needed some capacity for its own research that would focus on questions related to nursing interventions to create a coherent body of tested knowledge and improve care.

Now we think of doctoral curricula as including introductory course work in theory development and appraisal, orientation to various approaches to analytical and interpretive research, and opportunities to become conversant with major programs of research and the overall shape of the nursing discipline, particularly as these relate to a student's particular region of interest. But even more important is an apprenticeship in one or more ongoing research programs, and mentored sponsorship into becoming an active member in the relevant scholarly subcommunity(ies) with the skills and experience that entails. Specialized course work specific to the student's research interest provides the final piece of the foundation for the student's dissertation research, which is mentored and supported by a group of faculty members. All of this is "the curriculum" of a doctoral program. The requisite complex of interdependent resources and structures that make the doctoral program of 2004 a possibility were created in the 40 years before 1990, with especially intense activity in the 1960s and 1970s.

Both the nursing education department at Teachers College, Columbia University (TCCU) and nursing at New York University (NYU) had offered arrangements with their education departments for nurses to do doctoral-level study before the 1950s, but numbers of graduates were small. TCCU revised its program in the 1950s but continued to grant the EdD. With the coming of Martha Rogers as chair of the Department of Nursing Education at NYU in 1954, the doctoral program was redirected to become a PhD in Nursing. The University of Pittsburgh established a PhD with a focus in pediatric or maternal nursing in 1954. In contrast to Martha Rogers' view that theory was the starting point that would lead to knowledge development in the "applied" field of nursing, Florence Erickson and Reva Rubin at Pittsburgh believed that extensive exposure to clinical phenomena, along with skilled faculty guidance, would develop a truly nursing science (Paretti, 1979). In the West, in the early WICHE/WICHEN conversations, the temporary need for help from other disciplines for research training was posited as a mechanism to build nursing knowledge and a critical mass of investigators (WICHE, 1956). The journal *Nursing Research* became available in 1952 as a mechanism for systematic communication (Bunge, 1962).

In 1955 the Nursing Research Grants and Fellowship Program of the Public Health Service allocated $500,000 for research grants and $125,000 for fellowships, the first such funding for nursing. From 1955 to 1970, 156 nurses were supported by special predoctoral research fellowships for doctoral study, and from 1959 to 1968, 18 schools of nursing received federally funded faculty research development grants to stimulate research capacity. The Nurse Scientist Graduate Training programs, which provided federal incentive funding to disciplines outside of nursing to accept nurses as students and provided fellowships to them, were designed to create a critical mass of faculty and a climate conducive to establishing doctoral programs in nursing (Grace, 1978). The programs continued from 1962 to 1976 and funded more than 350 nurse trainees (Murphy, 1981; Berthold, Tschudin, Peplau, Schlotfeldt, & Rogers, 1966).

Three additional doctoral programs were established in the 1960s—Boston University, 1960, DNSc, psychiatric/mental health focus; University of California San Francisco, 1964, DNSc, multifocus; and Catholic University, 1968, DNSc, medical–surgical and psychiatric–mental health foci. The Boston program took a clinical immersion approach analogous to the University of Pittsburgh. UCSF's program was structured as a research degree, but identified clinical involvement as the base for knowledge development, influenced both by nurse faculty with a strong clinical identity and by the grounded-theory perspectives of the several social scientists who were a part of the faculty.

A federally funded series of nine annual ANA-sponsored research conferences was initiated in 1965, and WICHEN sponsored the first of its annual Communicating Nursing Research conferences in 1968, creating space for face-to-face research exchange. MEDLARS made its debut in 1964, the first in a series of databases that would aid dissemination. Essential components for school of nursing research centers were identified (Gunter, 1966). A series of three federally funded conferences on nursing theory in Kansas City from 1969 to 1970 provided further opportunity to work through the divergent views of the relationships of theory, practice, and research to one another (Murphy, 1981).

In 1971, the Division of Nursing and the Nurse Scientist Graduate Training Committee (NSGTC) convened an invitational conference to address the type(s) of doctoral preparation. In this setting, Joseph Matarazzo, chair of the NSGTC, presented a paper arguing that nursing as a discipline was ready to launch PhD study, citing its body of knowledge and the qualifications of trainees (Matarazzo & Abdellah, 1971; Murphy, 1981). Comprehensive information about the state of nursing doctoral resources became available by the mid-1970s (Leininger, 1976), and by the late 1970s, National Doctoral Forums, open to schools with established programs, provided a mechanism for exchange of viewpoints about doctoral education. Three additional research journals began publication in 1978 (Gortner, 1991). "The Discipline of Nursing" (Donaldson & Crowley, 1978) was a milestone paper. It differentiated the discipline of nursing from the practice of nursing, but related the two as well, and proposed a productive interrelationship of research, theory, and practice. It shifted the terms of debate away from the dichotomous basic/applied categories.

The body of knowledge in nursing was still, relative to the old disciplines, rather modest in the late 1970s, but the progress in 2 decades and the infrastructure to support further development was substantial (Gortner & Nahm, 1977). Students were focusing their dissertation research on nursing clinical issues (Loomis, 1984). But the DNSc and PhD degrees (the two dominant degree titles), though differently named were indistinguishable in their objectives and end products (Grace, 1978). Finally, themes related to the challenge of mentoring students who are dealing with what is not known and fostering "humanship" between students and faculty to encourage student growth were beginning to come to print at the end of this decade (Downs, 1978).

Fifteen additional doctoral programs opened their doors during the 1970s (Cleland, 1976; Parietti, 1979). From 1980 to 1989 the number of programs grew from 22 to 50, prompting editorial comment, "As dandelions in spring, more and more doctoral programs are appearing" (Downs, 1984). Other observers surveying the situation recommended regional planning to sponsor joint programs, but conceded that the resources were in individual universities and states and that the mechanisms for making such efforts were nonexistent. They predicted stormy waters for programs that launched without adequate internal and external supports in place (McElmurry, Krueger, & Parsons, 1982). At the end of the 1980s, the doctoral educators were examining the balance between theory and research methods on the one hand and "knowledge" or "substance" in the curriculum on the other (Downs, 1988).

Programs expanded from 50 to 70 from 1990 to 1999. By the early 1990s, as the research programs were more numerous and robust in the older and larger schools, greater emphasis on research team participation (Keller & Ward, 1993) and mentoring into the range of activities doctoral graduates became visible themes (Meleis, 1992; Katefian, 1991). Postdoctoral study became more feasible and attractive (Hinshaw & Lucas, 1993).

The perennial question of the 1960s to 1980s, that is, whether nursing should adopt the PhD or DNSc, was answered by the hundreds of individual choices of applicants and the program choices of numerous schools: By 2000, only 12% of nursing doctoral programs conferred the DNSc, or variants thereon (McEwen & Bechtel, 2000). Perhaps less clear, however, was the answer to the other ongoing question: What is the difference between the two? Questions about a true professional doctorate have been raised perennially, most recently related to a new title, the Doctor of Nursing Practice (DNP) (Mundinger et al., 2000). Concerns about attention to "substance," that is, organized analysis of the body of nursing knowledge, the adequacy of research programs to provide student experience, and preparation for the teaching component of graduates' expected academic roles, occupy curriculum planners as they look to the future (Anderson, 2000).

Best-Laid Plans?

Given this survey of nursing curricula, can one say that the curriculum plans of nursing have indeed been "best-laid"? The answer depends on the angle of the lens through which one views the scene. Certainly with narrow focus, one could point to Isabel Hampton's detailed plan for the Johns Hopkins curriculum, or the ever more specific *Curriculums* of the NLNE, or the endless curriculum massage characteristic of the 1960s and 1970s as examples of planning. But the uncertainties of nursing's external environment, its status as a predominantly women's field, and its limited access to major financial support apart from governmental funding have limited its "planning" in a comprehensive sense. More characteristic has been incremental or directional planning together with persistent activity to create openings and constant alertness for unexpected opportunities. Perhaps in the last analysis, the measure of these plans lies not in the elegance of the plans themselves but in the outcomes of the plans, measured not solely in educational terms, but also in nursing's contribution to health.

▲ SUMMARY

Chapter 1 reviews the rich heritage and development of nursing curricula from the mid- to late-1800s to the 1990s. It discusses the influence that changes in society and the health care system, the Civil War, and international wars had on nursing education. The role of accreditation and the changes it brought about in nursing curricula are reviewed.

   The visions of nurse leader educators over the century who called for a unified approach to curriculum development in nursing are reviewed, and the discussion continues with a description of the rapid changes in nursing education during the latter half of the 20th century that included the development of nursing programs in community colleges and baccalaureate and higher degree programs. Advanced practice roles at the master's level came about as demands for higher levels of nursing practice evolved, patterns of physicians' practice changed, and technological advances created opportunities for the adjustment of nursing boundaries. Doctoral programs developed as nursing consolidated its professional identity and began to build the scientific body of knowledge through research.

DISCUSSION QUESTIONS

1. If NLNE had formed a joint committee with the American Association of State Colleges in 1950 (fictional name, but conceptually the group of former normal schools that were becoming comprehensive baccalaureate degree-granting institutions in the post–World War II period), would the characteristics of nursing education be different today? Whatever your answer, explain your reasoning.

2. With the exception of a few years in the early 1990s, the shortage of nurses to provide care in hospitals has been a chronic problem with intermittent acute exacerbations since the 1930s. What effects at both macro level (e.g., public opinion, social policy) and micro level (e.g., individual schools, courses) has this had on nursing education? Has the net balance of positive and negative effects been positive for nursing education? Why?

LEARNING ACTIVITIES

Student Learning Activity

1. Choose teams and debate the wisdom and feasibility of setting the master's degree as the minimum marker for the professional segment of the nursing continuum. Given our 20/20 hindsight gained from the debacle of the 1965 Position Paper, how would you advise national nursing organizations to go about changing this definition, if it were to be changed?

Faculty Learning Activity

1. Trace your school of nursing's history and link major curriculum changes to events external to the nursing program.

I want to thank Joan E. Lynaugh, University of Pennsylvania Center for the Study of the History of Nursing, for her chapter review comments that drew from her seasoned historical perspective and knowledge.—MEF.

REFERENCES

Aikens, C. A. (Ed.) (1911). *Hospital management.* Philadelphia: Saunders. (Facsimile copy republished by New York: Garland, 1985.)

American Association of Colleges of Nursing. (1986). *Essentials of college and university education for professional nursing.* Washington, D.C.: Author.

American Association of Colleges of Nursing. (1996). *The essentials of master's education for advanced practice nursing.* Washington, D.C.: Author.

American Nurses' Association. (1965). *Educational preparation for nurse practitioners and assistants to nurses: A position paper.* New York: Author.

Anderson, C. A. (2000). Current strengths and limitations of doctoral education in nursing: Are we prepared for the future? *Journal of Professional Nursing, 16,* 191–200.

Armeny, S. (1983). Organized nurses, women philanthropists, and the intellectual bases for cooperation among women, 1898–1920. In Lagemann, E. C. (Ed.), *Nursing history: New perspectives, new possibilities* (pp. 13–46). New York: Teachers College Columbia.

Baldwin, D. O. (2002). Discipline, obedience, and female support groups: Mona Wilson at the Johns Hopkins Hospital School of Nursing, 1915-1918. In E. D. Baer, P. O. D'Antonio, S. Rinker, & J. E. Lynaugh (Eds.), *Enduring issues in American nursing* (pp. 85–105). New York: Springer.

Berthold, J. S., Tschudin, M. S., Peplau, H. E., Schlotfeldt, R., & Rogers, M. E. (1966). A dialogue on approaches to doctoral preparation. *Nursing Forum 5,* 48–104.

Bevis, E. O. (1989). *Curriculum building in nursing: A process.* New York: National League for Nursing.

Bevis, E. O., & Watson, J. (1989). *Toward a caring curriculum: A new pedagogy for nursing.* New York: National League for Nursing.

Bridgman, M. (1949). Consultant in collegiate nursing education. *American Journal of Nursing, 49,* 808.

Bridgman, M. (1953). *Collegiate education for nursing.* New York: Russell Sage Foundation.

Brimmer, P. F., Skoner, M. M., Pender, N. J., Williams, C. A., Fleming, J. W., & Werley, H. H. (1983). Nurses with doctoral degrees: Education and employment characteristics. *Research in Nursing and Health, 6,* 157–165.

Brown, E. L. (1948). *Nursing for the future.* New York: Russell Sage Foundation.

Brown, J. M. (1978). Master's education in nursing, 1945-1969. In J. Fitzpatrick (Ed.), *Historical studies in nursing* (pp. 104–130). New York: Teachers College.

Bullough, B. (1976). Influences on role expansion. *American Journal of Nursing, 76,* 1476–1481.

Bullough, V., & Bullough, B. (1978). *The care of the sick: The emergence of modern nursing.* New York: Prodist.

Bunge, H. L. (1962). The first decade of nursing research. *Nursing Research, 11,* 132–137.

Burns, P. G., Nishikawa, H. A., Weatherby, F., Forni, P. R., Moran, M., Allen, M. E., et al. (1993). Master's degree nursing education: State of the art. *Journal of Professional Nursing, 9,* 267–277.

Cleland, V. (1976). Developing a doctoral program. *Nursing Outlook, 24,* 631–635.

Committee of the Six National Nursing Organizations on Unification of Accrediting Services. (1949). *Manual of accrediting educational programs in nursing.* New York: National Nursing Accrediting Service.

Committee on the Grading of Nursing Schools. (1931). *Results of the first grading study of nursing schools.* New York: Author.

Conant, L. H. (1968). On becoming a nurse researcher. *Nursing Research, 17,* 68–71.

D'Antonio, P. O. (1987). All a woman's life can bring: The domestic roots of nursing in Philadelphia, 1830-1885. *Nursing Research, 36,* 12–17.

D'Antonio, P. O. (1993). The legacy of domesticity. *Nursing History Review, 1,* 229-246.

Diers, D. (1976). A combined basic-graduate program for college graduates. *Nursing Outlook, 24,* 92–98.

Dodd, D. (2001). Nurses' residences: Using the built environment as evidence. *Nursing History Review, 9,* 185–206.

Donaldson, S. K., & Crowley, D. M. (1978). The discipline of nursing. *Nursing Outlook, 26,* 113–120.

Downs, F. S. (1978). Doctoral education in nursing: Future directions. *Nursing Outlook, 26,* 56–61.

Downs, F. S. (1984). Caveat emptor. *Nursing Research, 33,* 59.

Downs, F. S. (1988). Doctoral education: Our claim to the future. *Nursing Outlook, 36,*18–20.

Egenes, K. J. (1998). An experiment in leadership: The rise of student government at Philadelphia General Hospital Training school, 1920–1930. *Nursing History Review, 6,* 71–84.

Eisenmann, L. (2000). Reconsidering a classic: Assessing the history of women's higher education a dozen years after Barbara Solomon. In R. Lowe (Ed.), *History of education: Major themes, Vol.1,* (pp. 411–442). New York: Routledge & Falmer.

Elder, R. G., & Bullough, B. (1990). Nurse practitioners and clinical nurse specialists: Are the roles merging? *Clinical Nurse Specialist, 4,* 78–84.

Faddis, M. (1973). *A school of nursing comes of age.* Cleveland: Howard Allen.

Fairman, J., & Lynaugh, J. E. (1998). *Critical care nursing: A history.* Philadelphia: University of Pennsylvania.

Gage, N. D. (1918). Organization of classwork and student life at the Vassar training camp. *American Journal of Nursing, 19,* 18–22.

Geolot, D. H. (1987). NP education: Observations from a national perspective. *Nursing Outlook, 35,* 132–135.

Goldmark, J. (1923). *Nursing and nursing education in the United States.* New York: Macmillan.

Goodnow, M. (1934). *Outlines of nursing history* (5th ed.). Philadelphia: Saunders.

Gortner, S. R. (1991). Historical development of doctoral programs: Shaping our expectations. *Journal of Professional Nursing, 7,* 45–53.

Gortner, S. R., & Nahm, H. (1977). An overview of nursing research in the United States. *Nursing Research, 26,* 10–33.

Grace, H. (1978). The development of doctoral education in nursing: An historical perspective. *Journal of Nursing Education, 17,* 17–27.

Graham, P. A. (1978). Expansion and exclusion: A history of women in higher education. *Signs, 3,* 759–773.

Gunter, L. (1967). Notes on a proposed center for nursing research. *Nursing Research, 16,* 185.

Gunter, L. M. (1966). Some problems in nursing care and services. In B. Bullough & V. Bullough (Eds.), *Issues in nursing* (pp. 152–156). New York: Springer.

Haase, P. T. (1990). *The origins and rise of associate degree nursing education.* National League for Nursing and Durham: Duke University.

Hampton, I. A. (1893). *Nursing: Its principles and practice. For hospital and private use.* Philadelphia: Saunders. (Facsimile re-published by Saunders, 1993.)

Hanson, K. S. (1991). An analysis of the historical context of liberal education in nursing education from 1924 to 1939. *Journal of Professional Nursing, 7,* 341–350.

Harms, M. T. (1954). *Professional education in university schools of nursing.* Unpublished doctoral dissertation. Stanford University, Stanford, CA.

Hine, D. C. (1989). *Black women in white: Racial conflict and cooperation in the nursing profession, 1890–1950.* Indianapolis: Indiana University.

Hinshaw, A. S., & Lucas, M. D. (1993). Postdoctoral education—a new tradition for nursing research. *Journal of Professional Nursing, 9,* 309.

JAMA. (1927, March 12). Hospital service in the United States. *Journal of the American Medical Association, 88,* 789–812.

James, J. W. (2002). Isabel Hampton and the professionalization of nursing in the 1890s. In E. D. Baer, P. O. D'Antonio, S. Rinker, & J. E. Lynaugh (Eds.), *Enduring issues in American nursing* (pp. 42–84). New York: Springer.

Kalisch, P. A., & Kalisch, B. J. (1978). *The advance of American nursing.* Boston: Little, Brown.

Katefian, S. (1991). Doctoral preparation for faculty roles: Expectations and realities. *Journal of Professional Nursing, 7,* 105–111.

Keller, M. L., & Ward, S. E. (1993). Funding and socialization in the doctoral program at the University of Wisconsin-Madison. *Journal of Professional Nursing, 9,* 262–266.

Lavine, D. O. (1986). *The American college and the culture of aspiration, 1915–1940.* Ithaca, NY: Cornell University.

Leininger, M. (1976). Doctoral programs for nurses: Trends, questions, and projected plans. *Nursing Research, 25,* 201–210.

Loomis, M. (1984). Emerging content in nursing: An analysis of dissertation abstracts and titles: 1976-1982. *Nursing Research, 33,* 113–199.

Lynaugh, J. E. (2002). Nursing's history: Looking backward and seeing forward. In E. D. Baer, P. O. D'Antonio, S. Rinker, & J. E. Lynaugh (Eds.), *Enduring issues in American nursing* (pp. 10–24). New York: Springer.

Lynaugh, J. E., & Brush, B. L. (1996). *American nursing: From hospitals to health systems.* Cambridge, MA: Blackwell.

Matarazzo, J., & Abdellah, F. (1971). Doctoral education for nurses in the United States. *Nursing Research, 20,* 404–414.

McElmurry, B. J., Krueger, J. C. & Parsons, L. C. (1982). Resources for graduate education: A report of a survey of forty states in the Midwest, West, and Southern regions. *Nursing Research, 31,* 5–10.

McEwen, M., & Bechtel, G. A. (2000). Characteristics of nursing doctoral programs in the United States. *Journal of Professional Nursing, 16,* 282–292.

Meleis, A. I. (1992). On the way to scholarship: From master's to doctorate. *Journal of Professional Nursing, 8,* 328–334.

Melosh, B. (1982). *"The physician's hand": Work culture and conflict in American nursing.* Philadelphia: Temple University.

Mundinger, M. O., Cook, S. S., Lenz, E. R., Piacentini, K., Auerhahn, C., & Smith, J. (2000). Assuring quality and access in advanced practice nursing: A challenge to nurse educators. *Journal of Professional Nursing, 16,* 322–329.

Murphy, J. F. (1981). Doctoral education in, of, and for nursing: An historical analysis. *Nursing Outlook, 29,* 645–649.

National Commission for the Study of Nursing and Nursing Education. (1970). *An abstract for action.* New York: McGraw Hill.

National Commission for the Study of Nursing and Nursing Education. (1971). *Nurse clinician and physician's assistant: The relationship between two emerging practitioner concepts.* Rochester, NY: Author.

National League for Nursing Council of Baccalaureate and Higher Degree Programs. (1969). *Extending the boundaries of nursing education—the preparation and roles of the clinical specialist.* New York: Author.

National League of Nursing Education. (1917). *Standard curriculum for schools of nursing.* Baltimore: Waverly.

National League of Nursing Education. (1927). *A curriculum for schools of nursing.* New York: Author.

National League of Nursing Education. (1937). *A curriculum guide for schools of nursing.* New York: Author.

National Nursing Accrediting Service Postgraduate Board of Review. (1951). Some problems identified. *American Journal of Nursing, 51,* 337–338.

Obituary. (1940). Mrs. Clara S. Weeks Shaw. *American Journal of Nursing, 40,* 356.

Parietti, E. S. (1979). *Development of doctoral education for nurses: An historical survey.* Ann Arbor: University Microfilms International.

Petry, L. (1937). Basic professional curricula in nursing leading to degrees. *American Journal of Nursing, 37,* 287–297.

Petry, L. (1943). U. S. Cadet Nurse Corps. *American Journal of Nursing, 43,* 704–708.

Petry, L. (1949). We hail an important first. *American Journal of Nursing, 49,* 630–633.

Plummer, E. M., & Phelan, J. J. (1976). College graduates in nursing: A retrospective look. *Nursing Outlook, 24,* 99–102.

Reitt, B. B. (1987). *The first 25 years of the Southern Council on Collegiate Education for Nursing.* Atlanta: Southern Council on Collegiate Education for Nursing.

Reverby, S. (1984). "Neither for the drawing room nor for the kitchen": Private duty nursing in Boston, 1873–1914. In J. W. Leavitt (Ed.), *Women and health in America* (pp. 454–466). Madison, WI: University of Wisconsin.

Reverby, S. M. (1987). *Ordered to care: The dilemma of American nursing, 1850–1945.* New York: Cambridge University.

Reverby, S. M. (2002). A legitimate relationship: Nursing, hospitals, and science. In E. D. Baer, P. O. D'Antonio, S. Rinker, & J. E. Lynaugh (Eds.), *Enduring issues in American nursing* (pp. 262–281). New York: Springer.

Rines, A. (1977). Associate degree education: History, development, and rationale. *Nursing Outlook, 25,* 496–501.

Robb, I. H. (1907). *Educational standards for nurses.* Cleveland: E. C. Koeckert.

Roberts, M. M. (1954). *American nursing: History and interpretation.* New York: Macmillan.

Robinson, T. M., & Perry, P. M. (2001). *Cadet Nurse stories: The call for and response of women during World War II.* Indianapolis: Center Press.

Schubert, W. H. (1986). *Curriculum: Perspective, paradigm, and possibility.* New York: Macmillan.

Scott, J. (1972). Federal support for nursing education, 1964–1972. *American Journal of Nursing, 72,* 1855–1860.

Sheahan, D. A. (1980). *The social origins of American nursing and its movement into the university: A microscopic approach.* Ann Arbor, MI: University Microfilms.

Smith-Rosenberg, C. (1985). *Disorderly conduct.* New York: Oxford.

Smoyak, S. A. (1976). Specialization in nursing: From then to now. *Nursing Outlook, 24,* 676–681.

Solomon, B. (1985). *In the company of educated women.* New Haven, CT: Yale University.

Styles, M. M. (1989). *On specialization in nursing: Toward a new empowerment.* Kansas City: American Nurses' Foundation.

The President's Commission on Higher Education. (1948). *Higher education for American democracy: A report of the president's commission on higher education.* New York: Harper.

Tomes, N. (1984). "Little world of our own": The Pennsylvania Hospital Training School for Nurses, 1895-1907. In J. W. Leavitt (Ed.), *Women and health in America* (pp. 467–481). Madison, WI: University of Wisconsin.

Tyack, D. (1974). *The one best system: A history of American urban education.* Cambridge, MA: Harvard University.

Veysey, L. R. (1965). *The emergence of the American university.* Chicago: University of Chicago.

Vogel, M. J. (1980). *The invention of the modern hospital: Boston 1870–1930.* Chicago: University of Chicago.

Weeks-Shaw, C. (1902). *A text-book of nursing: For the use of training schools, families, and private students* (3rd ed.). New York: D. Appleton.

Western Interstate Commission for Higher Education. (1956). *Toward shared planning in western nursing education.* Boulder, CO: Author.

Western Interstate Commission on Higher Education in Nursing. (1967). *Defining clinical content: Graduate programs, 1–4.* Boulder, CO: Author.

Wolf, G. A. (1990). Clinical nurse specialists: The second generation. *Journal of Nursing Administration, 20,* 7–8.

Wu, C. Y., & Connelly, C. (1992). Profile of nonnurse college graduates in accelerated baccalaureate nursing programs. *Journal of Professional Nursing, 8,* 35–40.

Responsibilities of Faculty in Curriculum Development and Evaluation

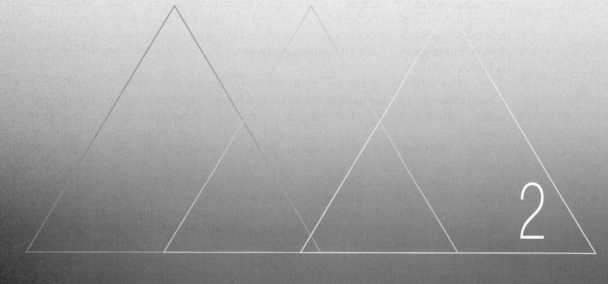

Julie E. Johnson, PhD, RN, FAAN

OBJECTIVES

Upon completion of Chapter 2, the student will be able to:

1. Describe the process involved in obtaining approval to implement the curriculum.
2. Analyze the faculty's role and responsibilities in curriculum development, revision, and evaluation.
3. Analyze current issues that impact curriculum development.
4. Analyze the linkages between the institution's mission/philosophy and the development of the nursing curriculum.
5. Evaluate the role of students, alumni, employers, and consumers in the development of the curriculum.

▲ OVERVIEW

When joining the faculty of a school of nursing, a person should orient him- or herself to the curriculum's mission, philosophy, goals, organizing framework, and objectives to ascertain if they are in congruence with his or her own conceptual base of nursing education. If there is a major lack of compatibility, then it is advised that the person seek a faculty role in another school that corresponds with his or her philosophies and beliefs about nursing education.

As a member of the faculty, a person should continually monitor the curriculum to maintain its integrity as it is implemented through instructional processes. This includes theory classes, laboratory practice, and clinical experiences. If incongruence occurs, the faculty member who identifies a problem has a responsibility to work with other members of the faculty to bring the course(s) into line or to consider and implement changes in the curriculum through the appropriate channels.

It is the responsibility of nursing faculty to continually assess the components of the curriculum, its processes, and outcomes to ensure quality education in nursing. Ways in which faculty can participate in this process are to join committees that pertain to the curriculum, to collaborate with other faculty members at various levels to observe the curriculum plan in action, to identify problems or potential problems, and to offer ideas for their resolution.

Nursing faculty must know the health care system and changes that occur to prepare graduates to meet the needs of that system and the people they serve. This requires looking into the future and collaborating with nurses and other health care providers to obtain an overall picture of the current and future health needs of the populace and how the system will meet those needs. The most efficient method for accomplishing this mandate is to invite consumers and members of the health care system to curriculum planning meetings and ask them to participate in the evaluation of educational programs and their products.

Nursing faculty must collaborate with other disciplines to provide interdisciplinary education to imbue in their graduates a sense of teamwork in meeting the needs of the people they serve. The knowledge base and clinical experiences for students should include in-depth experiences in a variety of health care settings, to prepare nurses who can provide interdisciplinary as well as nursing services to clients who move in and out of various levels of care.

The information age and high technology require that faculty members keep abreast of changes and gain the knowledge and skills required for facilitating learning, conducting research and other scholarly activities, and transmitting new knowledge and theories to students. Faculty should view students as partners in the teaching and learning processes and ensure their participation in the evaluation of the curriculum and program outcomes.

Curriculum development, evaluation, and revision are outcome-directed processes that are faculty driven. This chapter provides a detailed discussion of the levels of approval needed in adopting the curriculum and describes the faculty and administrator's roles and responsibilities in its development. It also examines the multiple factors that must be considered in the construction of a scholarly, creative, flexible, and cost-effective curriculum that is responsive to the needs of communities, consumers, and the financial resources of the parent institution. This chapter describes the mission and philosophy of the university and the expected objectives, competencies, and outcomes based on the philosophical beliefs of faculty integral to this process. It also addresses formative and summative evaluation strategies that are key to curriculum development/revision and the assurance of desired outcomes.

▲ LEVELS OF CURRICULUM APPROVAL

College and university governance includes curriculum committees of elected faculty members. Depending on the overall organizational structure, there may be several committees functioning at different levels. For example, if the nursing program is housed in a school or department within a larger college, approval of the curriculum will proceed through the school/department, college, and university committees. If it is a freestanding school or college, the curriculum will need approval from the curriculum committees at the school/college and university levels. After the curriculum receives approval from the appropriate committees, it may need to be forwarded to the academic vice president or provost and then to a governing board for the college or university for final approval. For example, it may be necessary to receive approval from a Board of Regents or Coordinating Board of the institution or educational system prior to implementing the curriculum. See Figure 2.1 for a flow chart of the levels of curriculum approval.

▲ CURRICULUM COMMITTEE MEMBERSHIP

Typically, members of the school of nursing's curriculum committee are elected as representatives of the faculty. In smaller nursing programs, all faculty members may serve as the curriculum committee. Senior tenured faculty, junior faculty on the tenure track, and clinical faculty bring unique perspectives to the process of curriculum development and evaluation that are based on their clinical specialties and practice experiences, academic experiences, and participation in professional organizations and continuing education. In addition, the presence of senior faculty provides opportunities for them to mentor new members of the faculty. Student representatives are elected by their peers to the committee and depending upon the program, represent various levels or tracks in the program. They may or may not have voting privileges as determined by the program's governance.

The committee elects its chair from the faculty membership. Standing or consultative membership can exist on the curriculum committee from representatives of alumni, employers of graduates, consumers, and/or faculty from departments from which collaboration is important in developing interdisciplinary educational experiences. The latter may include representatives from disciplines such as social work, nutrition, psychology, gerontology, human development and family studies, ethics, law, and medicine. These standing memberships can be part of the committee's bylaws or functions or can be created from a request by faculty or the nursing program administrator in consultation with the committee chair.

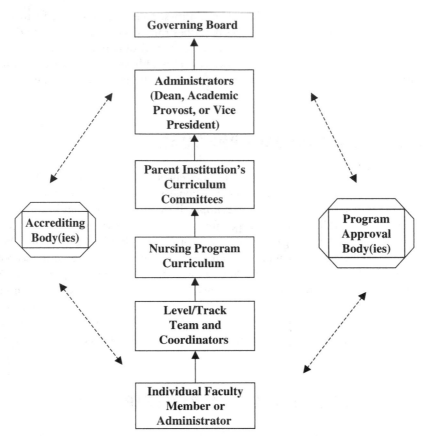

FIGURE 2.1 Flow diagram: Levels of curriculum approval.

Functions of the Curriculum Committee

A curriculum committee may either initiate curriculum development or revision on its own, or undertake it at the request of the administrator. Either way, it is essential that both the faculty members and the administrator seek the support and input of the faculty and key constituents. Suggested ways to gather information are described later in this chapter.

As the nursing curriculum committee engages in its activities, it is important that it keeps faculty informed of its progress and seeks continued input from faculty. The nursing administrator should provide ample time for discussion of curricular matters at faculty meetings. The size of the committee should be limited to ensure efficiency and effectiveness; thus, ad hoc committees or taskforces may be appointed by the faculty or administrator in collaboration with the faculty to examine particular issues of concern, or those that require more detailed examination.

When the committee has reached consensus on its plan for the curriculum, the curriculum is brought to the faculty for a final discussion and vote of approval or disapproval. If the faculty does not approve the proposed curriculum, the curriculum is returned to the committee for revision. If it is accepted by nursing faculty, the curriculum is forwarded to the next appropriate level for approval. It is very helpful to have the administrator of the school of nursing and/or a member of the curriculum committee present at subsequent levels to respond to questions or concerns related to the proposal.

External Program Approval

Once it has proceeded through the necessary institutional levels and received their endorsement, the curriculum must be formally presented to state boards of nursing for approval. In most states in the United States, only entry-level (prelicensure) programs must be approved by the state board of nursing. Graduate programs are not subject to review, although some states must approve advanced-practice programs for certification purposes (e.g., clinical specialists, nurse anesthetists, nurse midwives, and nurse practitioners). It is wise to inform the agency that the development of a new curriculum or revisions of an existing program are underway and to seek the agency staff's consultation as the work progresses. These actions help to avoid pitfalls and facilitate approval when the work is completed.

The purpose of state boards of nursing is to protect the safety of the public by ensuring that those they license are qualified to practice. As such, they set curriculum standards that must be met if programs are to be approved by them. Lack of approval means that graduates of the school are ineligible to take the licensure examination to become registered nurses. While regulations may vary by state, they usually include essential content that must be included in the curriculum, the minimum number of hours that students must spend in clinical areas, and the skills and competencies they must demonstrate upon completion of the nursing program (Finke & Boland, 1998). To learn how to contact a specific state board of nursing and obtain information regarding its curriculum requirements, visit the National Council of State Boards of Nursing (NCSBN, 2003) website at http://www.ncsbn.org. A challenge to nurse educators and staff members of state boards is to work together to understand the curricular changes needed to prepare students to function competently in the current and future dynamic health care environment (Larsen, 2000).

If the faculty chooses to become nationally accredited, the nursing curriculum must meet the criteria for accreditation by either the Commission on Collegiate Nursing Education (CCNE) or the National League for Nursing Accrediting Commission (NLNAC). Both of these bodies are approved at the federal level by the Department of Education to accredit schools of nursing. The CCNE accredits baccalaureate and master's degree programs. The NLNAC accredits licensed practical/vocational nursing, associate, baccalaureate, and master's degree programs. Approval of the curriculum by the state's board of nursing is a necessary prerequisite to obtaining accreditation from either organization. Therefore, attending to their criteria is essential to curriculum development. For national accreditation, nursing faculty must show that they developed the curriculum and that learning experiences for students flow from the school's mission and expected program outcomes (Finke & Boland, 1998).

Specific requirements of national accrediting bodies that affect curriculum development can change as needed to keep pace with the dynamic health care environment.

The most current criteria can be obtained by visiting the websites for CCNE (2004) at http://www.aacn.nche.edu/Accreditation/index.htm and for NLNAC (2004) at http://nlnac.org/home.htm. See also Chapter 12 for details on accreditation.

Faculty Role and Responsibilities in Curriculum Development

Faculty in higher education has the responsibility for developing, evaluating, and revising curriculum; teaching, guiding, and evaluating students; and mentoring faculty. Traditionally, faculty's right to self-governance gives them the needed academic freedom to meet these responsibilities. Academic freedom allows faculty members to investigate new theories and ideas and permits them to express opinions in the classroom that are relevant to the course being taught (Finke, 1998). The individual faculty member has the right to modify objectives, content, and teaching methods in the courses in which he or she teaches in response to changes in the discipline and practice. However, major changes in the overall objectives, content, and course sequencing must take place in consultation with other faculty members and within the protocols listed in the curriculum approval process.

Self-governance includes the right to develop policies and procedures that affect students' and faculty's conduct and curriculum, to advise administrative and student groups on educational issues, and to participate in administrative actions that affect the institution and broader community (Finke, 1998). Typically, these activities are accomplished by participating on elected or appointed department, school, and university committees and taskforces.

According to Ratliff (1997), a major responsibility of the faculty as it develops the curriculum is to ensure that content and related learning experiences are sequenced in such a way that students attain the expected educational outcomes. A framework for the curriculum is essential to this process because it allows the faculty to conceptualize and organize "the knowledge, skills, values, and beliefs critical to the delivery of a coherent curriculum that facilitates the achievement of the desired curriculum outcomes" (Boland, 1998, p. 135). The framework reflects the mission and philosophy of the faculty and its beliefs about teaching, learning, and nursing.

Because faculty members are experts in their discipline and the specialty areas within it, the curriculum has traditionally "belonged to them." They must decide what content should be conveyed to students, and the best teaching and learning methods to be used in delivering it. Inherent in this process is the creation of ways to evaluate student competencies and outcomes, as well as the effectiveness of the curriculum in preparing graduates to function in a rapidly changing and complex health care environment.

This process often results in feelings of territoriality because faculty members try to protect the inclusion of content that is in their specialty areas and that they believe is essential to positive student outcomes (Hull, St. Romain, Alexander, Schaff, and Jones; 2001). Resulting emotions such as fear, anger, insecurity, and loss of identity may interfere with curriculum development. A primary responsibility of the faculty is to develop strategies that facilitate the exchange of ideas and decision making in an effort to overcome these emotions (Dillard & Laidig, 1998) while attending to the other factors that influence their charge to develop a meaningful curriculum. See Box 2.1 for a list of faculty responsibilities in curriculum development.

▲ **BOX 2.1**   **Responsibilities of Faculty in Curriculum Development**

- ▲ Develop policies and procedures that affect students' and faculty's conduct and the curriculum.
- ▲ Advise administration and students on educational issues.
- ▲ Participate in administrative actions that affect the institution and community.
- ▲ Ensure that content and learning experiences are sequenced toward educational outcomes.
- ▲ Collect and analyze relevant information pertaining to the need for curriculum development and revision.
- ▲ Prepare graduates to function in the changing and complex health care environment.
- ▲ Develop strategies to facilitate the exchange of ideas and decision making relevant to curriculum development and revisions.

Strategies for Faculty Participation in Curriculum Development

The six C's of Lancaster's (1985) formula for collaborative research can be applied to the exchange of ideas to begin the process of curriculum development. These are commitment, compatibility, communication, contribution, consensus, and credit. The investment of time, energy, and resources demonstrates commitment and is required of faculty and administration. The dean/director/chair commits financial, space, time, and personnel resources to the endeavor. A committee of experienced and novice faculty may be appointed or elected to develop or revise the curriculum.

Since students will not practice as licensed nurses while in school, it is necessary to project future changes in nursing and health care to prepare them for practice upon graduation. To accomplish this, the committee seeks input from faculty, students, and the health care community regarding the essential content to be included in the curriculum. This may be accomplished via mailed surveys and/or face-to-face meetings depending upon available resources for collecting the information. The key, however, is to ensure that all constituents have an opportunity to voice their ideas and concerns (Hull et al., 2001). Once the descriptors for the future are collected, broad categories of essential content are developed and applied to the program goals, objectives, and course content and their sequencing. This information is then integrated into the curriculum to meet the actual environmental changes as the student progresses toward graduation.

Compatibility requires that a diverse group of individuals function as a whole (Lancaster, 1985). The curriculum committee must engage in open discussion that encourages its members to examine their beliefs and attitudes about nursing education and how they affect their charge to develop the curriculum. It is imperative that committee members remember that while they represent an area of expertise, they must view the curriculum as a whole (Hull et al., 2001). Communication among committee members may be facilitated by the use of a gatekeeper (Marriner-Tomey, 1996). This individual ensures that everyone has the chance to be heard, eases strain, and maintains harmony. As a time-effective measure, it may be helpful to form subcommittees to enhance communication within the larger group.

Each member of the committee is an expert within a given specialty and should have the opportunity to contribute to the development of the curriculum (Hull et al., 2001). Experienced faculty members provide a historical perspective and can guide the committee's work. Novice faculty members bring a fresh perspective to the curriculum that can result in creativity and innovation. Committee members with additional skills, such as recording minutes or acting as facilitator or mediator, contribute to the process.

Through commitment, compatibility, communication, and contribution, consensus is reached and committee members are given credit for their accomplishments. Consensus implies that the majority has reached agreement on key points and that all committee members will abide by those decisions. All committee members should be acknowledged and given credit for their contributions to a curriculum that required hard work and compromise (Cleary, 2001; Hull et al., 2001).

Faculty Mentoring

The mentoring of faculty members by experienced colleagues means that individuals are helped to reach their potential as members of the academic community (Lieb, 1995). It is an all-inclusive activity and not limited to those who are new to the world of university education. Mentoring includes guiding those who are inexperienced in their faculty role and supporting experienced faculty who are new to the institution. For example, inexperienced faculty members may need help in developing effective teaching skills with small and large groups, learning how to assign grades, planning meaningful clinical experiences, and serving as an academic advisor. Experienced faculty members may need assistance in how to adapt those skills to the expectations of a new institution. Faculty mentoring means helping those who are adjusting to teaching in a changing health care environment, and/or learning to use new information technologies (Riner & Billings, 1999).

Issues Impacting Curriculum Development

The current health care system is driven by the financial concerns of managed care companies. Hospital admissions are delayed and individuals who are admitted are often critically ill and discharged much sooner than in the past. Consequently, nursing care in community-based settings, such as home and school health, has been become predominant. Faculty development in community-based nursing, cultural diversity, health promotion and disease prevention, and the economics of health care is essential so that the needed knowledge and skills to deliver safe and appropriate nursing care is included in the curriculum.

Delivery of the curriculum by various distance technologies, such as the Web and video-conferencing, is current practice. Yet, many faculty members are not comfortable with these approaches to education. They need support from administration to ensure that they have the necessary skills to develop curricula that are compatible with teaching in these modalities and to evaluate their outcomes. See Chapter 14 for a detailed discussion of these types of modalities.

To develop a dynamic curriculum that is pertinent to the needs of society, faculty must be aware of national and global trends in health care, as well as the skills and competencies needed by nurses to be successful in the practice environment (Rains, 1998). These factors are interrelated, complex, and in a constant state of flux. They include changes in demography, family structure, economics, environment and delivery of health care (Klineberg, 1994).

Demographic trends that demand attention in curriculum development include the rapid population growth in developing countries, the increasing number of elders in America, and the growth of an ethnically diverse population (Rains, 1998). While specific content related to specialty areas is not specified in the majority of state board approval or accreditation criteria, the health care needs of vulnerable populations must be addressed in the curriculum. For example, it is critical that gerontology content is infused in the curriculum and that it addresses the health promotion and disease prevention needs of elders (Alford & Futrell, 1998). The health care needs of grandparents raising grandchildren, single parents, dual-career families needing child care, and end-of-life issues are examples of changes in family structure that need consideration in the development of a socially relevant curriculum.

Examples of environmental considerations to be addressed in the curriculum include the multiple sources of pollution and the threat of bio-terrorism. A word of caution is appropriate at this point related to the tendency for faculty to add content to the curriculum without equivalent reduction in other content. In these instances, faculty must review the curriculum to determine essential versus nonessential content.

Historically, the 1986 recommendations from the National League for Nursing and Society for Research in Nursing Education and the 1991 Pew Health Care Commission Report called for massive changes in nursing curricula (Mawn & Reece, 2000). They urged nursing faculty to recognize that health care is market driven and that the curriculum should reflect the multiple needs of culturally diverse consumers from a cost-effective, community-based, health promotion, and disease prevention perspective. They also suggested that students needed to acquire skills in information management, interdisciplinary collaboration, and involving families and patients in decision making (Barger, 1994). The 1999 Pew Health Professions Commission forecast continued changes in health care and recommended that all health education programs prepare their graduates with population and organizational skills (Larsen, 2000). These approaches to curriculum development challenge faculty to revise its philosophical approach to nursing education (Hamner & Wilder, 2001) and relinquish many long-standing traditions, such as only providing students with hospital experiences (Mawn & Reece, 2000), mandating skills check-offs, and requiring medical–surgical nursing as a prerequisite to specialty experiences (Larsen, 2000).

Community-based nursing focuses on partnering with individuals, families, and groups in any setting and helping them to move between systems (Hunt, 1998). Therefore, the curriculum must prepare students in the skills needed to develop these partnerships, value those of different cultures, and provide continuity of care in collaboration with other health care providers (Huston & Fox, 1998). As faculty incorporates these approaches to care in the curriculum, it gives them an opportunity to be innovative and futuristic in the inclusion of classroom content and clinical experiences offered. For example, they may wish to ensure that students receive a substantial amount of clinical learning experiences in settings such as home health, hospice, schools, industry, homeless shelters, beauty shops, providers' offices, prisons, and motels where low-income families rent by the week. The curriculum that faculty develops should also incorporate the use of creativity and innovation by students, and prepare them to function in an independent and self-directed manner. The inclusion of interdisciplinary classroom and clinical learning experiences in the curriculum is critical.

The Role of Mission and Philosophy in Curriculum Development

The mission statement of the institution delineates its unique purpose for existing and describes the population it serves (Newsom & Hays, 1991). It is the foundation for the institution's philosophy, goals, and educational programs. As faculty begins the process of curriculum development, it must reach consensus on how the school of nursing will enhance and support that mission. Elements of the mission statement that should be considered include the teaching, research, and service goals of the institution; the population to be served and its geographic area; and the desired outcomes for its graduates (Csokasy, 1998). Agreement among these elements and the desired curriculum must be reached by the faculty.

The philosophical foundation of the curriculum reflects the beliefs of the institution and faculty about education and people, as well as the influence of politics and society on what is taught (Csokasy, 1998). It supports the exploration of values and guides the development of curricular objectives, the outcome assessment plan, and methods of evaluation.

To create a sound basis for the curriculum, the mission and philosophy must be consistent with each other. Accrediting agencies, such as the Commission on Collegiate Nursing Education (CCNE), National League for Nursing Accrediting Commission (NLNAC), and state boards of nursing, ask that schools show how these documents guide the curriculum in achieving its outcomes.

Once faculty has reached consensus on how to contribute to the institution's mission and states its philosophy, expected program outcomes and course objectives are explicated. Course objectives reflect the faculty's philosophy about behaviors and competencies that are essential to functioning as a nurse (Bevis, 1989). They delineate what the student can do at the conclusion of each course; culminate in the program outcomes, or what is expected of students when they graduate; and are derived from the philosophical foundations of the curriculum.

The Role of Students and Consumers in Curriculum Development

In today's educational and health care environment, it is essential to gather thoughts and ideas about the curriculum from diverse sources to ensure that it meets current and future needs in a meaningful way. Important sources of information include nursing students, alumni, employers of graduates, health care consumers, and faculty from other disciplines with whom collaborative student learning experiences are important. The latter may include social work, nutrition, human development and family studies, psychology, gerontology, ethics, law, and medicine. There are several ways to involve these groups in the process of curriculum development.

Students can serve as elected or appointed representatives on the curriculum committee to ensure that their voice is heard regarding needed content and effective ways of delivering it. The faculty and administration of the school may also choose to invite representatives of alumni, employers of graduates, consumers, and other disciplines to participate on the committee. They may become standing members of it, or may be asked to attend at specific times to provide input as the curriculum is developed, revised, and evaluated.

Input regarding the curriculum may also be obtained through the use of surveys. These provide a means of collecting information in a highly structured way. The resulting data can be subjected to statistical analysis, such as determining frequency of response and measures of central tendency (Rains, 1998). Including a self-addressed stamped envelope for survey returns (if the questionnaires are mailed to participants) increases the response rate. Cost-saving alternatives for collecting information include distribution of surveys by faculty and students in the clinical agencies with which they affiliate and annual advisory board meetings whose members represent various constituencies.

Survey questions can be crafted to the particular population that is surveyed. For example, students may be asked to respond to questions about the usefulness of prerequisite courses in the nursing major and to suggest changes to them, the need for additional required courses or content in the nursing major, and the competencies they view as essential to their functioning after graduation (Mawn & Reece, 2000). Alumni and employers can be asked to respond to questions about the education needed to function in today's health care environment. Within that context, faculty may seek specific responses to prerequisites that should be required for entry into the nursing major, essential content to be included in nursing courses and its sequencing, the best methods to deliver content, and recommended clinical placements for students. Health care consumers can be queried about the skills and competencies they expect a nurse to possess.

Input from the various constituencies can also be obtained using a Delphi survey, which is an efficient, though expensive, way of obtaining information from a large group. This technique asks participants to respond to a series of questionnaires about their opinions on a specified topic (Polit & Hungler, 1995). Responses to each questionnaire are analyzed, summarized, and returned to participants with the next questionnaire. This gives them the chance to respond to group feedback regarding the topic. Usually, three rounds of questionnaires are needed to reach consensus.

Another effective way to gather information needed for curriculum development is the use of focus groups (Polit & Hungler, 1995). Five to 15 people participate in a group discussion on the topic of concern. A moderator guides the discussion using a predetermined set of questions to be addressed. In the case of curriculum development, the focus group may consist of a mixed group of members from each constituency (students, alumni, consumers, and employers), or may be composed of only members from one group.

Faculty Responsibilities in Curriculum Evaluation

While Section 5 of this text addresses program evaluation and accreditation, the role of faculty in the process of curriculum evaluation bears review as to its place in curriculum development. Chapter 11 describes the purpose and process for developing a master plan of evaluation for an educational program. It provides a conceptual framework for the discussion that follows.

According to Applegate (1998), curriculum evaluation is "the process of delineating, obtaining, and providing information useful for making decisions and judgments about a program of learning" (p. 179). It is an integral part of curriculum development and revision, and must be planned carefully to ensure that the data it generates are useful in guiding decisions about the curriculum and its expected outcomes. It is the responsibility of faculty to see that curriculum evaluation is carried out at regularly scheduled intervals. However, it may also be accomplished at the request of the administrator when it appears that there are concerns regarding student progression and/or completion of the program.

For evaluation to be effective, faculty must delineate the standards that will be used to measure intended outcomes versus actual outcomes. Faculty must also choose an evaluation model that is appropriate to their needs, as well as to the curriculum. According to Doll (1992), all models help distinguish the intended curriculum from the one that is implemented. They also have common elements that are required. These include clearly stated objectives, the use of measurements that are congruent with the objectives so that actual and intended outcomes can be determined, the use of standards against which data are measured, the analysis of the data that are obtained, and the documentation of decisions that are made based on the findings (Applegate, 1998).

It is the responsibility of the curriculum committee to evaluate individual courses as well as the total curriculum. Courses are evaluated to determine if they are placed appropriately in the curriculum and to assess if students had the necessary prerequisites to be successful in them (Applegate, 1998). Faculty must decide if the content, learning activities, methods of evaluation, and outcomes are congruent with the course objectives.

When evaluating the total curriculum, faculty must determine if courses and their content are sequenced in a way that makes sense. They must ensure that concepts and learning activities are ordered from simple to complex as students progress through the curriculum. Faculty should also determine if students have the needed knowledge from previous levels to be successful in the next one and to demonstrate the expected outcomes at the completion of the program.

Formative and summative evaluation measures are essential to determining course and program effectiveness. Formative evaluation occurs as courses are taught and the curriculum unfolds (Reilly & Oermann, 1990). It determines progress toward the achievement of the purpose, goals, and outcomes of the course or program. Data are used to make adjustments in the course or program as needed in an effort to ensure that it is effective. Summative evaluation takes place at the end of the course or program (Reilly & Oermann, 1990). It looks at the entire entity to determine its effectiveness in meeting the expected outcomes. Data are used to revise the curriculum as needed.

▲ SUMMARY

Chapter 2 reviewed the responsibilities of faculty in developing, revising, and evaluating the curriculum. Factors that were examined included the levels of approval needed to adopt a curriculum and the faculty and administrator's roles and responsibilities in its development and evaluation. These factors are addressed within the context of the institution's mission and philosophy as well as the philosophical beliefs of the faculty regarding the expected competencies and outcomes of the school of nursing's graduates. Chapter 2 also described effective communication strategies for accomplishing the curriculum development and revision processes.

This chapter emphasized the importance of including students, alumni, and consumers in the development of the curriculum and provided several methods to accomplish this. Finally, it discussed the importance of engaging in formative and summative evaluation of the curriculum.

DISCUSSION QUESTIONS

1. How does academic freedom apply to the process of curriculum development?
2. What global and societal trends are likely to affect the development of nursing curricula in the next 5 to 10 years?

3. How much influence should regulatory bodies, such as state boards of nursing, CCNE, and NLNAC, have on curriculum development?

4. To what extent should the NCLEX pass rates of graduates of a school of nursing dictate the need for curricular revision?

5. As faculty members plan the curriculum, should provisions be made for students to receive hospital experiences in all clinical specialty areas? Why or why not?

LEARNING ACTIVITIES

Student Learning Activity

1. Conduct a focus group composed of your classmates to determine what content should be included in a curriculum that you might develop.

Faculty Development Activity

1. Compare the accreditation criteria for baccalaureate programs set forth by the CCNE and the NLNAC. What are the similarities and differences between the two? Decide which set of criteria you will use as you develop/revise the curriculum. Provide a rationale for your decision.

REFERENCES

Alford, D., & Futrell, M. (1998). Wellness and health promotion of the elderly. In J. A. Alexander & C. L. Rector (Eds.), *Readings in gerontological nursing.* Philadelphia: Lippincott.

Applegate, M. H. (1998). Curriculum evaluation. In D. Billings & J. Halstead (Eds.), *Teaching in nursing: A guide for faculty.* Philadelphia: WB Saunders.

Barger, S. (1994). Educating nursing students for community-based practice. *Dean's Notes, 15,* 1–3.

Bevis, E. O. (1989). *Curriculum building in nursing: A process.* Boston: Jones and Bartlett.

Boland, D. L. (1998). Developing curriculum: Frameworks, outcomes, and competencies. In D. Billings & J. Halstead (Eds.), *Teaching in nursing: A guide for faculty.* Philadelphia: WB Saunders.

Cleary, K. K. (2001). Using the nominal group technique to reach consensus. *Acute Care Perspectives, 10*(3), 16–9.

Commission on Collegiate Nursing Education. (2004). *Home Page.* Retrieved October 11, 2004, from http://www. aacn.nche.edu/Accreditation/index.htm

Csokasy, J. (1998). Philosophical foundations of the curriculum. In D. Billings & J. Halstead (Eds.), *Teaching in nursing: A guide for faculty.* Philadelphia: WB Saunders.

Dillard, N., & Laidig, J. (1998). Curriculum development: An overview. In D. Billings & J. Halstead (Eds.), *Teaching in nursing: A guide for faculty.* Philadelphia: WB Saunders.

Doll, R. G. (1992). *Curriculum improvement: Decision making and process.* Boston: Allyn & Bacon.

Finke, L. M. (1998). Teaching in nursing: The faculty role. In D. Billings & J. Halstead (Eds.), *Teaching in nursing: A guide for faculty.* Philadelphia: WB Saunders.

Finke, L. M & Boland, D. L. (1998). Curriculum designs. In D. Billings & J. Halstead (Eds.), *Teaching in nursing: A guide for faculty.* Philadelphia: WB Saunders.

Hamner, J., & Wilder, B. (2001). A new curriculum for a new millennium. *Nursing Outlook, 49*(3), 127–131.

Hull, E., St. Romain, J., Alexander, P., Schaff, S., & Jones, W. (2001). Moving cemeteries: A framework for facilitating curriculum revision. *Nurse Educator, 26*(6), 280–282.

Hunt, R. (1998). Community-based nursing: Philosophy or setting? *American Journal of Nursing, 98,* 44–47.

Huston, C. J., & Fox, S. (1998). The changing health care market: Implications for nursing education in the coming decade. *Nursing Outlook, 46,* 109–114.

Klineberg, S. L. (1994). Envisioning the next fifty years: Six revolutionary trends. In T. Mullen (Ed.), *Witness in Washington: Fifty years of friendly persuasion.* Richmond, IN: Friends United Press.

Lancaster, J. (1985). The perils and joys of collaborative research. *Nursing Outlook, 33*(5) 231–232, 238.

Larsen, P. D. (2000). Community-based curricula: New issues to address. *Journal of Nursing Education 39*(3), 140–142.

Lieb, M. (1995). Mentoring: Making a difference in nursing education. In B. Bayles & T. Parks-Doyle (Eds.), *The web of inclusion: Faculty helping faculty.* New York: National League for Nursing.

Marriner-Tomey, A. (1996). *A guide to nursing management* (5th ed). St. Louis, MO: Mosby Year Book.

Mawn, B., & Reece, S. M. (2000). Reconfiguring a curriculum for the new millennium: The process of change. *Journal of Nursing Education, 39*(3), 101–108.

National Council of State Boards of Nursing. (2004). *Home Page.* Retrieved October 11, 2004, from http://www.ncsbn.org

National League for Nursing Accrediting Commission. (2004). *Home Page.* Retrieved October 11, 2004, from http://nlnac.org/home.htm

Newsom, W., & Hays, C. (1991). Are mission statements worthwhile? *Planning for Higher Education, 19*(2), 28–30.

Polit, D. F., & Hungler, B. P. (1995). *Nursing research: Principles and methods* (5th ed.). Philadelphia: JB Lippincott.

Rains, J. W. (1998). Forces and issues influencing curriculum development. In D. Billings & J. Halstead (Eds.), *Teaching in nursing: A guide for faculty.* Philadelphia: WB Saunders.

Ratliff, J. L (1997). What is a curriculum and what should it be? In J. G. Gaff & J.L Ratliff & Associates (Eds.). *Handbook of the undergraduate curriculum.* San Francisco: Jossey-Bass.

Reilly, D. E., & Oermann, M. H. (1990). *Behavioral objectives: Evaluation in nursing.* New York: National League for Nursing.

Riner, M. E., & Billings, D. M. (1999). Faculty development for teaching in a changing health care environment: A statewide needs assessment. *Journal of Nursing Education, 38*(9), 427–431.

Learning Theories, Education Taxonomies, and Critical Thinking

▼

Sarah B. Keating, EdD, RN, FAAN

2

▲ OVERVIEW

Section 2 introduces learning theories, educational taxonomies, and critical/creative thinking concepts that faculty must consider when developing or revising curricula. They serve to guide educators when they develop program statements for the mission (or in newer terminology, vision) and the philosophy (sometimes called values or belief statements). Learning theories, concepts, models, educational taxonomies, and critical/creative thinking theories and concepts apply to the processes of instructional design and evaluation that follow curriculum development and are considered again in detail at that time.

Learning Theories

Chapter 3 reviews five major categories of learning theories commonly accepted in today's education system and applies them to various levels of nursing education. It raises the continuing issue in nursing that faces educators—that is, nursing continues to rely upon the behaviorist theories of learning that focus on the teacher as the transmitter of knowledge instead of the learning needs and characteristics of the learners. Behaviorist models of learning are appropriate for students to gain basic knowledge and skills; however, to facilitate the critical and creative thinking skills necessary for nursing practice, the newer models of learning are better suited to the learner and to the needs of the health care system and profession.

Additional categories of learning theories are reviewed in Chapter 3, pointing out their contributions to learning strategies that are student focused. Several times the author of the chapter alludes to a need for the learner to be involved in planning learning experiences, including the choice of objectives or goals for learning experiences, content, and methods for achieving the goals. Throughout the chapter, learning theories are linked to various education programs in nursing that best suit the levels of student in gaining new knowledge and skills.

Familiarity with the major categories of learning theories and philosophical discussion among faculty members are essential parts of curriculum development, early in the process. The theories set the stage for how the curriculum will be organized and how its students will achieve program goals in preparing nurses for the profession. Furthermore, the choice of learning theories as part of a conceptual or organizing framework provides direction for the implementation of the curriculum and instructional strategies.

Education Taxonomies

Chapter 4 reviews the traditional educational taxonomies and domains of learning as they apply to nursing education. While nursing adopted and continues to use modified models based on Tyler (1949) for organizing the curriculum, there is a need to examine newer taxonomies that integrate the domains of learning and foster students' dispositions toward the development of critical and creative thinking. The newer taxonomies lift objectives from previous expectations related to rote or recall memorization to higher orders of understanding and conceptualization. The modalities of problem solving, critical and creative thinking, and decision-making are suited to today's changing health care system. There is a need for professionals who can respond to health care needs with strategies that utilize evidence-based and innovative solutions to health care problems and that foster health promotion and prevention of disease. Changes in the way the curriculum is developed and implemented through instructional designs that focus on the leaner and, ultimately, the consumer of nursing care are in response to NLN's latest call for curriculum reform (NLN, 2003).

Critical Thinking

An essential part of curriculum planning is the recognition by faculty of critical/creative thinking and the role it plays in the development of clinical decision-making skills for nursing practice. Thus, critical/creative thinking must be part of faculty's planning for the curriculum and how it will be integrated into courses and their instructional designs. Chapter 4 reviews definitions of critical thinking as they apply to nursing education. Integrated throughout the discussion are examples of teaching–learning strategies and ways in which to assess student learning that assist the educator when developing goals and objectives. The focus on the learner by using newer pedagogical modalities other than lecture is discussed. The issues raised in Chapter 4 include to what extent nursing curricula should change to meet health care demands by continuing to use taxonomies and domains of learning models without "throwing out the baby with the bath water." The second issue relates to critical and creative thinking and the application of existing definitions to nursing and its measurement. Some current definitions do not seem to apply to nursing; thus, the challenge to educators and the profession is to develop its own.

Learning Theories Applied to Nursing Curriculum Development

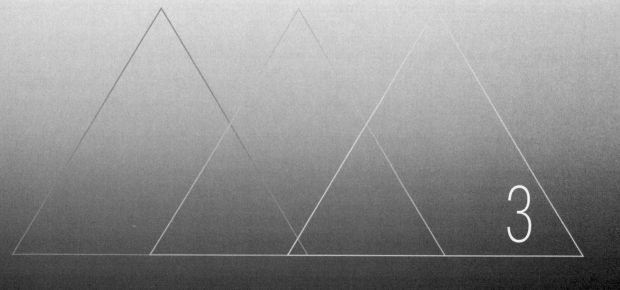

Mary Ann Haw, PhD, RN

OBJECTIVES

On completion of Chapter 3, the reader will be able to:

1. Evaluate learning theories for their potential usefulness in developing nursing curricula and instructional design at all levels of nursing education from vocational to doctoral degree programs.
2. Apply select learning theories judged as appropriate to a framework for nursing curriculum development and instructional design within a given nursing educational level, student population, and social context.
3. Evaluate the application of classic learning theories, concepts, and models to newer ideas in the development of nursing education programs.
4. Develop a plan for evaluating the effectiveness of specific theories in facilitating learning and building requisite nursing knowledge and competence among students at a given level of nursing education and within a given social context.

3

▲ OVERVIEW

As discussed in Chapter 2, the faculty holds the ultimate responsibility for curriculum development. In that role, faculty members must reach consensus on their beliefs about the learning processes their students undergo to master the knowledge and skills necessary for practicing as nurses. Identifying their beliefs about the teaching and learning processes is one of the earliest activities that faculty members take when revising or developing the curriculum. The Bureau of Health Professions (2002) reported that the average age of graduate nurses from associate degree programs—the largest producers of nurses—was 33 in 2000. With a preponderance of adult learners in nursing education programs and the need to continue to educate the existing and future nursing work force, it is important that faculty members include adult learning theories in their repertoire.

The application of learning theories in the curriculum is based on the students' needs and the nature of the program, and it should be included in the mission and philosophy statements. Learning theories are often identified by major categories and include classic theories, newer applications of them to the learning environment, and more recent theories and concepts. A synopsis of the major learning theories can be found at the Theory into Practice (TIP) website at http://tip.psychology.org/index.html.

Beginning in the 1920s and 1930s, there has been progressive development and refinement in learning theories from classic stimulus-response theory to the more progressive constructivist/transformational theoretical approach for guiding curriculum development in educational settings. These theories generally can be categorized under one or more of five learning paradigms: behaviorism, cognitivism, humanism, constructivism, and organizational learning. The organizational learning paradigm emerged in business settings and relates to theories appropriate for the development and education of employees in organizational settings using advanced technology (Leonard, 2002). Most educators agree that we are shifting from an industrial-age teacher-centric educational paradigm in which students passively receive a preset body of knowledge from the teacher to an active learning paradigm in which students participate in setting objectives, selecting content, and exercising choice over learning methods.

This chapter focuses on learning theories drawn from the five learning paradigms that can be used for guiding curriculum development and instructional design in nursing. Each learning paradigm is defined followed by a brief description of theories representative of the learning paradigm that either have been applied to nursing curricula development or instructional design or are promising new theories for application in the future. The definitions of the learning paradigms and descriptions of their representational theories are drawn primarily from Leonard's comprehensive text, *Learning Theories From A to Z* (2002). The potential strengths and weaknesses of major learning paradigms and their representational learning theories are summarized and highlight potential good matches with particular nursing education learning contexts and student learning needs across all levels of nursing education from the licensed vocational program to the doctoral degree.

▲ THE FIVE LEARNING PARADIGMS AND REPRESENTATIONAL THEORIES

Behaviorism

Stemming from Thorndike (1949) (connectionism), Watson (behaviorism) (1924), and Skinner (operant conditioning) (1938), it was proposed that learning occurs through close associations between stimuli and responses. A mechanistic approach, the stimulus–response association was believed to guide all behavior, including learning. The theory was based on Skinner's research on mice and later on humans involving control of the environment and pacing of reinforcements to foster consistent behavior (1953).

Behaviorism today is based on the belief that "instruction is achieved by observable, measurable and controllable objectives set by the instructor and met by students" (Leonard, 2002, p. 16). Instructors using a behaviorist approach develop learning objectives, identify content, structure learning from simple to complex, and assess achievement of learning outcomes by observing a set of behavioral outcomes. Behaviorism is not concerned with the creativity or autonomy of learners nor with their internal mental states. Instead, behaviorism is concerned only with behavioral change outcomes. Assessment of learning is based solely on demonstrated achievement of preset learning objectives. This learning paradigm has been criticized for constricting students' learning to a small set of objectives. Despite the limitations of this theory, it has been widely used in nursing education over the last 2 decades with increasing disfavor among progressive nurse educators. Spearheaded by Em Olivia Bevis, a noted expert in curriculum development in nursing, the call for a "new age curricular paradigm in nursing" based on "human caring and an emancipatory, liberating education" (Bevis, 1989) is a paradigm that is progressively being adopted by the profession.

Theorists representative of the behaviorist-learning paradigm are Gagne (1970) and Bandura (1976). Gagne, who is claimed by both behaviorists and cognitivists, developed the conditions of learning theory that involve "a hierarchy of different types of learning which require different instructional strategies and instructional designs based on specific learning outcomes" (Leonard, 2001, p. 36). According to Gagne (1970), there is a hierarchical set of cognitive processes that are associated with the nine instructional events. The nine instructional events and their respective cognitive processes (in parenthesis) are as follows: (1) gain learners' attention to focus on the task at hand (reception), (2) inform learners of the learning objective to let the learners know the projected learning outcomes (expectancy), (3) stimulate recall of prior learning to stimulate prior knowledge previously remembered and gained (retrieval), (4) present the stimulus to initiate new information (selective encoding), (5) provide learning guidance so that new information can be stored and remembered (semantic encoding), (6) elicit performance to stimulate learner recall through the learner's active responses (responding), (7) provide feedback to ensure that learning has occurred (reinforcement), (8) assess performance to determine that the learner's performance is appropriate, correct, and in line with projected learning outcomes (retrieval), and (9) enhance retention and transfer to place the new knowledge gained into long-term memory (generalization) (Gagne, 1974). These hierarchies provide a rationale for sequencing of instruction. Gagne's theory is suggested for application to vocational nursing students and those entering associate degree programs without any background or knowledge base in nursing. The sequencing of instruction provides a logical structure and sequence for acquiring and mastering foundational knowledge in nursing.

Bandura's social learning theory (1976) is based on a belief that learning occurs through imitation of others. Focusing on behavior modeling, a learner observes another and imitates the behavior of those around him or her, particularly those with whom the learner identifies and who are observed to achieve rewarding outcomes (Bandura, 1976). This theory has been tested in a variety of patient education contexts as well as nursing education contexts.

Support groups established for patients wanting to change health behavior such as weight loss, smoking cessation, and alcohol and drug addiction often learn from others who have been successful in changing health behavior (Glanz, Lewis, & Rimer, 1997). Bandura's theory is particularly well suited for learning in the clinical setting. Nursing students often learn from competent and expert role models such as faculty, nursing mentors, and preceptors in clinical practice. Potential role models should be evaluated and chosen carefully to ensure that nurse mentors and preceptors model positive behaviors for nursing students (Lockwood-Rayermann, 2003).

Cognitivism

Cognitivism is "the belief that human thinking and learning are similar to that of computer information processing" (Leonard, 2002, p. 29). This learning paradigm focuses on learning inputs and outputs that are processed by the human mind. In education, cognitivism focuses on the accurate transmission of knowledge of the objective reality of the world from the viewpoint of the teacher (expert) to students. Teaching methods involve required readings in preparation for class and lecture as a means of transmitting knowledge. Learning assessment involves determining the extent to which the learners' viewpoints match that of the teacher. The weakness of this model lies in determining whose construction of reality is an accurate depiction of reality, student or teacher (Leonard, 2002). Examples of cognitivist learning theorists are Ausubel (1963), Carroll (1963, 1989), and Merrill (1983).

Ausubel's subsumption theory (1963), expository and instructor-centric in nature, states that new material learned in a school setting should be related to previously presented ideas and concepts that become processed and extant in the cognitive structures of the learner's brain. Ausubel believes that teachers must provide contextual information to students, as well as advanced organizers such as abstracts, outlines, and introductions to a large body of content. These advanced organizers act as bridges between previously learned material and new material. Examples of teaching strategies using Ausubel's theory include concept-mapping, mind-mapping, and knowledge-mapping techniques. Concept mapping has been successfully used in teaching neophyte nursing students the nursing process, including how to gather and group clinical data meaningfully, diagnose nursing problems, specify relationships among the diagnoses, and develop appropriate interventions (Schuster, 2002). Subsumption theory may be effective with first-level bachelor of science in nursing (BSN) students who have mastered fundamental concepts and may need a bridge to facilitate advancing to a more complex level of clinical practice. The same holds true for nurses who have completed an associate degree in nursing (ADN) program and are accelerating through a BSN completion program.

Merrill's (1983) learner-centric component display theory (CDT) emphasizes that the learner should have control over the sequencing of learning, based upon the instructional components provided by the lesson. Merrill's theory has two learning dimensions: content and performance. Along the performance continuum, Merrill includes "find," "use," and "remember." Along the content continuum, Merrill includes "fact," "concept," "procedure," and "principle." Merrill's theory identifies four primary presentation forms for lessons: "(1) expository presentation of generality, (2) expository presentation of instances, (3) inquisitory generality, and (4) inquisitory instance, as well as four secondary presentation forms: (1) prerequisites, (2) objectives, (3) helps and mnemonics, and (4) feedback (Leonard, 2002, p. 33)".

The cognitive bases of Merrill's theory are associative memory (a hierarchical network structure) and algorithmic memory (using schema) (Merrill, 1983).

Merrill, Li, & Jones (1991) and Merrill (1996), later developed an instructional transaction theory, an enhancement of the component display theory, which can be used to individualize a learning sequence suitable to the learner's needs. Learners interact with a set of knowledge objects, also referred to as learning objects. Knowledge objects contain information, often presented in multimedia form, regarding a particular topic or subject. The container may include multiple files on the topic that are in the forms of text, graphics, audio, and video. The knowledge object is usually focused on acquisition of information to perform a specific job and contains a set of highly interactive instructional sequences that progressively build competence. The component display theory and variety of presentation forms is well suited for undergraduate nursing students and new BSN graduates being oriented to a new clinical setting and client population, particularly those students and graduates who wish to have some control over the direction of learning and whose learning style preferences include self-selection of a variety of media.

According to Leonard (2002), Carroll's mastery learning theory "shifts the learning from the teacher to the student in terms of the student being able to master certain content and skills within the instruction specified by the instructor," (p. 123). Mastery learning emphasizes the individual learning needs and pace of each learner. "Within the mastery learning method, teachers provide an instructional strategy within the curriculum design that permits all learners to be successful. Four activities are involved: (1) specify to the learner the goal of the learning in terms of what is to be learned and how the learning activity will be evaluated, (2) permit learner self-pacing whereby each learner can learn at his/her own pace, (3) monitor student progress and provide immediate feedback to keep students on the learning path, and (4) evaluate to ensure that the final goal of the learning activity is achieved by each student" (Leonard, 2002, p. 123–124). Although Carroll's model has been criticized for the amount of time it takes and that learners do reach different levels of achievement (Carroll, 1989), mastery learning theory seems well suited to anxious students, including those with test anxiety, students needing structure, or those for whom English is a second language.

Humanism

"Humanism is the belief that human thinking and learning are not driven by information processing theory, nor by the enhancement of schemas through the creation of new knowledge structures nor by conditioned responses to various stimuli. Rather, human thinking and learning are driven by the growth of the self as a whole, mature, and complete human being, who has a strong character and an ability to make decisions that positively influence others" (Leonard, 2002, p. 86). Learning theorists of behaviorist and cognitivist persuasions often dismiss humanism as a major learning theory. As a philosophy, "Humanism is the belief that humans have the freedom and autonomy to make choices that positively affect others as well as the ability to advance themselves morally, spiritually, emotionally and mentally" (Leonard, 2002, p. 86). Humanism is consistent with the emerging paradigm in nursing education of human caring and an emancipatory, liberating education. Examples of humanistic theories of psychology and education are Maslow (1970), Rogers (1961), and Wertheimer (1959).

Maslow's hierarchy of needs (1970) identifies seven levels that humans seek to achieve, from basic survival needs, such as food, water, and shelter, to self-actualization, "a state of full use and exploitation of talents, capacities and potentialities of the individual (Leonard, 2002, p. 86)." Within this context, "individual knowledge centers on the personal learning experiences of the learner, all leading toward a state of self-actualization" (Leonard, 2002, p. 86). Maslow's hierarchy is based on several assumptions about human needs: (1) basic needs must be at least partially satisfied before higher-order needs can be met; for example, one cannot focus on learner self-esteem needs if he or she is a single parent and has significant financial problems and job responsibilities; and (2) individuals perceive their own needs and meet them in different ways (Maslow, 1970). What is regarded as a perceived need and hoped-for outcome for one person may be quite different for another individual; therefore, an assessment of the student's needs and goals, as he or she perceives them, should be conducted. Many students entering nursing are employed and have family and community responsibilities. Maslow's theory may be applied pragmatically by linking the student with resources, such as financial aid, work-study programs, and on-campus child-care, as a step toward fulfilling the basic needs of the learner.

Rogers (1961), a mid-20th century psychologist/humanist, developed a theory of "personhood" based on the idea that people are constantly adapting, growing, and discovering themselves. Rogers was a great proponent of experiential learning, which had as its focus "the personal involvement and personal experience of the learner as the primary shaping influence over the individual's learning activity" (Leonard, 2002, p. 68). Roger's experiential learning theory is based on four basic principles: (1) personal involvement of the learner, (2) learner-initiated activity, (3) self-assessment and self-evaluation, and (4) learning situations that have real meaning to the individual (Rogers, 1961). Rogers' theory of personhood is well suited to students at any levels of nursing study but particularly to those who are at the graduate and doctoral levels of nursing education. Learning situations, clinical practice opportunities, and research opportunities that are real and compelling for graduate students are strategies for helping them to advance their practice, pursue fulfilling careers, and contribute to improve nursing outcomes.

In a similar vein, Wertheimer (1959), working in concert with colleagues Kohler and Koffka, began a movement that opposed behaviorism, particularly for its focus on empiricism and objective analysis, and favored a holistic subjective approach to how humans learn— gestalt theory (also referred to as phenomenology). This theory focuses on describing how individuals perceive the world as a meaningful whole rather than isolated stimuli. "In gestalt theory, no event nor single part can be separated from the whole. Whatever occurs to that individual human shapes that individual and influences all aspects of that person. In gestalt theory, the focus is on the totality, not the individual parts. *Consciousness* determines behavior. Human values, beliefs, and attitudes influence tremendously human conscious experience. Learning occurs through insight. After pondering a problem for a while, a human reaches a solution all at once" (Leonard, 2002, pp. 148–149). Gestalt theory is particularly well suited to collaborative learning among graduate and doctoral students in which human values, beliefs, and attitudes are articulated and subjected to scrutiny among peers and nursing scholars.

Constructivism

Constructivism is "the belief that learners, having had some prior knowledge and experience as a basis from which to test their hypotheses, build their own set of content to solve a particular problem posed by the instructor. Constructivism is a learner-centric educational paradigm, in which content is constructed by the learners in a team-based, collaborative learning, constructivist learning environment rather than by the instructor" (Leonard, 2002, pp. 37–39). Among the constructivist theorists are Knowles (1975), Bruner (1960, 1961), and Mezirow (2000).

Knowles' (1975, 1998) theory of adult education suggests that there are three principles to consider when working with adult learners: (1) the self-concept of the learner, (2) accumulated life experience, and (3) the purpose he or she has in mind for the material being learned. A person's self-concept may either enhance or impede learning. Someone who had successful learning experiences in the past will more likely have a positive self-concept regarding learning that facilitates new learning opportunities. Another person's negative experiences may present a barrier to learning. Becoming aware of a person's self-concept provides direction in selecting appropriate learning strategies that either build upon prior success or counter prior negative experiences and foster self-confidence in one's ability to learn in a new situation. Adult learners seek out learning when they have a specific learning goal in mind, which may or may not coincide with the teacher's goals. Unlike children, adult learners approach a learning situation with their accumulated life experiences and rich reservoirs of knowledge. As a consequence, adult learners want to have control over their own lives and have some say over the content and direction of their learning. Because nearly all who enter nursing as a profession are adult learners, it follows that adult learning theory should apply throughout all levels of nursing education from vocational programs through the doctoral level.

Bruner's discovery learning theory (1960, 1961) is based on the premise that "learners are more likely to remember concepts if they discover them on their own, apply them to their own knowledge base, and structure them to fit their own backgrounds and life experiences" (Leonard, 2002, p. 38). The emphasis is on the learner who sets the objectives and creates and structures the knowledge set to be learned. The students may make errors in the process, but they learn from their mistakes. A key assumption of this learner-centric theory is that learners are "mature enough, self motivated enough and experienced enough to actively take part in the learning formation and structuring of learning content. The instructor's role is as a facilitator, a coach, and a guide who points the way and assists the learners through their active learning activities" (Leonard, 2002, pp. 216–217). Discovery learning theory has been used in many different learning contexts. Because of the assumptions underlying this theory, teachers and instructors should assess and validate learners for requisite maturity, self-motivation, and experience for discovery learning.

Mezirow's (2000) transformative learning theory is based on the assumption that individuals have their own expectations about the world, framed within their own cultural backgrounds and presuppositions, which directly influence the meaning derived from personal experiences. Transformative learning theory addresses the *revision* of meaning structures (in other words, changing one's perspective). Perspective transformation explains the process of how adults revise their meaning structures. Mezirow's theory identifies experience, critical reflection on experience, and rational discourse with others as the process for changing one's meaning structures. Experience provides the grist for critical reflection. Each learner constructs meaning through personal reflection. The individual and others then subject these meanings to scrutiny. Critical reflection involves questioning the integrity of one's assumptions and beliefs, which results in transformation or change in one's perspective

(Taylor, 1998). In applying this theory to nursing education, emphasis should be placed on learning through clinical experience. Students should be encouraged to reflect on their clinical experiences to make their own interpretations of meaning (purposes, beliefs, judgments, and feelings) in nursing practice. Students should also be encouraged to articulate their own assumptions underlying their interpretations of clinical experiences and to subject these interpretations to their own and others' scrutiny.

Organizational Learning

Organizational learning concerns "learning theories and environments that are currently specific to industry education and training. Organizational learning as a term itself refers to learning that occurs by individuals and by groups and teams within the business enterprise (Leonard, 2002, p. 144)." Schein (1995) and his colleagues at the Massachusetts Institute of Technology (MIT) Center for Organizational Learning developed a set of guiding principles helpful in understanding what is meant by organizational learning as a paradigm for change in business:

> "(1) all humans have a drive to learn, which organizations should strive to encourage; (2) learning is a social activity and requires a learning community that should exist within the organization; (3) learning communities are the nucleus and the source of successful organizations; (4) successful organizations are set up to be in harmony with human, social and natural needs and requirements; (5) organizations must foster individual and collective capacities to resolve complex, interdependent issues that continually recur within the enterprise; (6) learning communities that include multiple organizations increase the capacity for organizational change and development. These principles of organizational learning are key drivers for guiding learning organizations and for creating business transformation and organizational change" (Schein, 1993, 1995 p. 144).

Representational theorists for organizational learning include Senge (1990), Mager (1975, 1997), and de Bono (1990).

While not a learning theory per se, Senge's (1990) text entitled, *The Fifth Discipline*, identified "a new way for companies to perceive themselves, grow, and develop a sense of self-awareness" (Leonard, 2002, p. 74). Senge's fifth discipline is "systems thinking," in which the entire organization and its constituent parts are analyzed, including all relationships among the parts, a process that must be completed for the organization to become a learning organization. Systems thinking enables the organization to "make informed decisions based on an understanding of how the entire organization operates within a social context" (Leonard, 2002, p. 74). This particular approach is potentially valuable for graduate program curriculum development in schools of nursing and hospital staff development programs for preparing nurses for top-level positions such as nurse managers, administrators, and executives.

Mager's Criterion-Referenced Instruction (CRI) (1975, 1997) focuses on the job activities of the learners and seeks to determine the specific competencies (knowledge and skills) needed to perform the job successfully. The CRI process includes the following activities in preparation for teaching students: (1) perform a task analysis of content to be learned; (2) determine learner performance objectives and outcomes; (3) set up tests and evaluations of learner outcomes based on performance objectives, and (4) develop the content. The CRI learning approach is particularly well suited to any level of nursing in which nursing students and/or practicing nurses need to master a new area of knowledge and requisite skills for advancing to a particular nursing position, nursing unit, and patient population.

According to Leonard (2002), de Bono (1990) is one of the most prolific learning theorists who explored extensively the creative learning process. De Bono's lateral thinking approach focuses on the process of generating creative ideas to solve problems. The thinking process outlines four steps to creativity: (1) focus on dominant ideas that come to mind to polarize perception of the problem, (2) look at multiple perspectives of the problem, (3) relax the logical thinking process taught in schools as part of the scientific method, and (4) allow "outside of the box" ideas to come to mind and be considered even if they do not fit into the logical, scientific pattern. De Bono's lateral thinking theory is particularly well suited to preparing nurses for management, administration, and executive levels.

▲ ANALYZING AND SELECTING LEARNING THEORIES FOR CURRICULUM DEVELOPMENT

Learning theories may be selected as an overall guide to the curriculum and for developing pedagogical approaches within specific programs of study and course offerings. In selecting learning theories for curriculum development, the following factors need to be considered: the philosophy and mission of the educational institution and the school of nursing; the faculty's beliefs, values, and philosophy regarding how students learn at various levels of study; and the characteristics of the students, such as age, experience, tacit and formal knowledge, race/ethnicity, aptitude, self-concept regarding learning, and learning disabilities.

The philosophy and mission of the school of nursing should be congruent with the philosophy and mission of the educational institution. One of the most significant problems in curriculum development in nursing education today is the rift among faculty members between those who support the industrial-age teacher-centric educational paradigm versus those supporting the learner-centric active learning educational paradigm. Divergent faculty values and beliefs on how students learn may create difficulties in selecting an overall educational paradigm. Essentially, the major choices are: (1) a behaviorist learning paradigm involving teacher control over the content, learning objectives, and direction of the learning or (2) a constructivist paradigm involving student participation and choice in the setting of objectives, selection of content, and direction of learning. However, it may not need to be an either-or decision. It is possible to negotiate a balance between the two paradigms. Perhaps first-year vocational and BSN students without any background in nursing may benefit from a behaviorist approach until they have mastered fundamental knowledge and skills. These same students in subsequent semesters may benefit from a gradual shift to a constructivist approach in which they assume more responsibility for their learning by identifying learning objectives and methods and having a say over the direction of learning. However, until there is some agreement among faculty on how to proceed, a timely change in establishing a new curriculum may be difficult (Schreiber & Banister, 2002).

The characteristics of students should also be considered in selecting learning theories. The age of the student is likely to have an impact on learning. Students entering nursing directly from high school are likely to have less life experience and maturity than students entering nursing in their 20s, 30s, or 40s. On the other hand, older students with a large gap between high school completion and entry into a nursing program are more likely to have some difficulty transitioning into a program of study, particularly if they have experienced a sense of competence in a job and must start at the level of novice in nursing.

Minority students may be the first among generations of family members to enroll in college. Lacking the expertise of family members' experience in what it takes to successfully complete college, these students may benefit from coaching and "know-how" by culturally similar mentors and role models with whom they can identify. Students' prior learning experiences and self-concept regarding learning should be assessed as a preliminary step to selecting learning approaches suitable to the students' present abilities and attitudes toward learning.

Students whose prior experiences in learning have been of the behaviorist paradigm, in which they passively received information from faculty in the form of classroom lectures, may need to be oriented to the constructivist paradigm and its merits, such as learning in collaboration with faculty and fellow students and exercising greater choice over learning goals, content, and methods. Students for whom English is a second language may benefit from sharing insights in a small group as opposed to a large class and from having more time to complete written assignments, exams, and quizzes. Students with physical or learning disabilities or sensory deficits will need classroom-learning accommodations for their particular needs.

Learning theory selection for graduate students depends on the background of the student. Graduate students who have had significant postgraduation experience in nursing will benefit more from a constructivist learning model and an adult learning theory approach. These students are likely to have acquired a great deal of knowledge and skills as well as goal direction and independence from their experience. This type of graduate student often has specific goals in mind for graduate study and is able and eager to direct his or her own learning.

Generic MSN students (students with a BA or BS in a field other than nursing who accelerate through a BSN as a prerequisite to entering a master's degree program) may need a more behaviorist and cognitivist approach as they accelerate through the BSN part of their program. However, these students often can progress to a more constructivist model of learning as they advance through courses in the master's degree program, particularly if they have had some degree of nursing-related experience, such as certified nursing assistant, home health aide, health education, or social work background.

▲ SUMMARY

Nursing education is in transition from a teacher-centric model, in which nursing students passively receive information in the form of lectures, to a learner-centric active learning model, involving student collaboration with faculty and fellow students in constructing knowledge for nursing. The five major learning paradigms: behaviorism, cognitivism, humanism, constructionism, and organizational learning; their representative theories each have something to offer nursing educators in developing innovative and effective curriculum approaches that fit with the social context of learning and characteristics of students. Students will benefit from greater opportunities to participate with faculty and fellow students in selecting learning goals and learning methods and evaluating learning outcomes.

Prior to selecting a learning-specific learning paradigm or theory for developing curricula, faculty members need to analyze students' characteristics and learning styles so that a good fit can be made. Faculty members may likewise benefit from self-assessment of their own teaching and learning styles vis-à-vis the various learning paradigms and learning theories. For some faculty, it may provide a welcome opportunity to experiment with a new theoretical approach or a tailor-made combination of theories. However, no one learning paradigm or theory is going to be universally appropriate for all students, faculty, and learning contexts. As a final step in making the choices and decisions regarding curriculum development for the present and future, a review of the school of nursing's statement of philosophy and mission statement may provide clarity, direction, and resolve for the future.

DISCUSSION QUESTIONS

1. Explain why teaching and learning theories, concepts, and models apply to both curriculum development and instructional design. Compare and contrast how the utilization of these theories, concepts, and models differ between the two processes (curriculum development and instructional design).
2. Do you think that all faculty members need to be in agreement on a particular learning paradigm or theory before making final choices for curriculum development in the future? Why or why not? What other alternatives can you offer?

LEARNING ACTIVITIES

1. As a teacher or as a student, recall a teaching–learning encounter that was very memorable for you, either because it went very well or very poorly. Analyze the factors that contributed either to the success or failure of the encounter, including (if you know) the learning paradigm or theory used. What changes or enhancements would you make in the future?

Student Activities

1. As a small group of BSN students, you are placed in a shelter for homeless families for your community health practicum. What will you need to learn to serve this population? What learning theories are appropriate to this situation? Using these theories, how might you make a difference in the health and quality of life of this population?

Faculty Activities

1. In a group of your nursing faculty colleagues, analyze the characteristics of your entering BSN students. Select a learning paradigm and theory for application to this group of students and a particular course or clinical practicum in the BSN program. Select learning strategies consistent with the learning paradigm and/or theory for the students in the classroom and clinical setting.

REFERENCES

Ausubel, D. P. (1963). *The psychology of meaningful verbal learning*. New York: Grune & Stratton.
Bandura, A. (1976). *Social learning theory*. Englewood Cliffs, NJ: Prentice Hall.

Bevis, E. (1989). *Toward a caring curriculum.* New York: National League for Nursing.

Bruner, J. S. (1960). *The process of education.* Cambridge, MA: Harvard University Press.

Bruner, J. S. (1961). The act of discovery. *Harvard Education Review, 31,* 21–32.

Bureau of Health Professions. (2002). *Health workforce analysis: Projected supply, demand and shortages of registered nurses: 2000–2020.* Retrieved November 10, 2002, from http://bhpr.hrsa.gov/oldhealthworkforce/rnproject/default.htm

Carroll, J. M. (1963). *A model for school learning. Teachers College Record, 64,* 723–733.

Carroll, J. M. (1989). The Carroll model: A 25 year retrospective and prospective view. *Educational Researcher, 18*(1), 26–31.

de Bono, E. (1990). *Lateral thinking.* London: Harper Collins.

Gagne, R. M. (1970). *The conditions of learning* (2nd ed.). New York: Holt, Rinehart & Winston.

Gagne, R. M. (1974). Learning hierarchies. In H. F. Clarizio, R. C. Craig, & W. A. Mehrens (Eds.), *Contemporary issues in educational psychology* (pp. 224–239). Boston: Allyn & Bacon.

Glanz, K., Lewis, M. L., & Rimer, B. K. (Eds.). (1997). *Health behavior and health education: Theory, research and practice* (2nd ed.). San Francisco: Jossey-Bass.

Knowles, M. S. (1975). *Self-directed learning: A guide for learners and teachers.* New York: Cambridge Book Company.

Knowles, M. S., Holton, E. F., & Swanson, R. A. (1998). *The adult learner: The definitive classic in adult education and human resource development* (5th ed.). Houston, TX: Gulf Publishing Company.

Leonard, D. C. (2002). *Learning theories A to Z.* Westport, CT: Greenwood Press.

Lockwood-Rayermann, S. (2003). Preceptors, leadership style, and the student practicum experience. *Nurse Educator, 26*(6), 247–249.

Mager, R. (1975). *Preparing instructional objectives.* Belmont, CA: Fearon Publishers, Inc.

Mager, R. (1997). *The new Mager six-pack.* Atlanta, GA: Center for Effective Performance.

Maslow, A. H. (1970). *Motivation and personality* (2nd ed.). New York: Harper & Row.

Merrill, M. D. (1983). Component display theory. In C. Reigeluth (Ed.), *Instructional design theories and models.* Mahwah, NJ: Lawrence Erlbaum Associates.

Merrill, M. D., Li, Z. & Jones, M. K. (1991). Instructional transaction theory: An introduction. *Educational Technology,* 31, 7–12.

Merrill, M. D. (1996). Instructional transaction theory: Instructional design based on knowledge objects. *Educational Psychology,* 33, 30–37.

Mezirow, J. & Associates. (2000). *Learning as transformation: Critical perspectives on a theory in progress.* San Francisco: Jossey-Bass.

Rogers, C. (1961). *On becoming a person.* Boston: Houghton Mifflin.

Schein, E. (1993). On dialogue, culture and organizational learning. *Organizational Dynamics, 22*(2), 40–45.

Schein, E. (1995). *Building the learning consortium.* (Issue Brief No. 10.005). Paper presented at the 1995 annual meeting of the Center for Organizational Learning. MIT Sloan School of Management, Cambridge, M. A.

Schreiber, R.. & Banister, E. B. (2002). Challenges of teaching in an emancipatory curriculum. *Journal of Nursing Education, 41*(1), 41–45.

Schuster, P. M. (2002). *Concept mapping: A critical thinking approach to care planning.* Philadelphia: F.A. Davis.

Senge, P. (1990). *The fifth discipline.* New York: Doubleday.

Skinner, B. F. (1938). *The behavior of organisms.* New York: Appleton-Century-Crofts.

Skinner, B. F. (1953). *Science and human behavior.* New York: Macmillan

Taylor, E. W. (1998). *Theory and practice of transformative learning theory: An overview.* Columbus, OH: ERIC Clearinghouse on Adult, Career and Vocational Education.

Theory into Practice Data Base (TIP). (2002). *Home page.* Retrieved October 10, 2004, from http://tip.psychology.org

Thorndike, E. L. (1949). *Selected writings from a connectionist's psychology.* New York: Appleton-Century-Crofts.

Watson, J. B. (1924). *The ways of behaviorism.* New York: Harper & Row.

Wertheimer, M. (1959). *Productive thinking* (enlarged ed.). New York: Harper & Row.

Taxonomies and Critical Thinking in Curriculum Design

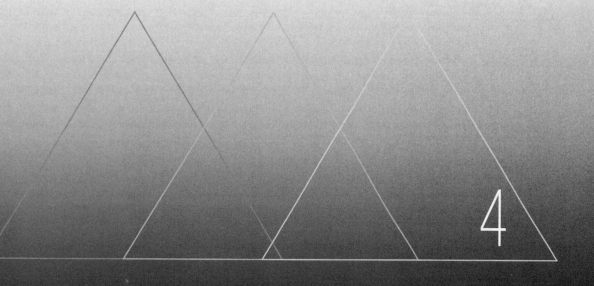

Therese A. Black, MS, RN, CNS

OBJECTIVES

Upon completion of Chapter 4, the reader will be able to:

1. Analyze educational objectives for "type of knowledge" indicators and the complexity of the cognitive processes involved to guide students to understand the scope and depth of the intended learning.
2. Critique the taxonomy lexicon to capture a deeper understanding of expression that is generative of rich and rigorous curriculum objectives.
3. Categorize objectives that progress from the simple to complex thinking processes commensurate with the levels of nursing program curricula.
4. Create taxonomy frameworks from the knowledge of the discipline (facts, theories, or concepts) and expected competencies from selected processes as they relate to nursing education.
5. Produce learning objectives and learning activities that demonstrate structured, higher-order thinking skills, and exemplify dispositions of critical thinking.

4

▲ OVERVIEW

Nurses practicing in the 21st century are continuously flooded with new information to assimilate as the spiraling explosion of technology and scientific discoveries stimulate change in health care. Educators need strategies to manage the vast amounts of information and data relevant to the preparation of new arrivals to the nursing profession. This chapter addresses educational taxonomies and critical thinking in curriculum development and instructional design. Taxonomies generate the architectural structure for objective learning statements, learning activities, and appropriate assessment methods to evaluate the teaching–learning process. Through a two-dimensional categorizing technique, aligning objectives with learning activities leads to increased student learning. Supplementing the structure with appropriate assessment methods permits a systematic review of the curriculum design. A panoramic view of the curriculum provides pragmatic opportunities for nursing educators to share the intent of teaching, determine curriculum comprehensiveness, and identify strategic weaknesses. With this proactive approach, identification of problems become easier to see and creatively resolved.

In the teaching–learning paradigm, whether it is the imparting of knowledge and stimulation of processes with a focus on the student or spotlighting the teacher, the choice of paradigm drives nursing education to be either a liberating or oppressive experience (Anderson et al., 2001; Bevis, 1989, 1993; Lowenstein & Bradshaw, 2001). Behaviorism uses a lens in which the teacher selects the knowledge, skills, and conditions to exactingly change a learner's behavior. Cognitive theorists' view points are that learning is the construction of meaning for the student; therefore, an educator's interest is more on the acquisition of knowledge and what it means for the student, rather than on changes in behavior (Billings & Halstead, 2004; DeYoung, 2003).

Learning occurs through transmission, acquisition, accretion, and emergence (Wilson, 2003). The transmission of information as knowledge, ideas, and skills occurs through purposive telling, demonstration, and guidance and is estimated to be 10% of acquired learning. Acquisition, on the other hand, accounts for about 20% of what is learned and is learning through conscious choice. This type of learning is acquired through exploration, experimenting, self-instruction, inquiry, or general curiosity. Learning by accretion is a subliminal or subconscious process to gain abilities like language, culture, biases, habits, and socially accepted behavior or respect for rules. This represents 70% of what an individual learns. Emergence results from patterning, structuring, and constructing new ideas not previously held that emerge from the brain through reflection, insight, and creative expression or through group interactions. The internal capacity for synthesis, creativity, intuition, wisdom, and problem solving flows from emergence. The influences on emergence are dependent on the allocation of time and opportunities to reflect and construct new knowledge (Wilson, 2003).

Critical thinking is a necessity for students as they apply prerequisite and nursing knowledge to the development of complex thinking skills that lead to clinical decision making in the practice setting. It is very important to nursing education and professional practice that critical thinking strategies and outcomes appear in the criteria for program approval and accreditation (Miller & Babcock, 1996). Scriven and Paul (2003), in their statement on defining critical thinking, state that, "Critical thinking is the intellectually disciplined process of actively and skillfully conceptualizing, applying, analyzing, synthesizing, and/or evaluating information gathered from, or generated by, observation, experience, reflection, reasoning, or communication, as a guide to belief and action." Additional explanations follow the definition and may be found at http://www.criticalthinking.org/University/univclass/Defining.html.

Several nurse educators conducted studies to evaluate the effectiveness of changes in the curricula of nursing programs to promote the development of critical thinking skills in students. Their findings demonstrated that deliberate changes in curricula to develop critical thinking skills in nursing students are effective (Angel, Duffey, & Belyea, 2000; Beckie, Lowry, & Barnett, 2001). Furthermore, one of the studies (Angel et al., 2000) pointed out that some existing assessment tools to measure critical thinking are useful; however, there is a need for evaluation tools that are specific to nursing. Critical thinking is an active process, within the larger teaching–learning picture. It is a process that educators should plan for and reinforce as students gain a base of knowledge and cultivate the heuristic skills of critical thinking. In this way, students develop an ability to pull the crucial essence of knowledge and skills together for the praxis of caring and lifelong learning. The ultimate outcome for students is the disposition to think critically, problem solve, and activate strategies for sound decision making—characteristics highly prized in the nurse.

▲ THE UTILITY OF EDUCATIONAL TAXONOMIES

A taxonomy is a form of classifying, categorizing, clarifying, and defining the features of elements found on a continuum from simple to complex. Creating order according to common or divergent qualities is an expected taxonomy characteristic. A learning domain is a class or category of knowledge and the learning processes involved in which abilities or types of knowledge are defined based on relative complexity or difficulty. Educators tap into the idea of using a classifying framework for educational objectives to communicate what is to be learned, how it will be executed, and, perhaps, to appreciate the underlying reason why.

By creating a means of communication through statements of learning goals and objectives, educators specify the intent of learning outcomes and how the learner will achieve them. The educator selects the knowledge and the processes upon which the student focuses. This knowledge is arrived at through research and consensus among the experts of the discipline. The levels of achievement among students is a function of individual differences, but at the outset, the curriculum plan, with its statements of learning goals and objectives, provides a map of understanding for all involved. External assessment agents such as accreditors seek evidence of program integrity from the flow of philosophical ideations, arrangement of educational objectives and course work, and appropriate internal assessments to demonstrate progression toward the learning outcomes.

▲ TYLERISM

In its effort to legitimize itself within academia, nursing took on the mantle of behaviorism for consistency with its parent educational structures. This learning philosophy served nursing education efficaciously through the 1950s until more recently. It was during the '50s that Tyler (1949) published his text *Basic Principles of Curriculum and Instruction,* the content of which was to significantly change the structure of education worldwide and which became the standard guideline for organizing curricula in schools of nursing (Bevis, 1989; Bevis & Watson, 2000).

Objectives utilize terms that reflect the students' expected or required behavioral changes and are stated in a format that guides teaching and selected learning experiences. The next steps in the Tyler model are purposive learning episodes (now referred to as active learning strategies), which are selected to promote attainment of the objectives and to organize activities into a plan of study consisting of courses and units for instruction. The final step addresses evaluation, which in Tyler's estimation, begins with the objectives of education and is measured by evidence of change in the student, thus accomplishing the behavior(s) sought (Bevis, 1989).

Bloom (1964) and Anderson et al. (2001) argue that Tyler's use of the term "behavior" was unfortunate. The predominant educational philosophy had spun away from the underpinnings of Dewey to the philosophy of "behaviorism," which valued the means employed to attain desired ends. Tyler's perspective, explain Anderson et al., was that a change in behavior was the result of instruction, and the specification of the behavior lent itself to make general and abstract learning goals more specific and concrete. Behavior became confused with behaviorism; thus, instrumental conditioning and formation of stimulus–response association beliefs were incorporated into the teaching–learning arena (Bloom, Englehart, Furst, Hill, & Krathwohl, 1956; Krathwohl, Bloom, & Masia, 1964; Anderson et al., 2001).

▲ OBJECTIVES

Objectives provide guidance to teachers, students, and assessors by focusing curricular efforts on nurse educators to teach and on nursing students to learn. A complete picture of the learning intended, the manner in which students are to make meaning of knowledge, and assessment of what actually transpires occurs through "formulation of ways in which students are expected to be changed by the educative process" (Bloom et al., 1956, p.26).

Establishing or revising the objectives of a nursing program is a time investment that requires considerable examination and planning. Objectives are ubiquitous in that they exist at every level of education with differing intentions communicated for each level of the educational process. Consider the levels of objectives as global, educational, or instructional guides (Anderson et al., 2001). Global objectives provide a visionary, philosophical perspective of the educational process, whereas educational objectives provide an overarching umbrella with more explicit and latent specifics of processes, content, and activities that are followed by the instructional objectives found in course study plans. The function of educational objectives is to provide suggestions for an overall structural design to the curriculum plan, influenced by criteria that come from a community-needs assessment, faculty ideation, accrediting agencies, and boards of nursing. When written at the global level, they connote a multiyear program, and ultimately and synonymously, resemble program terminal outcomes. Delineation of educational course and instructional objectives comes later, as each step of the structure of the curriculum reveals itself.

When composing program goals for nursing curricula, faculty members develop global goals or objectives that are broad statements of purpose, reflecting logical, thoughtful expression of well-defined community needs and desired outcomes. The goal may describe the desirable attributes of a professional nurse and how the study plan is designed to attain these characteristics. Global program goals, in contrast to instructional goals, do not reflect precise or even observable behaviors. Rather, they reflect a broad description of characteristics, using nonspecific terminology, and thus simultaneously sculpt a summative statement of intended student learning (Anderson et al., 2001; Bevis & Watson, 2000; Bevis, 1989; King, 1984; Krathwohl et. al., 1964; Bloom et al., 1956).

Tyler (1949) suggested "the most useful form for stating objectives is to express them in terms which identify both the kind of behavior to be developed in the student and the content... in which this behavior is to operate (sic)" (p. 30). Anderson et al. (2001) indicate that an objective possesses both a verb and a noun, with the term "verb" indicating the cognitive process to be used and the "noun" describing the knowledge students will acquire or construct. This latter description reflects a different educational philosophy (constructivism) from the underlying education in Tyler's time (behaviorism). Through the evolution of learning theory and research, Anderson and his colleagues replaced the historically used terms *behavior* and *content* with *cognitive process* and *knowledge*, respectively, to detach the taxonomy from the behavioral approaches that were predominant in the past.

Educational objectives may be written at three levels of specificity, according to Anderson et al. (2001). The levels include general achievement over the course of an academic year or determined length of time, a particular course or instructional unit within a course, or a particular lesson within an instructional unit. A taxonomy is most useful in the development of objectives at the course or unit level. After composing the objective, difficulties may arise when one is not able to visualize the outcome. For example, in a global objective stating, "The student will become an accountable member of the nursing profession," many ideas come forward, such as the intended learning to achieve the objective, the necessary factual knowledge that evolves into doing by knowing, valuing the quality of care, or, perhaps, a nurse who is proficient in completing records accurately. This example illustrates that specificity is required to describe exact levels of learning with respect to writing objectives. An important consideration in clarifying objectives is that they are written with an intended result for learning and that activities or behaviors are not the means to an end.

▲ THE OBJECTIVE TO LEARNING THEORY CONNECTION

Behaviorism encapsulates a belief that unless the desired behavior produced by education is observable and measured, learning has not occurred. Expecting specific behavior changes becomes problematic for nursing, in that not all learning can be overtly observed or manipulated directly when caring is the goal of nursing. While this presents a contemporary difficulty, the originators of the *Taxonomy of Educational Objectives* came to a consensus that virtually all objectives, when stated in behavioral terms, have their counterparts in student behavior (Bloom et al.,1956; Bloom, 1964). Learning for nurses expands daily with individual client information about unique problems and becomes lifelong due to whirlwind changes in technology and competing societal demands (Bevis & Watson, 2000; Dillard & Laidig, 1998). Despite this observation and whether it is consistent with newer learning theories and teaching and learning strategies, the use of behavioral objectives stands to this day.

Common criticisms of behavioral objectives are rooted in the belief that they are mechanistic and limit a student's involvement in learning (Krathwohl et al., 1964). Covert processes involved with complex mental processes such as concept formation, problem solving using critical thinking, and decision making are not as easily observed or measurable within the behaviorist paradigm (Norton, 1998).

The basic constructs of constructivism support the developmental concept of learning based on Piaget (1970a, 1970b, 1973). Fosnot (1996) holds that constructivism is developmental through assimilation, accommodation, and construction processes in learning. Learners build on previously erected and internalized representations of knowledge gained by personal interpretations, while striving to make sense of experiences. The paradigm of constructivism supports the view that knowledge constructs (structures) are amendable to change as new learning contributes knowledge to the existing foundation and connections.

While all nursing programs possess technical components for which behavioral objectives are ideal, the behaviorist model limits students' abilities to connect learning and construct knowledge. The praxis of nursing is the basic modality in which nurses care for clients with compromised health and ascends to the goal of health promotion for all. It involves constant change and asks the profession to engage in the challenge of transforming society through an emancipatory education for future nursing professionals (Bevis, 1993).

The model of tomorrow's professional is one who accepts a role of caring in professional reconstruction, demonstrates societal responsibilities, and participates in change needed for the future. The characteristics of the holistic nurse is one who thinks critically, is perpetually accountable and creative, and cares and shares power with clients, thus facilitating their ability to achieve higher states of health or peaceful conclusions to life. Directed to create curricula that meet the needs of students, nursing educators must diverge from traditions toward higher, more progressive forms of curricula for the learner. Discussion progresses, then, as to how recent changes in taxonomies and written objectives apply to preparing these curricula for the new model of student who is thinking critically and absorbing evolving knowledge.

▲ TAXONOMIES AND APPROACHES TO THE DOMAINS OF LEARNING

In the mid- to late 1940s, Bloom and selected colleagues held a cycle of meetings to discuss and resolve assessment difficulties that had been plaguing educators for years. What evolved from these brainstorm sessions was a classification system for educational objectives, published later in 1956 as the *Taxonomy of Educational Objectives*. (This text will be referred to as the "Handbook" throughout this discussion to differentiate it from subsequent work.) The results of their collective effort profoundly affected all levels of education. The group set about categorizing terms under three domains, that is, cognitive, affective, and psychomotor, to guide the objectification of learning goals. The first to be completed was the cognitive domain (Bloom et al., 1956). Work on the affective domain was published in 1964, with Krathwohl editing the manuscript for the collective contributors involved (Krathwohl et al., 1964). A void in the literature for the psychomotor domain existed until Simpson (1966) produced a multilevel structure in 1966, although others in the psychomotor domain were quickly published soon after (Dave, 1970; Harrow, 1972; Kibler, Barker, & Miles, 1970).

In the original work of Bloom et al. (1956), the taxonomy for the cognitive domain was arranged from simple to complex and concrete to abstract, and cut across all subject matters (Krathwohl et al., 1964). It was assumed to have a cumulative hierarchy to represent mastery of the lower levels before successful attempts at the complex levels were possible, thus reflecting the influence of Piaget's developmental approach (Bloom et al., 1956; Krathwohl et al., 1964; Piaget, 1970a, 1970b, 1973). As time elapsed, the original "Handbook" was primarily used to design instructional objectives and assessment techniques, disregarding the richness of its greater role in education. Research analyses of Bloom's taxonomy relied heavily on classified objectives that only studied recognition or recall. It failed to extend beyond the lowest level to realize the utility of the taxonomy above the category of knowledge (Bloom et al., 1956; Anderson & Sosniak, 1994; Anderson, 2002).

In the original "Handbook," knowledge of specifics, of ways and means of dealing with specifics, and of universals and abstractions in a field were subsumed under the first general category of knowledge (Bloom et al., 1956). Sosniak (1994) exposed the misuse of the hierarchy in the original one-dimensional structure by stating that the important goals of education are found in the categories above knowledge that involve understanding and the use of knowledge for comprehension or synthesis. Literature analyses concerning objective placement contribute to a greater understanding of the taxonomy and a base of impetus to move curricula and assessment toward the higher ranges of the taxonomy (Anderson et al., 2001; Krathwohl, 2002).

The primary purpose for establishing a taxonomy is to facilitate communication among faculty, colleagues, and students, and externally for reviewers or internally for the individual faculty member (Bloom, 1964). Communication at the individual faculty level involves internal consistency between the teaching plan and the learning intention. The classification system (taxonomy) assists in organizing and managing objectives around vast amounts of facts and concepts. The benefit of "being on the same page" for faculty, educational colleagues, and students enhances the shared beliefs and values among all stakeholders as stated in the mission and philosophy of the nursing program. Students have the advantage of knowing role expectations in the learning process, understanding the types and depth of knowledge to be acquired, and using the process to meet predetermined outcomes of learning. External reviewers profit from the classification when established competencies or standards are expressed visually as the program construct.

The Cognitive Domain of Bloom

The original taxonomy "Handbook" of the cognitive domain underwent considerable revision based on new understandings of dimensional knowledge in cognitive psychology and what the learner does in the process of using knowledge (Anderson et al., 2001; Krathwohl, 2002). The revised structure of the cognitive domain has a two-dimensional scaffolding. See Figure 4.1, which illustrates the vertical supports anchoring the four types of knowledge: factual, conceptual, procedural, and meta-cognitive. The horizontal dimension spans the cognitive processes of remembering, understanding, applying, analyzing, evaluating, and creating in ascending order within the hierarchy. The knowledge categories continue to traverse all subject matter lines (Anderson et al., 2001).

	THE COGNITIVE PROCESS DIMENSION					
THE KNOWLEDGE DIMENSION	**1. REMEMBER**	**2. UNDERSTAND**	**3. APPLY**	**4. ANALYZE**	**5. EVALUATE**	**6. CREATE**
A. FACTUAL KNOWLEDGE						
B. CONCEPTUAL KNOWLEDGE						
C. PROCEDURAL KNOWLEDGE						
D. META-COGNITIVE KNOWLEDGE						

F I G U R E   4 . 1   The taxonomy table.

The cognitive domain addresses intellectual skills and types of knowledge. A hierarchy develops as the student is able to first acquire and remember information and then restate the information to represent the retention of learned material before actually using it. Retention represents the minimum level of cognitive learning required, for example, for lay people to know and understand a medication regimen to improve health. In a similar way, this is the primary level of learning for individuals who are not encouraged to seek new understanding at the higher levels of cognitive ability. In the past, nursing curricula utilized this type of behaviorist model and purposive transmission that focused on factual knowledge. Now, the sole use of the lower level cognitive taxonomy is the least beneficial to gain knowledge relevant to nursing, develop critical thinking, and acquire the hands-on skills required in a practice profession.

Although a base of knowledge is necessary, the "knowing how," rather than the "knowing that," begins to occur above the understanding level and moves with increasing sophistication through applying, analyzing, evaluating, and creating. Transfer of learning is demonstrated by applying previously learned information in known or new situations (Anderson, 2001; Krathwohl, 2002). Understanding the relationships between concepts and using analysis begins an ascent into higher levels of cognition that are needed to apply learning to new situations, create meaning, and think critically. The synthesis of knowledge involves putting together bits of information to form larger concepts of knowledge, requiring the student to evaluate information and think and question whether all things have been taken into consideration. All of these processes come into use before creating the whole picture. The latter term, creating, is the pinnacle of the processes, where all of the lower levels of cognition are harvested for the production of meaningful learning. This is particularly true in clinical practice, where things learned are called upon for direct and immediate application to the care of patients.

In this regard, the role of the nursing instructor is most valuable. Nursing educators, in the role of facilitators, are present for students as guides in the process of learning. Facts, concepts, ways of doing things, and an awareness of personal thinking mean little if not placed in context, which for nursing is the clinical care of patients. Nursing educators help to build a cognitive infrastructure for students, who will eventually recall and transfer their knowledge at times of need. Skilled questioning by the instructor assists the student to focus on the "knowing how" to transfer knowledge from the theoretical stage to the clinical setting. With practice and continuous critical thinking about one's thinking processes, the student begins the transition to a novice practitioner. The types of knowledge within the revised taxonomy are utilized throughout the whole cognitive process, with increasing interlocking relationships that become the networking body of knowledge that nurses use to provide informed and safe clinical care.

TYPES OF KNOWLEDGE

Factual knowledge contains the basic elements students must know to be familiar with the discipline and to solve problems within it. For the general nursing curriculum, this type of knowledge includes facts, specific details, and technical terminology found in prerequisite and early course work covering such subjects as anatomy and physiology, chemistry, foundations of nursing, and pharmacology (Anderson et al., 2001).

Conceptual knowledge begins to define interrelationships among the basic elements within a larger context to enable the elements to function together in concepts (Anderson et al., 2001; Krathwohl, 2002). For example, the classification and categories of drugs and medication administration; principles and generalizations of concepts such as stress and coping; and nursing theories or models for understanding the health care system involve concepts that relate to baseline knowledge for nursing.

Procedural knowledge gives direction as to how to do something and provides methods of inquiry and criteria for using skills, algorithms, techniques, and methods (Anderson et al., 2002; Krathwohl, 2002). Skills used in sterile technique with rationales are exemplars of knowledge of subject-specific skills and algorithms, whereas knowledge of subject-specific technique is best demonstrated by knowing the difference between listening and open- or closed-ended questioning. Knowledge of criteria, the last knowledge type subsumed under procedural knowledge, involves knowing the criteria of when to apply a specific procedure, such as sterile technique, or the criteria of how to judge the feasibility of a particular method of cost containment in health care (Anderson et al., 2001).

Metacognitive knowledge is explained as cognition or thinking in general, with respect to an awareness of one's own thinking. It is the newest of the knowledge dimensions to be included (Anderson et al., 2001; Krathwohl, 2002). An important distinction in an awareness of metacognition is between the knowledge of cognition and its processes involving the monitoring, control, and regulation of cognition (Pintrich, 2002). Flavell's (1979) classic article on metacognition gives light to the knowledge of strategy, task, and person variables that are incorporated into the revised taxonomy as the subcategories of metacognitive knowledge. The subtypes of metacognitive awareness include strategies employed for different tasks, situational circumstances for which the strategies are most useful, the extent to which the strategies are successful or effective, and the knowledge of self that is gained (Pintrich, 2002). An example of a strategy is outlining subject matter by enumerating the supra-ordinate as well as the subordinate topics in units of instruction. Another example is the types of examinations a theory instructor uses to measure contextual or conditional knowledge as opposed to instructor-administered laboratory tests.

Self-knowledge is the final area of metacognition, in which knowing about personal strengths and weaknesses or one's own knowledge level is the focus. An incomplete knowledge base for performing procedures and seeking to rectify the weakness exemplifies an awareness of one's own knowledge level. Consistently, researchers demonstrate the importance of students being cognizant about their thinking activity and using this self-awareness to adapt their thinking to new contexts and needs (Anderson et al., 2001).

THE COGNITIVE PROCESSES

Retention and transfer of knowledge are two important goals of education related to the cognitive domain, with retention being the ability to remember material at a remote period in time. Transfer of learning is defined as the application of something learned in one situation carried over to another situation; therefore, transfer of knowledge is the ability to use meaningful learning in new situations, solve new problems, or answer new queries that facilitate new learning. The literature indicates that the ability to transfer learning from one context to another is not occurring as extensively as educators hope. "Near" transfer of knowledge occurs when new knowledge or a new skill is used in situations almost identical to the initial application, whereas "far" transfer occurs when new connections are made to contexts that appear different from the initial application (Perkins & Solomon, 2003).

Transfer is indicative of meaningful learning (Mayer & Wittrock, 1996). Although the literature is unable to clearly measure the time elapsed in far learning owing to the difficultly of instilling the ability in students, transfer of learning is of continuing concern because contexts or situations most often encountered by students for application of learning do not resemble the classroom setting or task (Perkins, 1990). In summary, retention requires the student to remember, and transfer has the added effect of requiring the student to not only remember, but also to make sense of and use what has been learned to apply learning to new and different situations (Bransford, Brown, & Cocking, 1999; Detterman & Sternberg, 1993; Mayer, 1995; McKeogh, Lupart, & Marini, 1995; Phye, 1997).

The facility for writing, instructing, and assessing educational objectives focused on retention is apparent, whereas writing objectives for transfer may entail more difficulty for educators (Baxter, Elder, & Glaser, 1996; Phye, 1997). The utility of the new educational taxonomy allows for expansion into previously undefined or unstated areas of knowledge and processes useful to nursing by objectifying the terms for students to explore meaning. Nursing students benefit from coaching by their educators to link facts, concepts, and procedural knowledge and to guide the development of metacognition in decision making. Nursing educators assist students in the recognition of knowledge that is essential to thinking, thus creating meaningful learning in the discovery process.

REMEMBERING

Remembering is defined as the retrieval of significant knowledge from long-term memory in the areas of factual, conceptual, procedural, and metacognitive knowledge. The associated subcategories are recognizing and recalling. When the intent of instruction is to promote retention, also considered rote memorization, the assessment of students' ability to retrieve material is in the same form as it was taught. When educators concentrate on promoting rote learning, teaching and assessing focus on remembering facts or fragments of knowledge in a narrow contextual view. Recalling is the retrieval of relevant material when asked to respond to a prompt. Recognizing is synonymous with identifying and locating knowledge in long-term memory for the purpose of comparison with current information. Remembering is essential to the development of meaningful learning at the application level and of more complex processes for problem solving. When meaningful learning is desired, remembering is embedded in the larger venue of new knowledge construction or problem solving. In the past, the overuse of this cognitive process became a barrier that neglected the use of higher levels of the taxonomy for learning and, therefore, inhibited the development of critical thinking in nursing students (Bowers & McCarthy, 1993; Brookfield, 1993).

Group discussion through sharing and clarifying students' knowledge of the content is a useful activity to promote remembering, especially when the exchange of ideas requires consensus of the group. This promotes affective valuing by raising consciousness about the importance of the material being covered. When educators prepare for assessment in the recognizing subcategory; verifying, matching, or forced-choice techniques are useful. Verification is the equivalent of true or false items. In matching requires the student selects an item from one list that exemplifies an item from the second list. When using a forced-choice technique, several possible answers are provided and the choice must be correct or the "best" answer; the most frequently used format for the latter is multiple-choice.

Assessment for recalling involves a prompt, usually in the form of a question, but it may vary according to the number and quality of cues given to students. Low cueing provides no clues, hints, or related information, whereas high cueing provides several hints. The amount of embedding or the extent to which items are situated in a larger meaningful context is flexible. Low embedding stipulates that the recall task is placed in an isolated, single event, whereas in high-embedded tasks, the recall question relates to a larger problem or scenario.

UNDERSTANDING

When the goal of instruction involves the desire of transference of learning, understanding is the first and largest level of the cognitive processes encountered. Understanding occurs when students are capable of constructing meaning from instructional messages, including oral, written, and graphic transmissions from whatever means are employed to convey the information (lecture, texts, or telecommunications). Student understanding becomes connected when links between the most recent information acquired and previously learned information are formed in schemas and cognitive frameworks. Concepts and frameworks are the building blocks of these schemas, so it follows that conceptual knowledge becomes the basis for understanding. Cognitive processes are subordinates of understanding and include interpreting, exemplifying, classifying, summarizing, inferring, comparing, and explaining (Anderson et al., 2001). A description of these processes follows:

▲ Interpreting may use alternate terms, such as *clarifying*, *paraphrasing*, *representing*, and *translating*, to describe the student's ability to change a representation from one form to another.

▲ Exemplifying is the ability to locate a specific example or illustration of a concept or principle and may use similar terms such as *illustrating* or *instantiating*.

▲ Classifying involves concluding that something belongs to a category. Alternate means for using this term may be *categorizing* or *subsuming*.

▲ Summarizing, abstracting, or generalizing consists of extracting a general theme or major points from a topic.

▲ Inferring or drawing a logical conclusion from material or information received is alternately named *concluding*, *extrapolating*, *interpolating*, and *predicting*.

▲ Comparing is the ability to detect linkage or nonlinkage between two objects, ideas, or similarities and may employ the alternate terms of *contrasting*, *mapping*, or *matching*.

▲ Explaining involves building the cause and effect of a system through construction of models.

Activities to promote learning in the area of "understanding" may require students to note abnormal assessment findings using underlying pathophysiology as a manifestation of the difference from expected findings. This differs from the higher cognitive process of analysis due to the lack of breakdown involved, especially if using lower-level taxonomy terminology in the objective. "Interpreting" involves conversion of words to words, pictures to words, words to pictures, numbers to words, etc., with an alternate arrangement of potential selections in significant contrast to those on the primary list. To ensure that the student task of interpreting is more than simply remembering, the manner in which information is asked must be new. If the task is identical to one used in the presentation, then assessment is most likely to measure remembering rather than interpreting, despite efforts to camouflage it. Anderson et al. (2001) warn educators that, "If assessment tasks are to tap into higher order cognitive processes, they must require that students cannot answer them correctly by relying on memory alone" (p. 71).

For assessment, tasks for "exemplifying" can be implemented as constructed responses. In this format, the student must supply an example as an answer or select the answer from a given set (multiple choice). For the category "classifying" the choice for assessment is a constructed response task asking the student to supply the related concept or principle. In a selected response, the student is given an instance and the answer is selected from a set of given concepts or principles. Sorting is a variation of this task, where a student is given a set of instances and then asked to determine which category relates to a specific category, to select multiple categories for placement, or to select the category to which it does not pertain. "Summarizing" assessment tasks are measured by using constructed responses or selection formats with the possible responses assuming themes or summaries. In a selection format, the student is required to read a passage and respond with a summarizing title. Assessment for the category of "inferring" utilizes a set or series of examples or instances in which a concept or principle accounts for them. Common tasks involve completion, analogy, and novel oddity tasks (selecting one that does not belong). To be able to insure that the task is measuring inferring, it must ask the student to state the underlying concept or principle.

Mapping is a major activity technique for the "comparing" category. The student is required to show how each object, idea, problem, or situation is linked to another. The final subcategory of "explaining'" employs several assessment tasks that include reasoning, troubleshooting, redesigning, or predicting. In reasoning, the student is asked to supply a rationale for a given event. Students asked to troubleshoot make a diagnosis of the problem in malfunctioning situations. Changing a system is a means of assessing a student's ability to redesign the system to achieve a goal. Predicting involves asking a student how a change in the system could effect a change in another part of the system.

APPLYING

To apply, the student uses procedures to perform executions or solve problems. Applying is selected for situations where there is some degree of understanding between the problem and the potential procedure. Applying is closely associated with the procedural knowledge dimension and is related to the task of executions with which the student is familiar prior to using the procedure; that is, the exercise has become routine. The two subcategories under applying consist of executing and implementing.

In executing, the student carries out a procedure as a result of clues that influence and guide the choice of the appropriate procedure. Execution is closely tied to the use of skills and algorithms. The sequencing of steps in a fixed order and performed correctly results in a predetermined outcome. Implementing (synonym for using) is a problem situation in which a student is not initially familiar and must engage in problem solving by locating and/or identifying the proper solution. To differentiate between these two processes, executing is a task when the exercise is familiar and implementing is a problem-solving task when the situation is unfamiliar. Little thought is needed for familiar tasks in executing, whereas for unfamiliar tasks in implementing, students must decide what knowledge is essential. Modifications in procedural knowledge may be necessary for implementing in situations where there is not an exact match for the problem situation. Implementation requires the student to understand conceptual knowledge as a prerequisite to enable application of procedural knowledge.

Assessment strategies for executing ask the student to supply the answer, select from a set of possible answers where appropriate, and/or show the work in the process of arriving at the answer. Implementing assessment tasks involve students being asked to solve problems with which there is no familiarity. This type of assessment begins with a format where a problem is presented with specifics and students are asked to identify procedures to solve the problem, use the selected procedure with modifications as needed to solve the problem, or both of the aforementioned.

ANALYZING

When asked to analyze, students are taking apart material into its constituents and examining each part to determine how it relates to another part. The processes in this category include differentiating, organizing, and attributing. Differentiating involves determining relevant messages or pieces of a message, the manner in which the pieces are organized (organizing), and the underlying purpose of the message (attributing). When viewed as an end in itself, analyzing may be more defensible when considered as an extension of understanding or as a precursor to evaluating or creating. Educators who set a goal of education to improve student skills in analysis ask students to:

▲ Distinguish fact from opinion and reality from fantasy.
▲ Connect conclusions with supporting statements.
▲ Distinguish relevant from extraneous material.
▲ Determine how ideas relate to each other.
▲ Ascertain the unstated assumptions involved in what is said.
▲ Distinguish dominant from subordinate ideas or themes.
▲ Find evidence in support of the author's purposes (Anderson et al., 2001).

Differentiating may be used synonymously with discriminating, distinguishing, focusing, and selecting. It may be clarified by distinguishing pertinent from nonpertinent parts or important from less important or unimportant parts of presented information. Organizing determines how elements depict the overall picture or function within the structure. Terms commonly used as alternate words are *finding, coherence, integrating, outlining, parsing,* and *structuring.* When determining the point of view, bias, value, or intent underlying the presented material, the student uses the cognitive subprocess of attributing.

Constructed response methods or selection tasks are appropriate for assessing students' ability to differentiate. Constructed response is when the student is supplied with a given topic matter and then asked to indicate the elements that are most important or to select parts most relevant to the whole. Because organizing entails structures such as outlines, tables, matrixes, or hierarchical diagrams, the assessment method for this category may be constructed response or selection tasks with slight variations. An assessment example for a constructed response is a student assignment to produce an outline of a procedure in a written format. An example of a selected response is for the student to examine several graphic representations of hierarchies and to select which one best represents the organization of a selected text. To assess attributing, the student must construct or select a description of an author's point of view or message intent in a selected text.

EVALUATING

Making judgments based on criteria and standards of performance is the defining element of the category evaluating. Evaluating uses criteria to judge the quality, effectiveness, and consistency of the items under evaluation. These measuring standards (or criteria) may be quantitative or qualitative. Cognitive processes for evaluating include checking and critiquing and are based on the use of standards and established criteria.

Testing for internal consistencies or fallacies in operations (e.g., performance of nursing care) is suggested by the subcategory of checking. Checking occurs when students determine whether a conclusion logically follows from the presented premises, whether hypotheses are supported or unfounded by the data, or whether there are conflicts or contradictions among parts of the premises. When combined with planning and implementing, checking assists students to see how accurate a plan is or if it is effectively working. Alternative terms for checking are *testing, detecting, monitoring,* and *coordinating.* To accomplish assessment for checking, the instructor observes or interacts with the student, looking for consistency of performance during the implementation of a solution or while performing a procedure that yields positive or negative consequences.

The synonym for critiquing is judging. The elements of critiquing involve imposing external criteria or standards on a product or operation. In the critiquing process, positive or negative features of a situation or product are judged. Critiquing is crucial for critical thinking leading to decision making in nursing. Students may be asked to objectively evaluate a proposed solution in light of its potential effectiveness. Other potential activities are to evaluate hypotheses for reasonableness or competing alternatives to solving problems effectively or efficiently. Another method to assess critiquing is to ask students to judge their personal work or that of others using established positive or negative criteria, or both methods combined.

CREATING

Within the revised taxonomy, creating involves assembling parts into a coherent or functioning whole or restructuring the parts into a new scheme or pattern. Subcategories of creating are generating, planning, and producing (Anderson, 2002). When using the term *creating,* first thoughts may go to a unique or previously unknown product produced by the student. In the revised taxonomy, creating has an alternate meaning that calls for a unique product derived from all a student can and will do within the context of a learning objective. When defining the learning activity, educators need to make explicit the meaning of *unique* or *original.* The objectives inherent in this category focus on the synthesis of dissimilar or divergent data into a whole. Examples of creating are those that direct students to assemble previously learned material into an organized presentation. Creating can be observed and is more than a student's ability to produce a repetition of previous work. Tasks requiring creating are likely to require several lower category processes, either by individual subcategory or collectively to produce the end product. Processes in the creative category involve three phases: problem presentation (generating), solution planning (planning), and solution execution (producing). Students seek and explore possible solutions for a workable plan in the solution–planning phase and successfully carry out the plan in the solution–execution phase.

Generating involves problem presentation with alternatives or hypotheses under certain criteria. A synonym for generating is to hypothesize. It requires a student to step over the boundaries of one's prior knowledge or personally held theories and use divergent thinking, also known as creative thinking. It is important to point out that generating is different in this context from the generative process inherent in understanding. Here it connotes divergent thinking, in contrast to the convergent process where it connotes understanding.

Planning is described as designing problem solutions or plans to solve a problem as a step prior to the implementation phase. Subgoals are established or deconstructed into a plan strategy with specific subtasks to be executed in the final problem solution phase. It is important to include the planning phase in the written objectives rather than assuming or implying its place when producing objectives.

The Affective Domain of Krathwohl

This domain of affective learning and its classification system of expected behaviors are symbolic of the original "Handbook's" method of categorizing objectives. The affective domain deals with individual feelings or emotions that are reflected in values and interests. A predominant portion of learning in this domain surrounds ethical and moral behavior in nursing. Krathwohl et al. (1964) developed five affective domain levels as follows:

▲ Receiving: being conscious of phenomena and to another's expressions of ideas or beliefs. The subcategories are awareness, willingness to receive, and controlled or selected attention.

▲ Responding: verbal and nonverbal reactions that indicate response to a phenomenon ranging on a continuum from compliance to satisfaction.

▲ Valuing: attaching worth to an object or belief; exhibiting commitment as a pattern of choice.

▲ Organizing: conceptualizing and building a consistent belief system.

▲ Characterizing: acting and responding, consistently; reflecting an internally consistent value system.

This portion of the taxonomy was completed before the paradigm shift to the learner as the focus of the teaching–learning relationship. For behavioral objectives, the educator indicates what the intended outcome of learning is to be, recognizing that a learner possesses previous "formal or informal" experiences. The focus is on the teacher who is made responsible for evoking the behavior from the student.

RECEIVING

Receiving as attending to phenomena or to expressions of another's beliefs or ideas has measurable behaviors such as listens attentively, attends to, and demonstrates awareness, sensitivity, and interest. It is explicated by the verbs *listens, attends, selects, prefers, shares, accepts, describes, follows, guides, identifies, locates, names, observes,* and *replies.* There are three subcategories to receiving. The subcategory of awareness is the cognitive behavior of becoming aware of something or becoming conscious of its presence, such as taking into account a situation, phenomenon, object, or state of affairs (Krathwohl et al., 1964). Suggestions for eliciting student behavior in this area are developing awareness of stressful stimuli for patients or a consciousness of different patient settings. Assessment for this type of behavior is basically cognitive and is the regurgitation of another's beliefs or values, for example, a student's reflection of readings in a text or journal article (King, 1984; Krathwohl et al., 1964).

Progressing a step upwards in the hierarchy, a "willingness to receive" is considered a cognitive behavior owing to the required ability to suspend judgment or maintain neutrality with regard to the stimulus and a willingness to attend to it (Krathwohl et al., 1964). Examples of a student behavior of willingness to receive is the appreciation or tolerance of cultural patterns exhibited by individuals or an increase in sensitivity to human need and the plight of the homeless. The educator is singularly satisfied with the student becoming aware of the phenomenon, not seeking it out or discriminating it from other phenomena, but just realizing it exists by giving it attention without judgment (King, 1984; Krathwohl et al., 1964).

Controlled or selected attention is a higher step in the receiving ladder of the affective domain. In controlled or selected attention, the differentiation of a given stimulus and the student selection of that stimulus are at the heart of this subcategory (Krathwohl et al., 1964). Alertness to human values and judgments about living wills by the student is an example. Examples for assessing controlled or selected attention is by teacher observation. Rating scales for assessing student behavior using a Likert scale to gauge the student's attention is a suggested methodology, with the scale reflecting little or no attention at the minimal level and consistency of the behavior at the maximum level (King, 1984; Krathwohl et al., 1964).

RESPONDING

Responding is the second level of hierarchy in the affective domain. It involves giving more than simple attention to a situation. Instead, students demonstrate compliance through the acquisition of some degree of satisfaction in response to stimuli. The subcategories of the continuum proceed from acquiescence in responding, to a willingness to respond, to satisfaction with the response (Krathwohl et al., 1964).

In acquiescence, the student complies with the desired behavior, but has not accepted the rationale for being asked to do so. Goals relevant to student behavior that connect with valuing patient health and safety are found at this level. The desired student behavior is "obedience" or, more acceptably, "compliance." Obedience implies a potential resistance or yielding unwillingly to the request, while compliance suggests more of the desired trait. The student makes the response, but is not yet accepting of the rationale to do so (Krathwohl et al., 1964). Examples of student behaviors that provide evidence in this area are compliance with required preclinical tuberculosis testing and adhering to traditional dress codes in the clinical area. Assessment of behaviors for compliance is found in the student's willingness to maintain isolation techniques or follow the preparation requirements for clinical practice (King, 1984; Krathwohl et al., 1964).

Behaviors corresponding to a willingness to respond are based on voluntary activity without student fear of recrimination or punishment (Krathwohl et al., 1964). The essential presence of consent or proceeding from one's own choice is necessary to differentiate this from acquiescence. Students may display this behavior by voluntarily reading material to gather additional information on health-related issues, surveying patients for ideas of leisure-time activities in the hospital setting, or accepting responsibility for personal health for the protection of others. A suggested assessment item for educators in this area includes an anecdotal record of the student's voluntary activities or similar methods of tracking the voluntary efforts of the student (King, 1984; Krathwohl et al., 1964).

Satisfaction in response encompasses a willingness to respond with the addition of expressing satisfaction as an emotional response. While this involves internalizing the emotional aspect of willingness, the precision for pinpointing internalization puts the authors of the affective taxonomy into a quandary as to whether it should be included as an objective for this domain (King, 1984; Krathwohl et al., 1964). The inclusion of the subcategory indicates that internalized feelings serve as an intrinsic reward that tends to increase the likelihood that the behavior will be repeated, and it gives the emotional component focus and importance in learning (Krathwohl et al., 1964). An example of an objective is, "The nursing students express enjoyment when participating in celebratory activities such as the

NICU graduate party" or "The nursing students take pleasure in planning leisure activities for mental health patients." Educators may assess these behaviors by including open-ended items as a projective technique in examinations (King, 1984).

VALUING

The third level of the affective domain is valuing. Individuals begin to make choices and to internalize the value of their selection. This level of valuing includes acceptance of a value, preference, and commitment. Valuing implies that something, a phenomenon or behavior, has worth (Krathwohl et al., 1964). Socialization into nursing by students becomes evident, so it is not surprising that many behavioral objectives are written at this level rather than below it. Nursing educators attempt to overtly demonstrate socially acceptable professional behaviors that are valued in nursing. Students emulate these behaviors, which instructors reinforce as acceptable ways of behaving. A vital understanding about valuing is the motivation underlying and guiding the behavior as determined by the student's internal commitment and not simply the desire to comply. Values can be defined as attitudes or beliefs, if the characteristics are manifested consistently in appropriate situations and that students hold as having worth (King, 1984; Krathwohl et al., 1964).

Acceptance of a value is reflected in a student's ability to consistently describe the worth of an overt behavior in a way that the value is identifiable by observers (King, 1984; Krathwohl et al., 1964). In objectifying this subcategory, students are asked to demonstrate a sense of responsibility for promoting quality health care for indigent patients. An activity to exemplify this objective is for students to read a case study and determine the position and action they will take. A student whose actions reflect Kohlberg's (1975) stages of moral development exemplifies affective achievement (King, 1984; Krathwohl et al., 1964).

To fill the gap between acceptance of a value and the subcategory of commitment, preference for a value implies more than the process of acceptance and less than beginning commitment (King, 1984; Krathwohl et al., 1964). Preference for a value is described as the active pursuit of a value by seeking it out to fulfill the desire for it. To demonstrate a measurable behavior in this category, educators seek evidence of a student's assuming responsibility and cooperating with, participating in, or accepting a commitment to values. An example of a student learning activity is letter writing to local, state, and federal service agencies regarding access to health care for the maternal–child population (King, 1984). Another example is asking students to develop, implement, and analyze a value activity, such as discussion of Oregon's "right to die" legislation in a group setting. Observing and listening to the students as they reveal a preference for particular values is an example of a method of the assessment of values by the instructor.

Emotional acceptance of a belief is activated as the student develops convictions and an unshakable certainty of the value to the extent that he or she attempts to convince others of the value (King, 1984; Krathwohl et al., 1964). Loyalty to a position, group, or cause is the premise of this category and the motivation is to act out the behavior. An example of commitment is active participation in the "right to life" or "right to choose" cause by distributing pamphlets or participating in informational meetings. Means of assessment include anecdotal notes on student participation or a student-authored position paper that expresses the conviction held as a "beyond a doubt" value.

ORGANIZING

With increasing numbers of internalized values, a learner is often faced with situations where more than one value is relevant. To manage the number of values, the student begins to determine the interrelationships among them, establishing the most significant and ever-present values, and then organizing the values into a system. This category consists two tiers, namely conceptualization of a value and organization of a value system (King, 1984; Krathwohl et al., 1964).

In the hierarchy of the affective domain, values development is progressive. Conceptualization of a value exemplifies the development. As noted in the valuing category, use of values with consistency and stability are the hallmarks of the internalization of a value. Similarly, the "organization" category of values takes on characteristics of abstraction and conceptualization, permitting the holder to appreciate how new and old personal values relate. Conceptualization will most likely be more symbolic in its abstractness (King, 1984; Krathwohl et al., 1964). Students display conceptualization of a value by forming moral judgments, such as what the responsibilities of society are to protect vulnerable populations. A sample activity for evoking this subcategory is a group discussion in which there is evidence of abstract thinking related to a conceptualized value. The situation is a delineated case scenario where a dilemma presents itself based on interpersonal family conflict. To assess the student's achievement "to conceptualize a value," the learner is asked to assume the role of the nurse, describe actions to take regarding the various family participants, share the plan with peers, and relate the plan to the nursing process. The educator must be cognizant of the limitations of the assessment due to a strong interdependence of knowledge and responsibility. The conceptualization of values requires a student to act upon internalized values.

Organizing a value system requires the student to assemble a potentially dissonant complex of values into a harmonious semblance of order. Among the relationships, the student may encounter conflicts or cognitive dissonance where equilibrium needs to be found to cope with internal or external environments. In the process of organizing, transformation of a new value or complex of higher-order values occurs (King, 1984). To prepare objectives relevant to organizing a value system, educators might have students contrast alternative actions with established or traditional health care policy. A suggested activity is a research paper comparing the alternatives of traditional and nontraditional policies concerning public health management of AIDS. Educator assessment of student performance is based on an analysis of the paper.

CHARACTERIZATION OF A VALUE OR VALUE COMPLEX

The highest level of the affective domain is identified as characterization of a value or value complex, with subcategories of general set and characterization. By the time a person arrives at this level, an individual's values have been internalized and placed in a personal hierarchy, organized in an internally consistent system, and set as a control of personal behavior to the extent that arousal of the evoked behavior ceases to stimulate emotion or affect unless provoked by fear or challenged. The individual's behaviors are consistent and in accord with the internalized values to the degree that generalized control tendencies influence the description and characterizing traits of the person. These beliefs, ideas, and attitudes are integrated into the personal philosophy or paradigm of the person (King, 1984; Krathwohl et al., 1964). It is unrealistic to think that an educational program is capable of stimulating a student to reach this pinnacle of affective behavior. Few ever attain this level, and it can be a lifelong endeavor. The "generalized set" subcategory describes the intensity to which internal consistency of the value and attitude system is maintained at any point in time. It is a selective and generalized response at a very high level. Characterization is a value system that reflects an individual's philosophy and maturity (King, 1984; Krathwohl et al., 1964).

Considering the implausibility of educators successfully evoking the highest order of the affective domain, objectives in the endeavor are more global for several reasons. An individual's philosophy of life and level of maturity are evolving, influenced by the developmental stage, internal and external factors, culture, and life circumstances (King, 1984). A sample objective to stimulate the student's aspirations to the higher level of response is to ask the student to develop a consistent philosophy of life, viewing problems in objective, realistic, and tolerant terms. A suggested activity to measure progression is to have the student compose a philosophy of nursing early in the education program, with formative additions along the way, and a summative philosophy upon graduation. Assessing progression is difficult but possible if educators are mindful that the written documents are highly personalized, without a sense of right or wrong answers, and will reveal the disposition and beliefs of the student. To assist educators in determining the level of student progress, it behooves faculty members to describe the superlative characteristics of a model student at this level of affective function and maturity, incorporating this desirable student profile into the philosophy and outcomes of the educational program.

The Psychomotor Domain of Simpson, Dave, and Harrow

As one would expect, the psychomotor domain is more discipline dependent, yet contains similar taxonomy terms depending on the educator's perspective and the skills expected in the various disciplines. Three primary psychomotor taxonomies are available to educators to guide objectives of learning.

Although the first two of the taxonomies are relevant to the acquisition of nursing skills and bear mentioning, the latter is most frequently utilized for learning objectives in nursing education. Simpson (1966) authored the final volume of the trivolume taxonomy originally proposed by Bloom et al. in 1956. The taxonomy verbiage is composed of perception, set, guided response, mechanism, complex overt response, adaptation, and origination, and is reproduced in *How to Write and Use Instructional Objectives* (Gronlund, 1991).

"Perception" involves the tuning into sensory cues to guide physical activity, and "set" denotes the learner's readiness to act by demonstrating alertness or knowledge of the behaviors essential for executing the skill. Suggested verbs for perception types of objectives are *distinguish, identify,* and *select*; those applicable to "set" include *assume a position, demonstrate,* and *show.* "Guided response" occurs in the early stages of a complex skill that includes imitation and indicates that the learner is capable of completing the steps in the skill. *Attempt, imitate,* and *try* are possible verbs for these objectives.

"Mechanism" is the ability to perform a complex skill gauged at an intermediate stage. The verbs applicable to this ability include *do, execute, act upon,* or *complete.* "Complex overt response" introduces correctness in the performance of a skill and verbs to introduce this include *carry out, operate,* and *perform.* "Adaptation" indicates that a learner is able to modify skills to a new situation and *adapt, change, modify,* and *revise* are appropriate verbs in this context. "Origination" is the creative ability to develop a unique, innovative skill that replaces the skill originally learned. Suggested terminology to employ in objectives for origination includes *create, design, derive,* and *invent* (Oermann, 1990).

In 1972, Harrow (1972) presented a taxonomy of behavioral terms to guide the composition of learning objectives that consists of reflex movement, basic fundamental movements, perceptual abilities, skilled movements, and nondiscursive communication. Harrow's taxonomy consists of ". . . observable voluntary human motions" (p. 31) that are heralded by forethought of the performer in the context of the consequences that are produced. Practice and reinforcement are required for the maintenance of skills (Bachman, 1990). Reflex movement is defined by segmental, intersegmental, and suprasegmental reflexes, and the verb *respond* may be used to develop the objectives for this taxonomy. Basic fundamental movements are classified as locomotor movements, nonlocomotor movements, and manipulative movements.

Perceptual abilities are categorized as kinesthetic, visual, auditory, tactile discrimination, and coordinated abilities, whereas physical abilities are described by endurance, strength, flexibility, and agility. Skilled movements are simple, compound, and complex adaptive skills. Those involving nondiscursive means of communication are expressive or interpretive. Appropriate verbs to use for Harrow's last category of the taxonomy are *arrange, compose, create, originate*, and *compose.*

Following a presentation at the International Conference of Educational Testing in 1967, Dave (1970) published his taxonomy as a construction of imitate, manipulate, precision, articulation, and naturalization. Dave's taxonomy is based on neuromuscular movement and coordination and underlies criteria proposed by Reilly and Oermann (1990), which are based on a developmental approach to competency. Using these criteria to write objectives or competencies commands an understanding of the criteria. The criteria for each level are (Reilly & Oermann, 1990):

- ▲ Imitation level: Occasional errors are apparent in the necessary actions of the skill and are accompanied by some weakness of gross motor actions, and the time required to complete the skill is dependent on the learner's need. (Verbs for this subcategory are *attempt, copy, duplicate, imitate*, and *mimic.*)
- ▲ Manipulation level: Coordination of movements occurs with some variation and in the time required to complete the actions of the skill. (Verbs for this subcategory are *complete, follow, play, perform*, and *produce.*)
- ▲ Precision level: A logical sequence carries activities through to completion, almost free of errors in noncritical actions, although the speed of completion continues to be a concern. (Verbs for this subcategory are *achieve automatically, excel expertly*, and *perform masterfully.*)
- ▲ Articulation level: Logic is evident in the coordinated actions, few errors are noted, and the time required to execute the skill is considered reasonable. (Verbs for this subcategory are *customize* and *originate.*)
- ▲ Naturalization level: Professional competence is noted in the skill performance that is automatic and well coordinated. (Verbs for this subcategory are *naturally performs* and *perfectly performs.*)

The Holistic Taxonomy of Hauenstein

Hauenstein (1998) objected to the sprawling number of categories and subcategories in Bloom's traditional taxonomy, favoring a streamlined, simplified taxonomy that supports constructivism characteristics. Hauenstein agrees that the education focus is to prepare students for productive places in society, but finds fault with the established taxonomies as being less than successful in assisting students to achieve this outcome. A holistic curriculum, supported by Hauenstein, includes the cognitive, affective, and psychomotor domains of learning and a unifying domain of behavior. According to Hauenstein, the traditional taxonomies lack integration, are separated into reductionary perspectives, and are unconnected entities. Incompatibility among these learning domains and the difficulty to apply them as a collective in the classroom are other shortcomings noted by Hauenstein.

The guidelines Hauenstein employed to restructure and define a holistic educational taxonomy consist of rules or criteria that oversee the architecture of its design. These rules are as listed as follows

Rule 1: The taxonomy must possess applicability or relevancy to the function for which it will be utilized.

Rule 2: Total inclusiveness must be apparent to represent all categories in a given context.

Rule 3: To prevent overlap between categories or within subcategories, the taxonomy must be mutually exclusive to preserve the independence of intent and function of each.

Rule 4: A principle of order allowing ready recognition of simple to complex, facility to difficulty, concrete to abstract, and prerequisite to requisite must be evident.

Rule 5: Terminology used to label categories and subcategories communicate the concepts or ideas that are generic and representative of the discipline being taught.

Hauenstein proposes revision of the taxonomy through reducing the categories to five objectives per domain, consolidating the subcategories to a limit of three to four per domain, with a unifying structure describing behavior (the fourth domain) as solutions to the aforementioned difficulties. The structure of this taxonomy can be seen in Figure 4.2.

The conceptual framework used by Hauenstein is a systems approach with information or content (knowledge from others) as the input to promote the integrity of the taxonomy, whether or not the domains are used individually or integrated for subject matter mastery by students. Output in his proposed systems approach is described as knowledgeable, acculturated, competent individuals. Monitoring, evaluation, and consequent revisions are regarded as the feedback components to the information inputs and process objectives.

Hauenstein is persistent in using the behavioral model to anchor learning for students by synthesizing the cognitive, affective, and psychomotor domains into a composite fourth domain entitled "behavioral" with five categories of objectives and limited to three subcategories. The claim is that through synthesis of the traditional domains of cognitive, affective, and psychomotor, the educator can focus on student-centered understandings, skills, and dispositions. According to Hauenstein, the benefit of such an instructional system is classification of objectives through their levels and identification of the developmental levels of the students resulting in appropriate objectives, lesson plans, and outcomes for students.

The definition of cognitive in this holistic taxonomy is the domain involving the process of knowing and the development of intellectual abilities and skills. Unknown knowledge from others to be acquired by students is identified as the external input for process objectives. This knowledge does not become true knowledge for students until it has become internalized through experiences. Hauenstein identifies these cognitive inputs as symbolic, prescriptive, and technological information/content. A redefinition of the affective domain is directed toward developing dispositions in relationship to feelings, values, and beliefs. Hauenstein describes the definition of the psychomotor domain as the development of physical abilities and skills that result from the input of information and content.

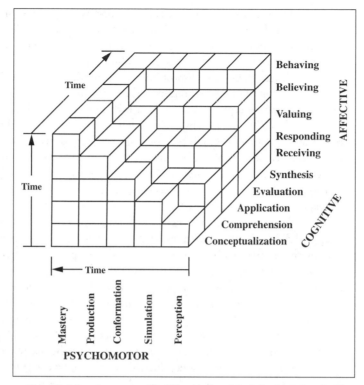

Fig. 4.2 shows the matrix of building blocks of the behavioral domain. One *behaves* or *acts* in relation to what one *knows*, *feels*, and *can do*. All three domains are essential for each block and level for *whole learning*. The time needed to develop understandings, skills, and dispositions is cumulative. Lower levels require more time because of the number of components. Higher levels require additional time because of the number of layers and blocks that are prerequisites for attainment.

FIGURE 4.2 Hauenstein's behavioral domain.

The behavioral domain, according to Hauenstein (1998), is the tempered demeanor that an individual displays as a reaction to a social stimulus, or an inner need, or combination thereof. This observable comportment is measurable in effect whether it is provided by external or internal stimuli. Hauenstein concludes his definition by stating, "it is the domain of knowledge involved with developing knowledgeable, acculturated, and competent individuals" (p. 3). The behavioral domain proposed by Hauenstein is a distinct departure from the traditional taxonomy of Bloom and others. The purpose of the behavioral domain proposed by Hauenstein is to provide an overall process of learning distinct from the process established by Anderson et. al. (2001) in the revised learning taxonomy of Bloom. Hauenstein suggests that the behavioral domain is a condensed framework of the cognitive, affective, and psychomotor domains that assists in learning level identification, classifying and composing objectives, and planning lessons, teaching, learning, and outcome measurement. The behavioral domain consists of acquisition, assimilation, adaptation, performance, and aspiration.

The acquisition objective is understood as the process for understanding, perceiving, and conceptualizing new information while being mindful of the context in which the information has specificity. The intention of this level is for students to learn new concepts, ideas, terminology, and information about symbolic, prescriptive, descriptive, and technological understandings, skills, and dispositions (Hauenstein, 1998). Assimilation is defined as the "comprehension of" and "responding to" in a learning situation. It enables a student to comprehend a new concept or mesh an idea with previously attained knowledge, and to respond to this intake of information by explaining it in his or her own verbiage or simulating an example or skill. Adaptation modifies knowledge, skills, and disposition to conform to a predetermined quality of level of performance, criterion, or standard. The purpose of an adaptation objective is to develop a degree of skill or competency in knowledge utilization and to problem solve real or imagined situations with similarities to the context in which first encounters are experienced (Hauenstein, 1998).

Performance, the process of evaluating situations and producing, includes the ability to appropriately analyze, qualify, evaluate, and integrate information with the values and beliefs held by the learner that become ingrained and are repeatable in new or routine situations. The purpose of a performance objective is to utilize knowledge, skills, and dispositions on a continuous basis that become components of the learner's current behavior. Aspiration is the process of synthesizing knowledge and mastering skills by continuously demonstrating these behaviors. An enormous part of this behavior is the valuing and incorporation of beliefs into the demonstrable performance using knowledge, skills, and dispositions proficiently and excelling in the ability to perfect and achieve through the mastery of complex problems or situations. It instills a desire to attain higher levels of knowledge and skills through advancement of disposition for independent learning. The ultimate purpose of an aspiration objective is to enable students to continuously strive for higher levels of expertise (Hauenstein, 1998).

▲ CURRICULUM ALIGNMENT USING A TAXONOMY TABLE

It is important to differentiate between knowledge and content for the purpose of instructional design. "Content domains," "disciplinary content" (Doyle, 1992), and "pedagogical content knowledge" (Shulman, 1987) exemplify typical definitions found in the literature. Anderson et al. (2001) use "substance" as a synonym for content. When applied to a specific subject matter, content becomes a curriculum's substance, but a nursing curriculum is a plan to achieve competencies and values, as well as the knowledge of nursing. Current concepts of learning focus on meaningful learning and include active, cognitive, and constructive processes to achieve the desired outcome. Students learn based on their construction of information that is meaningful and valuable to them. The curriculum plan has the task of organizing and exposing the student to the constructs of knowledge, values, and skills to meet the desired outcomes in nursing education. This moves the student away from a passive role of behaviorism into a more cognitive and constructivist mode of learning. The challenge, then, is for faculty to communicate what the intended learning is with consistency and clarity.

The systematic use of cognitive, affective, psychomotor, and behavioral domains provides design opportunities for activities that facilitate the achievement of course objectives, program competencies, and courses or units of learning toward the stated outcomes. The interdependence of the domains does more collectively to help accomplish this goal than each of the categories individually (Anderson et al., 2001; Bloom, 1956; Krathwohl, 2002; Krathwohl et al., 1964; Mayer, 2002; Reilly & Oermann, 1990). A faculty-designed curriculum that addresses each of the learning domains creates a comprehensive plan of study when the program outcomes are targeted.

After completing the phases of planning to meet the outcomes using appropriate taxonomy terms for objectives, activities throughout the course work are designed and strategically placed to foster increasingly complex learning by planned learning sessions. Nursing is a practice discipline requiring inclusive use of all levels of knowledge types as well as the cognitive processes demonstrated in the taxonomies. There are several cautions in developing a curriculum and plan of study based on the taxonomies. Be mindful that separation of the cognitive, affective, psychomotor, and behavioral domains for the purpose of classifying objectives and learning activities; the time lapse of publication history for the domains; and the emergence of newer learning theories may detract from amalgamating the domains as a framework for curriculum. Close interrelationships of behaviors in one domain may also be seen in the others. A holistic view of education comes into focus when all of the domains are represented in the objectives.

Logically, knowledge must first be possessed and then built upon through recognizing and valuing the role that this knowledge plays in the care of others. Thus, it becomes a necessary part of the application of knowledge in a meaningful way. For example, values of professional nursing and well-practiced skills expressed throughout the curriculum design become applicable and simultaneously internalized in student nursing practice only if addressed in holistically written objectives. Learning becomes transferable across a greater variety of practice situations when objectives are designed to progress from simple to complex and from the concrete to abstract. Faculty must heed these cautions to prevent selecting domain levels that are too low in the hierarchy for the intended outcomes of learning. First-semester students are capable of progressing through all of the cognitive processes if started with simpler concepts that are aggregated into larger, more complex pictures along the way.

Learning activities must be appropriate for each of the supra-ordinate and subordinate categories of the domains and explained in well-written objectives. It is acceptable that one activity may meet several objectives, which is especially true for the more broadly focused objectives. Sequenced learning activities based on expanding concepts provide continuity for students to base new learning on previous knowledge. Repeated use of conceptual matter is acceptable when the application involves increasingly complex situations. Learning activities can be designed to foster integration of concepts, rather than the parts, thus unifying knowledge, attitudes, and skills.

The educator must be mindful of the hierarchal order of simple to complex or concrete to abstract. The assumption is that each level builds on and integrates knowledge from the previous level. The cognitive domain, with the various types of knowledge, exemplifies progression of simple to complex when applying it to a conceptual model or theory. The affective (attitudes) domain joins the progression of simple to complex as in the cognitive domain. Examples of the two domains using the concept of change follows:

- ▲ **Cognitive:** identifies the steps in the process of change (factual, conceptual, and procedural knowledge)
  - *Affective:* listens for the patient's concerns for current level of wellness (attending)
- ▲ **Cognitive:** differentiates the steps in the change process (understanding)
  - *Affective:* accepts the client's concerns for health-related problems (responding)

▲ **Cognitive:** applies change theory to patient teaching (applying)
  • *Affective:* assumes responsibility for involving the patient in decisions about self-care practices
▲ **Cognitive:** relates the change process to health promotion for a patient (analyzing)
  • *Affective:* assumes responsibility for involving the patient in decisions about self-care (valuing)
▲ **Cognitive:** determines the priorities for health promotion based on the change process (evaluating)
  • *Affective:* develops a nursing care plan incorporating the patient's belief system (organization)
▲ **Cognitive:** proposes individualized nursing activities based on the change process and health promotion for the patient (creating)
  • *Affective:* revises nursing care plans in accordance with the patient's preferences (characterizes values)

The psychomotor domain is integrated into the cognitive base when learning "how" and knowing "why" the technical skills of nursing are performed. The adaptive nurse is capable of transferring conceptual knowledge to the practice arena for direct implementation of patient care. Nursing students who become well versed in the principles supporting their activities are able to adjust and recognize situations that require the skill. Rote learning, in contrast to meaningful learning, does not develop the flexibility needed for this adaptive ability for skill usage. Meaningful learning, which is the use of integrated knowledge, crosses over and links these two essentials (Smith, 1992).

Smith recommends the use of concept mapping and the Vee heuristic as tools to enhance the theoretical components of learning skilled activities that explicitly promote this ability. Concept maps link the learner's knowledge to the identified skill through the creation of a plotted diagram with general concepts linking to the subconcepts that depict the relationships and interactions. By seeing the student's imaged word, the instructor is able to fill in gaps and correct misconceptions in the learner's theoretical knowledge. Vee heuristics link theory and practice components of a skill together when nursing educators use focused questions for formative evaluation. This tool is designed with the theory components listed sequentially on the left side of the diagram and the corresponding practice elements on the right side, linked by the representative skill activity. Students answer questions from both the theoretical (why) and practice (how) point of view (Smith, 1992).

Using "what if" and "why" questions during the instruction of psychomotor skills in the laboratory is useful in the clinical setting. A simulation of unanticipated problems with a student in the laboratory environment, when probed by questioning from an educator, prompts the student to search cognitive stores for information necessary to problem solve. Being cognizant of the similar circumstances of one scenario to others helps to transfer information. The construct of meaningful learning can be tapped in the clinical setting when students are asked to recall and then transfer previously used knowledge and activities to the clinical setting. Sample questions are: "What would happen if...?"; "How can a nurse prevent this from happening?"; and "What if the patient is immobilized, how would you...?" Students in clinical situations find that the practice of self-stimulating questions, such as those mentioned above, stirs reflection on situations with similar applications. With practiced reflection and internal or external dialogues, the student is able to recognize that elements exist for using transferable knowledge, skills, and attitudes resulting in critical thinking. The curriculum that interweaves these opportunities by means of holistic objectives provides for these opportunities and more realistically informs the student of that intention, communicated through the objectives. Means to examine the curriculum for the inclusion of all the domains of learning and cognitive processes is possible by creating a taxonomy table to achieve this end.

As stated previously, the revised structure of the cognitive domain has two-dimensional scaffolding, the vertical supports anchoring the four types knowledge of factual, conceptual, procedural, and metacognitive, and the horizontal dimension of remembering, understanding, applying, analyzing, evaluating, and creating. The applications described previously for all knowledge types and the process dimensions give depth and breadth to the vertical and horizontal planes of the constructed two-dimensional table.

Figure 4.3 illustrates curriculum alignment with objectives linked to the taxonomy. The objective is placed within the vertical column to reflect the cognitive process designated in the stated objective as it intersects with the particular knowledge (noun) to be applied. The learning activities designed to enhance the learning for students are similarly fashioned into the two-dimensional grid, followed by the selected assessment method. The consistency with which the objective, learning activity, and evaluation method fall into the same intersecting square is an indicator of curriculum alignment and the integrity of that objective.

Evaluation of the curriculum is enhanced when the objectives possess the essential words that clearly communicate attributes of intended learning. Inconsistency is avoided, especially when the format of words (objectives) and actions (instructional activities and assessments/evaluation) reflect the faculty's intentions across the program. Voids in the tapestry of the curriculum, duplication, or repetition of knowledge (with the exception of building on basic concepts) in higher levels of the taxonomy and overlooked topical matters are visible by comparing the curriculum to the taxonomy. Through this assessment, the validity and defensible classification of objectives and actions are realized (Anderson et al., 2001).

▲ CRITICAL THINKING AND TAXONOMY

Content, activities, and assessment in nursing instruction are not hastily prepared in a conglomeration of material. A nursing education program is a carefully planned structure of knowledge with learning activities strategically placed within curricula, and the outcome is nurses prepared for professional practice. Recognized agencies such as the National League of Nursing (NLN) and the American Association of Colleges of Nursing (AACN) establish competencies for graduates of nursing educational programs. These agencies define essential knowledge, values, and professional behaviors expected of the graduate nurse. The NLN advises nursing educators to instill in future graduates a strong value for standards of professional practice, a responsibility for being accountable for personal actions and behaviors, and a responsibility to practice within legal, ethical, and regulatory frameworks. NLN descriptions of professional behaviors include demonstrating concern for others through caring, valuing the profession of nursing, and continuing professional development beyond matriculation (NLN, 2000).

The AACN (1998) describes similar expectations of graduate nurses upon completion of the educational program, advocating the design of "educational programs that allow

THE KNOWLEDGE DIMENSION	THE COGNITIVE PROCESS DIMENSION					
	1. REMEMBER	2. UNDERSTAND	3. APPLY	4. ANALYZE	5. EVALUATE	6. CREATE
A. FACTUAL KNOWLEDGE						
B. CONCEPTUAL KNOWLEDGE	Objective 1	Objective 1			Objective 3	
C. PROCEDURAL KNOWLEDGE						Objective 4
D. META-COGNITIVE KNOWLEDGE		Objective 2			Objective 2	

Key
Objective 1 = Acquire knowledge of a classification scheme of "appeals."
Objective 2 = Check the influences commercials have on students' "senses."
Objective 3 = Evaluate commercials from the standpoint of a set of principles.
Objective 4 = Create a commercial that reflects understandings of how commercials are designed to influence people.

FIGURE 4.3 Taxonomy table based on objectives.

the student to acquire the described knowledge, skills, competencies, and values, and to evaluate graduates to ensure the achievement of desired outcomes at graduation (p. 2)." The AACN supports the development and acquisition of an appropriate values and ethical framework for the professional nurse (AACN, 1998; Bevis & Watson, 2000; NLN, 2000). Critical thinking, strong communication/assessment skills, and demonstration of a balance of intelligence, confidence, understanding, and compassion are hallmarks of baccalaureate-prepared graduates.

Nursing professionals rely heavily on critical thinking to solve problems for clients experiencing altered health states leading to sound decisions for planned care. The NLN and AACN both hold that critical thinking is a valued skill essential for all practicing nurses and that the education of nursing students must promote the ability to use higher orders of thinking with consistency and exactitude to achieve these abilities (AACN, 1998; National League for Nursing Accrediting Commission, 2001).

Facione and Facione (1996) maintain that nursing education as a "fact loading" process is undesirable in itself; instead, it should develop the ability in nurses to identify problems, inquire rigorously and honestly, master selections of best possible interventions, and evaluate the efficaciousness of chosen interventions through critical thinking. Ford and Profetto-McGrath (1994) believe the capacity to achieve the recommendations by Facione and Facione is possible by shifting the teaching–learning paradigm to an emancipatory model of education as praxis.

"Critical thinking is integral to education and rationality and, as an idea, is traceable, ultimately to the teaching practices—and the educational ideal implicit in them—of Socrates of ancient Greece," offers Paul in a statement of principles concerning critical thinking (Paul, 2003). The message delivered by the National Council for Excellence in Critical Thinking included the following goals for education:

1. To articulate, preserve, and foster high standards of research, scholarship, and instruction in critical thinking;
2. To articulate the standards upon which "quality" thinking is based and the criteria by means of which thinking can be appropriately cultivated and assessed;
3. To assess programs that claim to foster higher-order critical thinking; and
4. To disseminate information that aids educators and others in identifying quality critical thinking programs and approaches, which ground the reform, and restructuring of education on a systematic cultivation of disciplined universal and domain specific intellectual standards (Paul, 2003).

These goals are based on the founding principles of the organization as listed in Box 4.1.

Using the principles as guidelines, educators acquire a sense of the concept of critical thinking and how it is possible to craft critical thinking as an integral element into curriculum substance. What is needed, though, is an operational definition of critical thinking.

Philosophers and educators have long sought a definition of critical thinking and have failed to reduce it to a single, epitomizing construct that informs nursing educators as to what critical thinking is and how to teach students to acquire it. Indeed, thinkers across all disciplines recognize the concept within their own intellectual spheres, settling on what seems reasonable and applicable for them. Thinking has been described as general, reflective, critical, creative, and reasoning with a purpose (Alfaro-LeFevre, 1999; Bandman & Bandman, 1995; Beyer, 1985; Brookfield, 1993; Ennis, 1985; Facione, 1990; Halpern, 1994; Kurfiss, 1988; Lipman, 1988; National Council for Excellence in Critical Thinking, 1992; Paul, 1993; Sheffer & Rubenfeld, 2000). Illuminating the role that critical thinking plays in the expansion of nursing knowledge and as a basis of sound decision making, nursing educators seek more insight into the connection of critical thinking to the education of students and performance as registered nurses. This begins with an understanding of what critical thinking is and what meaning it has for nursing educators.

▲ **B O X 4 . 1**   **Principles of Critical Thinking**

Founding Principles from the National Council for Excellence in Critical Thinking

1. There is an intimate interrelation between knowledge and thinking.
2. Knowing that something is so is not a matter of believing that it is so; it also entails being justified in that belief. (Definition: Knowledge is justified true belief.)
3. There are general as well as domain specific standards for the assessment of thinking.
4. To achieve knowledge in any domain, it is essential to think critically.
5. Critical thinking is based on articulable intellectual standards and hence is intrinsically subject to assessment by those standards.
6. Criteria for the assessment of thinking in all domains are based on such general standards as: clarity, precision, accuracy, relevance, significance, fairness, logic, depth and breadth, evidentiary support, probability, and predictive or explanatory power. These standards, and others, are embedded not only in the history of the intellectual and scientific communities but also in the self-assessing behavior of reasonable persons in everyday life. It is possible to teach all subjects in such a way as to encourage the use of these intellectual standards in both professional and personal life.
7. Instruction in critical thinking should increasingly enable a student to assess both his or her own thought and action and that of others by reference, ultimately, to standards such as those mentioned above. It should lead progressively, in other words, to a disciplining of the mind and to a self-chosen commetment to a life of intellectual and moral integrity.
8. Instruction in all subject domains should result in the progressive disciplining of the mind with respect to the capacity and disposition to think critically within that domain. Hence, instruction in science should lead to disciplined scientific thinking; instruction in mathematics should lead to disciplined mathematical thinking; instruction in history should lead to disciplined historical thinking; and in a parallel manner in every discipline and domain of learning.
9. Disciplined thinking with respect to any subject involves the capacity on the part of the thinker to recognize, analyze, and assess the basic elements of thought: the purpose or goal of the thinking; the problem or question at issue; the frame of reference or points of view involved; assumptions made; central concepts and ideas at work; principles or theories used; evidence, data, or reasons advanced; claims made and conclusions drawn; inferences, reasoning, and lines of formulated thought; and implications and consequences involved.
10. Critical reading, writing, speaking, and listening are academically essential modes of learning. To be developed generally they must be systematically cultivated in a variety of subject domains as well as with respect to interdisciplinary issues. Each are modes of thinking which are successful to the extent that they are disciplined and guided by critical thought and reflection.
11. The earlier that children develop sensitivity to the standards of sound thought and reasoning, the more likely it is that they will develop desirable intellectual habits and become open-minded persons responsive to reasonable persuasion.

▲ BOX 4.1   Principles of Critical Thinking (continued)

12. Education—in contrast to training, socialization, and indoctrination—implies a process conducive to critical thought and judgment. It is intrinsically committed to the cultivation of reasonability and rationality.

(Paul, 2004)

Dressel and Mayhew (1954) described "the ability to problem solve" as an early definition of critical thinking. Their definition included the selection of pertinent information needed for a solution; recognition of implicit or explicit assumptions; the statement of formulated or selected but relevant hypotheses that hold promise; arrival at valid conclusions; and an ability to judge the validity of inferences. At the time, their definition had little effect on nursing education. Another major influence for defining critical thinking came from Watson and Glaser in 1964. These quantifying pioneers in critical thinking measurement described critical thinking as a composite of skill development, knowledge of the subject, and attitude of the practitioner (Watson & Glaser, 1964). Many nursing researchers used their methodology to quantify critical thinking to assess students' acquisition of critical thinking skills. However, it is now believed by some that the methodology of Watson and Glaser does not measure critical thinking in nursing.

The definition of critical thinking is viewed as having two components, that is, a set of skills to process and generate information and beliefs and the habit, based on intellectual commitment, of using those skills to guide behavior (Scriven & Paul, 2003). Scriven and Paul offer that critical thinking will vary according to the underlying motivation. When immersed with self-centered motives, it is often characterized by skillful manipulation of ideas that are self-promoting for the individual or represent a group's vested interests. This type of critical thinking is often fraught with intellectual flaws despite how seemingly successful it might appear.

A higher order of rational thinking occurs when it is fair-minded and grounded in intellectual integrity. People are not consistently critical thinkers, and individuals may experience episodes of lethargic or irrational thought. The quality of an individual's critical thinking is a result of the degree and depth of experience in a domain of thinking or in respect to a specific class of questions. This can be seen in several other selected definitions of critical thinking. Some of these selected definitions of critical thinking are available for examination in Box 4.2.

Analysis of the definitions in Box 4.2 puts forward the idea that critical thinkers are nonbiased, reasoning people with a penchant for truth seeking. Critical thinking involves making decisions. It is considered critical only when the thinking process passes through criteria that are evaluative and linked to an affective belief or a purposeful action. Critical thinking is demonstrated in the cognitive processes and knowledge needed to give depth and breadth to the discipline. These are represented in the horizontal and vertical axes of the taxonomy table found in Figure 4.1.

The application of higher-order learning activities found in an educational taxonomy requires more than rote memory or recall and involves understanding conceptual connections, appropriate analysis, and evaluation of the situation's need, and decisional creativity to adapt information to similar or new scenarios. Over 40 years of research by cognitive psychologists

▲ **BOX 4.2**   **Definitions of Critical Thinking**

Critical thinking is:

▲ "[A] purposeful, outcome-directed (results-oriented) thinking . . . [that] requires knowledge, skills, and experience . . . [and helps one] constantly re-evaluate, self correct . . . , and strive to improve" (Alfaro-LeFevre, 1999, p. 9).

▲ "[A] rational investigation of ideas, inferences, assumptions, principles, arguments, conclusions, issues, statements, beliefs, and actions that covers scientific reasoning and includes the nursing process, decision making, and reasoning in controversial issues" (Bandman & Bandman, 1995, p. 7).

▲ "[R]eflective and reasonable thinking that is focused on deciding what to do or believe" (Ennis, 1995, p. 45).

▲ "[P]urposeful, self-regulatory judgment which results in interpretation, analysis, evaluation, an inference as well as explanation of the evidential, conceptual, methodological, criteriological, or contextual considerations upon which that judgment was based" (Facione, 1990, p. 3).

▲ "[T]hose skills (or strategies) that increase the probability of achieving a desirable outcome" (Halpern, 1994, p. 13).

▲ "[A]n investigation whose purpose is to explore a situation, phenomenon, question, or problem to arrive at a hypothesis or conclusion about it that integrates all available information and that can therefore be convincingly justified" (Kurfiss, 1988, p. 2).

▲ "[T]he intellectually disciplined process of actively and skillfully conceptualizing, applying, analyzing, synthesizing, and/or evaluating information gathered from, or generated by, observation, experience, reflection, reasoning, or communication, as a guide to belief and action" (National Council for Excellence in Critical Thinking, 1992, p. 201).

▲ "[T]hinking about your thinking while you're thinking in order to make you think better" (Paul, 1993, p. 91).

and philosophers, behaviorally oriented psychologists, and content specialists established that critical thinking exists at the higher levels of the educational taxonomy (Huitt, 1998). Recognition and recall are viewed as rudimentary demonstrations of knowledge in any subject. However, the comprehension of knowledge within its context is foundational to an understanding and application of information in any discipline, eventually requiring analysis, evaluation, and transfer of that knowledge to expanding spheres of knowing.

Prior to the revision of the taxonomy, two camps of thinking concerning synthesis (now referred to as creating) and evaluation existed. It was recognized that thinking processes leading up to these two highest levels are essential to create new pictures from the lower level pieces of information. Based on an analysis of a statement or proposition by means of information assessment or judgment, these two types of thinking were thought to have different purposes. Since the process of critical thinking is often equated to problem solving and decision making, similar linkages are observed for evaluative and creative thinking.

Huitt (1998) classified techniques for problem solving and decision making into similar creative/critical groups that are considered dichotomously as critical and creative. One set, critical thinking, is more linear and serial, with structure driving rational, analytical, and goal-oriented thinking. The second set, creative thinking, is a more global or holistic pattern of thinking. The latter is parallel and more emotive, intuitive, and creative, and paints a visual, tactile, or kinesthetic model of the creative-thinking process. Huitt contends that available definitions are problematic because creative thinking is often subsumed under critical thinking rather than as a separate, though related, process with its own distinctive standards. This goes hand in hand with beliefs that critical thinking is classified as "good thinking" and it expands "good thinking" definitions beyond the concept's intent, obfuscating its overall understanding. Good thinking requires both critical and creative thinking according to Huitt. Another difficulty noted with definitions for critical thinking is when authors confuse attitudes and dispositions toward thinking with an actual thinking process (i.e., emotion versus cognition, feeling versus reasoning). This contributes to the problems of separating out the skills of cognitive processing from attitudes or dispositions to use the skills (Huitt, 1998).

The introduction of attitudes and dispositions to the discussion of critical thinking is based on motivation, attitudes, values, and habits of mind typically utilized in "good critical thinking." These dispositions are identified as inclinations toward specific models of intellectual behavior. Ennis (1995) states that there is a propensity to do something under certain conditions in a reflective, purposeful manner. Norris (1992) further qualifies dispositions as not only predilections, but also as inclinations to habitually utilize abilities, selectively thinking, and choosing the thinking abilities to use. Solomon (1994) contributes to these notions by stating that dispositions go beyond this description of behaviors. He adds that a disposition is a cluster of preferences, attributes, and intentions and is also the capacity to follow thinking abilities through to fruition.

Tishman and Andrade (2003) offer a "triadic conception of thinking dispositions" that must be present and can be taught to students, which includes the concept of ability. The triad surrounds three psychological components cogent for dispositional behavior, sensitivity, inclination, and ability. When the engaged thinker uses sensitivity, he or she is appropriately perceptive of a particular behavior and feels an impetus toward carrying out that behavior. Finally, ability is identified as the capacity to follow through with the behavior (Tishman & Andrade, 2003). Examples of these elements in nursing can be found in students who seek balanced reason based on evidence or justification in situations. These may be students who are sensitive to occasions that call for supporting data, who are motivated or impelled toward seeking evidence, and who carry out an investigation to completion.

Each of the preceding contributors to the understanding of dispositions offers insight into what these dispositions entail. Perhaps the most relevant from educational philosophers in nursing and other related fields are those compiled by Facione and Facione (1996). These authors offer that critical thinkers are cautious, analytic, systematic, openminded, truth seeking, self-confident, and mature. Inquisitiveness is described as an eagerness to acquire knowledge and diligence in seeking information that is relevant to a situation, thus creating a well-informed state. The critical thinker engaged in decision making uses caution to focus on clarity in communication and uses reason to arrive at decisions. A critical thinker is clear about the issues enmeshed in a decision, analyzes the evidence, is alert for problem situations, and has the ability to anticipate the consequences of outcomes.

Critical thinkers who are open-minded demonstrate a willingness to reconsider their decisions and allow for their personal biases, especially if the biases have the potential to modify (positively or negatively) the decision. A systematic disposition guides the thinker to be orderly and focused in complex matters. Truth seeking requires results that are steeped in precision and reflect the most reliable or best knowledge, even in the shadow of equivocal support for preconceptions, beliefs, or self-serving purposes. The disposition of self-confidence develops as an internal trust of the thinker's personal reasoning skills. Prudence consists of formation, postponement, or reformulation of judgments and an awareness that multiple acceptable solutions are possible and open for consideration. Uncertainty is a fact of life even in reference to decisional situations and is part of mature critical thinking. It includes an acknowledgment that closure is possible without a complete knowledge of concerns relative to the situation (Facione & Facione, 1996).

▲ ACTIVE LEARNING STRATEGIES

Nursing educators often debate what strategy best suits the instillation of critical thinking dispositions in students through initial exposure to knowledge and refinement of novice skills. There is a plethora of suggested recommendations and activities from nursing education contributors (Billings & Halstead, 2005; DeYoung, 2003; Lowenstein & Bradshaw, 2001). However, the soundest recommendation relates to the preferred learning styles of students in a shared learning environment (Ford & Profetto-McGrath, 1994). In this approach, critical thinking is viewed as a cognitive process rather than a product of learning and requires a paradigm shift in the nature of student–teacher relationships. Educators have pondered how the experienced nurse achieves the transition of using information from one context of learning to another and attempt to duplicate and guide students to achieve this ability in the clinical environment. The development of critical thinking ability requires recognition, decision making, implementation, and evaluation. For students to gain this ability, educators need to review learning theory as it applies to critical thinking.

Perry's (1978) model of intellectual and ethical development addresses the learning stages for collegiate students based on cognitive theory and explains the nonstatic progression of students. Dualism, multiplicity, relativism, and commitment are the components of a developmental and explanatory model of how students move in intellectual and ethical progression. Dualism, the initial stage in which students perceive knowledge as an absolute (black or white) or concrete without regard to the gray areas of understanding, is the stage in which there is always a right answer, with all others being wrong. It is in this stage that students regurgitate facts without the ability to organize, prioritize, or interpret the data. The reinforcement of dualism underlies courses that ask little of students other than to repeat or use rote memory to demonstrate learning. Students in the dualism stage experience difficulty in seeing beyond the facts to the contextual nature of knowledge or the multiple perspectives in which it may be used (Perry, 1978).

Multiplism, the advancing stage from dualism, demonstrates growth in cognitive development in which the concrete recognition of facts and data is replaced by a realization that all knowledge is relative. Students appreciate that more than one interpretation of any issue may exist, but it is limited to their perspective as being valid; that is, it is based simply on the fact that it is their perspective and they have entitlement to that perspective. Students struggle and perceive personal affronts when asked to support opinions and perspectives, often desperately seeking out what the educator's position is to repeat what is thought to be the right position. Ironically, the students may maintain that their perspectives hold no more validity than the teacher's. Appreciation of supported or informed opinion is not yet valued by students and is often received by students as unjust challenges or personal criticisms when asked to provide support for that position (Perry, 1978).

The context in which students begin to understand the existence of multiple positions or perspectives on issues, contextualism, represents the third developmental stage of critical or analytical thinking. The students begin to understand that perspectives are based on the context in which they are recognized and that some responses hold more validity than others in that context. The "aha" moment moves the student to apply information from one scenario to another, which is satisfying instead of frustrating for the learner, and internalizes the lesson learned for reapplication in future events. Students are able to visualize in the mind's eye that the application of knowledge of a problem in the acute care setting has shades of variation, for example, application to the home care setting (Perry, 1978).

Informed commitment is the final stage of the model and is characterized by the ability to weigh the virtues of multiple positions, to understand the contextual nature of each, and to make a commitment to one based on the information available. This includes the capability of giving credence and respect to others' perspectives (Perry, 1978). Interesting differences have been noted at this point in the development of a predictable pattern based on gender in respect to how a perspective is evaluated and how decisions or commitments are made (Gillian, 1982).

The strategies to employ in teaching were discussed throughout this chapter specific to the taxonomy discussion; types of approaches for developing critical thinking will be the focus for the remainder of this chapter's discourse. Lecture is used most frequently by nursing faculty when the student is passively taking in information and the teacher is the active player. To influence the dispositions toward thinking, the role of the student is to take the active position in learning, especially when the tenets of constructivism are kept in mind. When learning is held to be a shared responsibility, learners define their own needs, take responsibility to explore the plethora of resources at their disposal, and evaluate changes to meet learning needs. It is the educator's responsibility to create and maintain an environment conducive to learning, facilitating the environment, and mentoring students in their achievement. This requires the facilitator to push students on occasion by challenging their thinking and at the same time supporting them throughout the learning process. An educator's goal is to alter close-minded student perspectives while opening students' thinking to alternatives and perspectives other than those previously held. The educator should consider instructional methods other than the traditional method of lecture to promote learning.

Writing-to-learn, concept mapping, and debate are alternatives worth consideration to achieve the desired outcomes. Documentation of ideas through writing serves as a stimulus for critical thinking by immersing the student in the subject matter available from the literature and seeking not only cognitive utilization of that knowledge, but also the affective absorption of values and beliefs. A caveat to this alternative is that students must be introduced to what is deemed as quality or worthy literature and provided directives for organizing the literature in a logical format to convey their affective beliefs, values, and commitments. This involves learning to make decisions based on what is assimilated from the literature to achieve the assignment's objective(s). The educator selects the format and provides adequate guidelines for the students to follow for grading purposes. Suggestions for this method include journal writing, formal papers, creative writing assignments, summaries of course content, summarizing collectives of research abstracts with a position statement, or poetic expressions of emotional reactions to situations.

At times, students consider the evaluation of such assignments as subjective and that the time invested to the assignment distracts from other areas of learning. Assignments can be as simple as requiring a 1-minute paper as proposed by Cross (1981). In this instance, students are asked to present an overall statement of what they found interesting or new information gleaned from a presentation or other educational exposure.

Other methods for involving students in writing-to-learn require them to prepare one- to two-page thought-papers written on controversial topics in health care. Journal writing helps students reflect on their experiences and infuse concepts into their knowledge base or contrast others' perspectives to their own thoughts. Evaluating these types of assignments is considered controversial or subjective unless teachers remember to set aside their own biases or positions.

Writing-to-learn programs and writing-across-the-curriculum projects were successful for several nursing programs with significant outcomes toward the development of dispositions in critical thinking (Bower & McCarthy, 1993; Crowles, Strickland, & Rodgers, 2001; Lashley & Wittstadt, 1993; Niedringhaus, 2001; Slimmer, 1992). Techniques and requirements for these programs are specific to each curriculum and course objectives, with the desired outcomes resulting in logical and consistent thought by students.

Concept mapping lends visual assistance to students when asked to demonstrate their thinking in a graphic manner to demonstrate the interconnectedness of concepts or data. In these instances, the educator assesses and makes suggestions related to faulty logic or inadequate information to facilitate the assimilation of information. With repeated exposure to concept mapping, students become more adept at creating and examining a map for connections and missing information. Eventually, the process of cognition requires less representation on paper and becomes more mentally oriented when problem solving or decision making. Inherent in this growth is the ability to self-evaluate thinking processes. Students need to support their thinking with evidence based on what is known through research or clinical practice. This process is evident in practicing nurses but has been elusive in the educational process. When attempting to measure critical thinking in students through curriculum or program assessment, many studies conclude that current methods for measuring critical thinking are inadequate. This is an area of continuing discussion, yet considered a mandatory requirement by accrediting agencies (NLN, 1996).

Concept mapping is adaptable to a variety of courses or topic matters. As an activity tool, it expands the students' abilities to examine their own thinking, support relationships within the data or evidence, note holes in the structure of their thinking, substantiate the connection of causes with effects, consider the context of situations, search out predisposing factors, and identify reasonable outcomes associated with the diagrams of their thinking. Contributors to concept mapping (or mind mapping) use it to teach subject matters such as pharmacology, enhancing clinical and theoretical class preparation, pathophysiology, and major conceptual components in care planning. Findings from studies of concept mapping demonstrate that it is an effective method for promoting critical thinking in students (Castellino & Schuster, 2002; Daley, Shaw, Balistrieri, Glesenapp, & Piacentine, 1999; King & Shell, 2002; Mueller, Johnston, & Bligh, 2001; Reynolds, 1994).

Debate as a strategy to foster critical thinking requires in-depth research of topic matters for supporting evidence and for developing a position on a controversial issue. It encourages analytical skills, recognizes the complex facets of issues or concerns, permits students to consider alternative posits with the freedom to change one's mind based on the preponderance of the information presented, develops an ear for listening to all aspects of an issue before arriving at a conclusion, and enhances communication skills. This feeds directly into the affective growth of the student with respect to the values and beliefs of the profession and develops empathy for alternative stances from those personally held. This strategy is more effective if utilized at high levels of cognitive thinking. It promotes teamwork to develop solid platforms, may be focused on timely ethical and moral issues, or revisits issues with implications that continue to the present.

At the same time, it requires a time investment on the part of the educator to teach the art of argument and on the student to prepare the debate. The latter investment of time may be overcome by introduction of the debate early in the course with an expectation that strategies incorporated during the term are utilized and demonstrated by the end of the course. This methodology is recommended for the promotion of critical thinking from the perspective of student preparation for weighing of the evidence. Lowenstein and Bradshaw (2001) add that debate provides the students with opportunities for objective analysis to arrive at a conclusion without bias. An advantage of debate is the rapid timeframe in which learners must consider and analyze information to arrive at conclusions. Candela, Michael, and Mitchell (2003) state that debate encourages students to respond to the conflicts between personal values, morals, opinions, professional responsibilities, and relationships, and to the perceived role of advocate for patients and family members. Ethical debate opens the students' thinking to others' positions, thus enabling the advocate role. Debates that require the use of evidence rather than personal opinion are more effective in developing critical thinking skills. Debate as a teaching strategy is considered most effective in the third or fourth stage of Perry's (1978) model for developing human thought and knowing processes when applied to critical thinking. These learning activities are but a few examples of teaching strategies for the development of critical thinking in nursing.

▲ SUMMARY

Chapter 4 reviewed the use of educational taxonomies and domains of learning in nursing education to guide the development of goals and objectives in the curriculum plan and their eventual implementation through instructional design. It traced the history of the taxonomies from Tyler's (1949) initial model, to Bloom et al.'s (1956) three domains of learning, Anderson's (2001) update of Bloom et al.'s work, and Hauenstein's (1998) recent work on the behavioral domain of learning as an integration of the taxonomies toward a holistic curriculum. The application of these models to nursing curricula was reviewed, and educators were exhorted to analyze the objectives and their relationship to the mission and philosophy of the program and their flow from the selected taxonomies for appropriate levels and expected outcomes. Examples of activities to demonstrate the cognitive processes were presented and instances of factual, conceptual, and procedural knowledge were tied to the domains of learning. Suggested teaching and assessment strategies for learning outcomes were interspersed throughout the discussion.

A discussion of critical thinking and its definitions were presented with their connection to the preparation of nursing students for the profession and clinical decision making in practice. The importance of critical thinking in the development and evaluation of curricula and its relevance to accreditation criteria were reviewed. A comparison of critical thinking and creative thinking exposed new vistas for the preparation of rational professionals who are open to innovative ideas for practice and research in nursing. Several strategies for teaching–learning activities to promote critical thinking concluded the chapter.

DISCUSSION QUESTIONS

1. What are your beliefs about the use of educational taxonomies in curriculum development and their application to instructional design? If you were to analyze existing nursing education and staff development/patient education curricula for the use of these taxonomies and domains of learning, is it your belief that educators set outcome expectations at appropriate levels? Explain your answers and link them to the expected outcomes for learners.
2. The nursing profession places great emphasis on the application of critical thinking skills. How do you define critical thinking and what do you see as the building blocks toward the development of these skills? Explain why critical thinking skills are essential to nursing practice and research.
3. To what extent do you believe writing ability influences critical thinking ability?

LEARNING ACTIVITIES

Student Learning Activities

1. Select one piece of nursing knowledge and the skills with which it is associated. Using one or several educational taxonomies and associated domains of learning, develop an overall goal and objectives that you expect the learner to accomplish. Explain how the objectives relate to the goal and give the rationale for your choice of taxonomy(ies) and domains.
2. From your experience as a nurse, analyze a situation in which critical thinking took place. Explain how critical thinking led or did not lead to clinical decision making. What previous knowledge and skills served as the foundation for these critical thinking and clinical decision-making skills? What types of learning activities and experiences would you have a student or new graduate engage in to build upon critical thinking and decision-making skills?

Faculty Learning Activities

1. Analyze your curriculum's end-of-program and level objectives for evidence of educational taxonomies. What domains of learning can you identify? Link them to the type of learning outcomes that you expect from your students and graduates in nursing knowledge and skills. Are there relationships and logical sequences from level objectives to end-of-program objectives and are they at the appropriate level within the educational taxonomies and domains? How do they relate to the mission, philosophy, and conceptual framework of your curriculum?
2. Examine the most recent accreditation self-study report for your program's response to criteria that relate to critical thinking. How does your program define critical thinking?

How does it purport to measure the development of critical thinking in your students and demonstration of these skills in your graduates?

REFERENCES

Alfaro-LeFevre, R. (1999). *Critical thinking in nursing: A practical approach* (2nd ed.). Philadelphia: Saunders.

American Association of Colleges of Nursing (1998). *The essentials of baccalaureate education*. Washington, DC: Author.

Anderson, L. W. (2002). Curriculum alignment: A re-examination. *Theory into Practice*, 41(4), 255–260.

Anderson, L. W., Krathwohl, D. R., Airisan, P. W., Cruickshank, K. A., Mayer, R. E., Pintrich, P. R., et al. (Eds.). (2001). *A taxonomy for learning, teaching, and assessing: A revision of Bloom's taxonomy of educational objectives*. San Francisco: Longman.

Anderson, L. W., & Sosniak, L. A. (Eds.). (1994). *Bloom's taxonomy: A forty-year retrospective*. Chicago: University of Chicago Press.

Angel, B. F., Duffey, M., & Belyea, M. (2000). An evidence-based project for evaluating strategies to improve knowledge acquisition and critical thinking performance in nursing students. *Journal of Nursing Education, 35*(9), 213–218.

Bachman, K. (1990). Using mental imagery to practice a specific psychomotor skill. *Journal of Continuing Education in Nursing, 21*(3), 125–128.

Bandman, E. L., & Bandman, B. (1995). *Critical thinking in nursing* (2nd ed.). Norwalk, CT: Appleton & Lange.

Baxter, G. P., Elder, A. D., & Glaser, R. (1996). Knowledge-based cognition and performance assessment in the science classroom. *Educational Psychologist, 31*, 133–140.

Beckie, T. M., Lowry, L. M., & Barnett, S. (2001). Assessing critical thinking in Baccalaureate nursing students: A longitudinal study. *Holistic Nursing Practice,15*(3), 18–26.

Bevis, E. O. (1989). *Curriculum building in nursing: A process* (3rd ed.). Boston: Jones and Bartlett.

Bevis, E. O. (1993). All in all, it was a pretty good funeral *Journal of Nursing Education 32*(3), 101–105.

Bevis, E. M., & Watson J. (2000). *Toward a caring curriculum. A new pedagogy for nursing*. Boston: Jones and Bartlett.

Beyers, B. K. (1985). Improving thinking skills; Defining the problem. *Phi Delta Kappa, 65*(7), 486–490.

Billings, D. M., & Halstead, J. A. (2005). *Teaching in nursing: A guide for faculty* (2nd ed.). St. Louis, MO: WB Saunders.

Bloom, B. S., Englehart, M. D., Furst, E. J., Hill, W. H., and Krathwahl, D. R. (1956). *Taxonomy of educational objectives: The classification of educational goals*. New York: Logmans, Green & Co.

Bloom, B. S. (1964). Reflections on the development and use of the taxonomy. In L. W. Anderson & L. A. Sosniak (Eds.), *Bloom's taxonomy: A forty-year retrospective*. Chicago: University of Chicago Press.

Bowers, B., & McCarthy, D. (1993). Developing analytic thinking skills in early undergraduate education. *Journal of Nursing Education, 32*(3), 107–114.

Bransford, J. D., Brown, A. L., & Cocking, R. R. (1999). *How people learn: Brain, mind, experience and school*. Washington, DC: National Academy Press.

Brookfield, S. (1993). On impostership, cultural suicide, and other dangers: How nurses learn critical thinking. *Journal of Continuing Education, 24*(5), 197–205.

Candela, L., Michael, S. R., Mitchell, S. (2003). Ethical debates: Enhancing critical thinking in nursing students. *Nurse Educator 28*(1), 37–39.

Castellino, A. R., & Schuster, P. M. (2002). Evaluation of outcomes in nursing students using clinical concept map care plans. *Nurse Educator 27*(4), 149–150.

Cross, K. P. (1981). *Adults as learners*. San Francisco, CA: Jossey-Bass.

Crowles, K. V., Strickland, D., & Rodgers, B. L. (2001). Collaboration for teaching innovation: Writing across the curriculum in a school of nursing. *Journal of Nursing Education, 40*(8), 363–367.

Daley, B. J., Shaw, C. R., Balistrieri, T., Glesenapp, K., & Piacentine, L. (1999). Concept maps: A strategy to teach and evaluate critical thinking. *Journal of Nursing Education 38*(1), 42–47.

Dave, R. H. (1970). Psychomotor levels. In R.J. Armstrong (Ed.), *Developing and writing behavioral objectives*. Tucson, AZ; Educational Innovators Press.

Detterman, D. L., & Sternberg, R. J. (1993). *Transfer on trial: Intelligence, cognition, and instruction*. Norwood, NJ: ABLEX.

DeYoung, S. (Ed.). (2003). *Teaching strategies for nurse educators*. Upper Saddle River, NJ: Pearson Education.

Dillard, N., & Laidig, J. (1998). Curriculum development: An overview. In D. M. Billings & J. A. Halstead (Eds.), *Teaching in nursing: A guide for faculty*. Philadelphia: WB Saunders.

Doyle, W. (1992). Curriculum and pedagogy. In P. W. Jackson (Ed.), *Handbook of research on curriculum*. New York: Macmillan.

Dressel, W., & Mayhew, L. B. (1954). *General education: Exploration in evaluation.* Washington, DC: American Council on Education.

Ennis, R. (1985). Critical thinking and the curriculum. *National Forum, 65,* 28–31.

Ennis, R. (1995). A logical base for measuring critical thinking skills. *Educational Leadership, 43*(2), 44–48.

Facione, P. A. (1990). *Critical thinking: A statement of expert consensus for purposes of educational assessment and instruction (the Delphi Study Report of the American Philosophical Association).* Millbrae, CA: California Academic Press. (ERIC Document Reproduction Service No. E0315423)

Facione, P. A., & Facione, N. (1996). Externalizing the critical thinking in knowledge development and clinical judgment. *Nursing Outlook, 44*(3), 129–136.

Flavell, J. (1979). Metacognition and cognitive monitoring: A new area of cognitive-developmental inquiry. *American Psychologist 34,* 906–911.

Ford, J. S., & Profetto-McGrath, J. (1994). A model for critical thinking within the context of curriculum as praxis. *Journal of Nursing Education, 33*(8), 341–344.

Fosnot, C. T. (1996). *Constructivism: Theory, perspectives, and practice.* New York: Teachers College Press.

Gillian, C. (1982). *In a different voice.* Cambridge, MA: Harvard University Press.

Gronlund, N. E. (1991). *How to write and use instructional objectives* (4th ed.). New York: Macmillan.

Halpern, D. F. (1994). Critical thinking: The 21st century imperative for higher education. *The Long Term View, 2*(3), 12–16.

Harrow, A. (1972). *A taxonomy of the psychomotor domain. A guide for developing behavioral objectives.* New York: McKay.

Hauenstein, A. D. (1998). *A conceptual framework for educational objectives: A holistic approach to traditional taxonomies.* New York: University Press of America.

Huitt, W, (1998). *Critical thinking.* Retrieved March 21, 2002, from Kibler, R. J., Barker, L. L., & Miles, D. T. (1970). *Behavioral objectives and instruction.* Boston: Allyn. http://chiron.valdosta.edu/whuitt/col/cogsys/critthnk.html

King, E. C. (1984). *Affective education in nursing: A guide to teaching and assessment.* Rockville, MA: Aspen.

King, M., & Shell, R. (2002). Teaching and evaluating critical thinking with concept maps. *Nurse Educator 27*(5), 214–216.

Kohlberg, L. (1975). The cognitive-developmental approach to moral education. *Phi Delta Kappa, 56*(10), 670–677.

Krathwohl, D. R., Bloom, B. S., & Masia, B. B. (1964). *Taxonomy of educational objectives: The classification of educational goals II: Affective domain.* New York: Longman.

Krathwohl, D. R. (2002). A revision of Bloom's taxonomy: An overview. *Theory in Practice, 41*(4), 221–218.

Kurfiss, J. (1988). *Critical thinking: Theory, research, practice, and possibilities (ASHE-ERIC Higher Education Report, No 2).* Washington, DC: Association for the Study of Higher Education.

Lashley, M., & Wittstadt, R. (1993). Writing across the curriculum: An integrated curricular approach to developing critical thinking through writing. *Journal of Nursing Education, 32*(9), 422–424.

Lipman, M. (1988). *Critical thinking—What can it be?* (Resource Publication Series 1. No. 1). Montclair, NJ: Institute for Critical Thinking, Montclair State College.

Lowenstein, A. J., & Bradshaw, M. J. (2001). *Fuzzard's innovative teaching strategies in nursing.* Gaithersburg, MD: Aspen.

Mayer, R. E. (2002). Rote versus meaningful learning. *Theory in practice, 41*(4), 226–232.

Mayer, R. E., & Wittrock, M. C. (1996). *Problem-solving transfer.* In D. C. Berlenir & R. C. Colfee (Eds.), Handbook of Educational Psychology. New York: Macmillan.

Mayer, R. E. (1995). *The promise of educational psychology: Learning in the content area.* Upper Saddle River, NJ: Prentice-Hall.

McKeogh, A., Lupart, J., & Marini, A. (Eds.). (1995). *Teaching for transfer.* Mahwah, NJ: Erlbaum.

Miller, M. A., & Babcock, D. E. (1996). *Critical thinking applied to nursing.* St. Louis, MO: Mosby.

Mueller, A., Johnston, M., & Bligh, D. (2001). Mind-mapped care plans; a remarkable alternative to traditional nursing care plans. *Nurse Educator 26*(2), 75–80.

National Council for Excellence in Critical Thinking. (1992). *Proceedings of the 12th annual International Conference on Critical Thinking and Educational Reform (August 9-12, 1992)* (pp. 197–203). Rohnert Park, CA: Center for Critical Thinking and Moral Critique, Sonoma State University.

National League for Nursing. (2000). *Educational competencies for graduates of associate degree nursing programs.* Sudbury, MA: Jones and Bartlett.

National League for Nursing (1996). *Criteria guidelines of baccalaureate and higher degree programs.* New York: Author.

National League for Nursing Accrediting Commission. (2001). *Accreditation manual and interpretive guidelines by program type for post secondary and higher degree programs in nursing.* New York: Author.

Niedringhaus, L. K. (2001). Using student writing assignments to assess critical thinking skills: A holistic approach. *Holistic Nursing Practice, 15*(3), 9–17.

Norris, S. (1992). Testing for the disposition to think critically. *Informal Logic 2/3,* 157–164.

Norton, B. (1998). Teacher to learner. In D. M. Billings & J. A. Halstead (Eds.), *Teaching in nursing: A guide for faculty.* St. Louis: W. B. Saunders.

Oermann, M. H. (1990). Psychomotor skill development. *Journal of Continuing Education in Nursing, 21*(5), 202–204.

Paul, R. (1993). *Critical thinking: How to prepare students for a rapidly changing world.* Santa Rosa, CA: Foundation for Critical Thinking.

Paul, R. (2004). *The National Council for Excellence in Critical Thinking: A draft statement of principles.* Retrieved June 6, 2003, from http://www.criticalthinking.org/

Perkins, D. N. (1990). The nature and nurture of creativity. In B. F. Jones & L. Idol (Eds.), *Dimensions of thinking and cognition instruction.* Hillsdale, NJ: Erlbaum.

Perkins, D. N., & Solomon, G. Transfer of learning. Retrieved June 7, 2003, from http://learnweb.harvard.edu/alps/thinking/docs/trancost.doc

Perry, W. (1978). Growth in the making of meaning: Youth into adulthood. In A. Chickaring (Ed.), *The future of American colleges.* San Francisco: Jossey Bass.

Phye, G. D. (Ed.). (1997). *Handbook of educational assessment.* San Diego: Academic Press.

Piaget, J. (1970a). Piaget's theory. In P. H. Musen (Ed.), *Carmichael's manual of psychology.* New York: Wiley.

Piaget, J. (1970b). *Structuralism.* New York: Basic Books.

Piaget, J. (1973). *To understand is to invent: The future of education.* New York: Grossman.

Pintrich, P. R. (2002). The role of metacognitive knowledge in learning, teaching, and assessing. *Theory into Practice, 41*(4), 219–225.

Reilly, D. E., & Oermann, M. H. (1990). *Behavioral objectives: Evaluation in nursing* (3rd ed.). New York: National League for Nursing.

Reynolds, A. (1994). Patho-flow diagramming: A strategy for critical thinking and clinical decision making. *Journal of Nursing Education, 33*(7), 333–336.

Scriven, M., & Paul, R. (2003). *Defining critical thinking.* Retrieved October 10, 2004, from http://www.critical-thinking.org/University/univclass/Defining.html

Sheffer, B. K., & Rubenfeld, M. G. (2000). A consensus statement on critical thinking in nursing. *Journal of Nursing Education, 39*(8), 352–360.

Shulman, L. (1987). Knowledge and teaching: Foundations of the new reform. *Harvard Educational Review, 567,* 1–22.

Simpson, B. J. (1966). The classification of educational objectives: Psychomotor domain. *Illinois Journal of Home Economics, 10*(4), 110–144.

Slimmer, L. W. (1992). Effect of writing across the curriculum techniques on students' affective and cognitive learning about nursing research. *Journal of Nursing Education, 31*(2), 75–78.

Smith, B. E. (1992). Linking theory and practice in teaching basic nursing skills. *Journal of Nursing Education, 31,* 16–23.

Solomon, G. (1994). *To be or not to be (mindful).* Paper presented at the Annual Meeting of the American Educational Research Association, April 4–8, 1994, New Orleans, LA.

Sosniak, L. A. (1994). The taxonomy, curriculum, and their relations. In L.W. Anderson & L. A. Sosniak (Eds.), *Bloom's taxonomy: A forty-year perspective.* Chicago: The University of Chicago Press.

Tishman, S., & Andrade, A., (2003). *Thinking dispositions: A review of current theories, practices, and issues.* Retrieved June 7, 2003, from http://learnweb.harvard.edu/alps/thinking/docs/Dispositions.htm

Tyler, R. W. (1949). *Basic principles of curriculum and instruction.* Chicago: University of Chicago Press.

Watson, G., & Glaser, E. M. (1964). *Critical thinking appraisal.* Orlando: Harcourt, Brace, and Jovanovich.

Wilson, L. (2003) *Different types of learning. Current Index of Topics. Different types of learning- transmission, acquisition, accretion and emergence.* Retrieved June 6, 2003, from http://www.uwsp.edu/education/lwilson/

Conducting a Needs Assessment for Reviewing and Developing Curricula

Sarah B. Keating, EdD, RN, FAAN

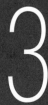

▲ OVERVIEW

When contemplating a new education program or revising an existing curriculum, a needs assessment is indicated. There are two purposes for conducting an assessment. The first is to validate the currency, academic and professional relevance, and continued need for an existing program. The second is to establish the feasibility for a new nursing program including the demand for it, available resources, academic soundness, and financial liability.

Even though justification for current programs usually exists, it is wise to survey constituents and collect information relative to the same factors that are examined in a needs assessment for a new program. This information either reaffirms assumptions about the curriculum on the part of the program planners or identifies gaps or problems that indicate a need for change. It is also useful for accreditation and program review purposes and can serve as an organizing framework for a master plan of evaluation. (See Section 5.)

▲ THE FRAME FACTORS MODEL

Johnson (1977) presented a conceptual model for curriculum development, instructional planning, and evaluation that is similar to the nursing process. Although it is a simple and linear model, (P [planning], I [implementation], E [evaluation]), Johnson expands it into a complex step-by-step logical process for curriculum development and evaluation. The process includes examining the frame factors or context within which the program exists, setting goals, identifying curriculum content, structuring the curriculum, planning for instruction, and finally, evaluation. Johnson speaks of frame factors as the context in which the curriculum exists. Furthermore, he classifies the context into natural, cultural, organizational, and personal elements. This author chose the terms of frame factors, external and internal, from Johnson's discussion and adapted them to curriculum development in nursing. Included are the elements that Johnson identified, and it adds other components that specifically apply to nursing education, health care systems, and the nursing profession.

Frame factors for this text are defined as the external and internal factors that influence, impinge upon, and/or enhance educational programs and curricula. As a conceptual model, it serves to collect, organize, and analyze information that is useful for the development and evaluation of curricula. There are two major categories of frame factors, external and internal. External frame factors are those that influence curriculum development in the larger environment and outside the parent institution. Internal frame factors are those that influence curriculum development and are within the environment of the parent institution and the program itself. The figure on page 107 illustrates the frame factors conceptual model.

While the principal activities of faculty in curriculum development and evaluation are on the curriculum plan itself and the need for improvement based on evaluation of the processes of implementation and the program outcomes, the needs assessment should become part of the education repertoire of the faculty. Even if faculty is not involved in the details of the needs assessment, it should be aware of all of the factors that have an influence on the curriculum. Faculty members sophisticated in the assessment of external and internal frame factors have an advantage in viewing the curriculum and its place in the scheme of financial security, position

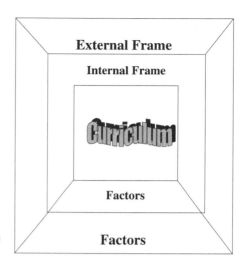

Frame factors conceptual model.
Adapted with permission from Johnson
(1977).

within the health care system and the profession, role in meeting the health care needs of the community and industry, and significance to the parent institution.

It is recommended that nurse educators in both the academic and practice settings use this model when evaluating education programs, considering revisions of existing programs, or initiating new programs. While administrators may take the leadership role in conducting needs assessments, faculty should participate in the decisions for what type and how much data to collect and what decisions are made that affect the curriculum.

External Frame Factors

Chapter 5 describes the factors in the external environment outside of the parent institution and the nursing education program that influence the curriculum. They include the community, population demographics, the political climate and body politic, the health care system and the health needs of the population, the characteristics of the academic setting, the need for the (nursing) program, the nursing profession, regulation and accreditation standards, and external financial support. All of these factors can influence the curriculum in positive and negative ways, and while they may not be in the control of the faculty, they are important to recognize and analyze for their impact on the program. They can make or break a program. For example, lack of accreditation for a nursing program can prohibit its graduates from career opportunities and continuing education. Each external factor is discussed in detail and a table provides guidelines for collecting and analyzing data for informed decision- making. Chapter 5 initiates a case study based on an actual feasibility study that utilized the conceptual frame factors model and guidelines. The case study continues into Chapters 6 and 7.

Internal Frame Factors

Chapter 6 discusses the internal frame (environmental) factors within the parent institution and the nursing program that influence the curriculum. The frame factors model identifies the following internal frame factors: description and organizational structure of the parent academic institution; mission, philosophy and goals of the parent institution; economic situation and its influence on the curriculum; resources within the institution (laboratories, classrooms, library, student services, etc.); potential faculty and student characteristics; and a description of the health care system that supports the curriculum. Similar to the external frame factors, these internal factors influence the curriculum and play a major role in developing, revising, or expanding programs. As with the external frame factors, faculty use the information gleaned from an assessment of these factors for arriving at decisions regarding the curriculum. The same data collected for a needs assessment are, in fact, related to total quality management of the curriculum and contribute to the evaluation of the program.

▲ RELATIONSHIP OF NEEDS ASSESSMENT TO TOTAL QUALITY MANAGEMENT OF THE CURRICULUM

Establishing a new program is not an exercise that occurs in a vacuum. Somehow, preliminary information had an impact on the key stakeholders and program planners that indicated a possible need for the program. The same is true for the need to revise a program or expand its offerings; that is, there are trigger mechanisms that initiate the change process. Rather than responding to these external stimuli in a reactive way, faculty and nurse educators should have a master plan of evaluation in place that continuously monitors the program and provides the data needed for planning for changes both that are timely and that look to the future. Such activities are part of a total quality management process that provides the data for analysis and decisions leading to the continuous improvement and quality of the educational program. The factors discussed in the frame factors model in this section of the text apply to evaluation strategies as well. While Section 5 discusses program and curriculum evaluation at great length, it is useful to incorporate the notion of evaluation as a continuous process when conducting a needs assessment, not only in terms of the present plans for program start-up and changes, but also for planning for the future.

REFERENCE

Johnson, M. (1977). *Intentionality in education.* Albany, NY: Center for Curriculum Research and Services.

External Frame Factors: Influence and Assessment

Sarah B. Keating, EdD, RN, FAAN

OBJECTIVES

Upon completion of Chapter 5, the reader will be able to:

1. Evaluate the essential external frame factors for a needs assessment when developing or revising a curriculum.
2. Analyze external frame factors in the Frame Factors Conceptual Model for their application to a needs assessment for curriculum development and evaluation purposes.
3. Examine a case study that illustrates a needs assessment of external frame factors for a curriculum development project.
4. Apply the Guidelines for Assessing External Frame Factors in a simulated or real curriculum development situation.

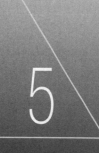

▲ OVERVIEW

Most nurse educators work in an established academic setting or in a health care agency that has a major plan for staff development and client education. Thus, the process of curriculum development usually relates to revision of the curriculum based on feedback from staff, clients, students, faculty, administrators, alumni, and consumers of the program's graduates. It is rather infrequent that new programs are initiated. Whether curriculum development involves a new program or revisions of an existing curriculum, program planners and faculty must evaluate both external and internal frame factors that affect the curriculum, their impact on the current program, and what role they play in forecasting the future.

Chapter 5 provides detailed information for conducting a needs assessment of external frame factors for the development of a new program and its curriculum or for revising an existing curriculum. *A needs assessment for curriculum development is defined as the process for collecting and analyzing information that can influence the decision to initiate a new program or revise an existing one.* The first step in curriculum development for faculty and program planners is to examine the environmental and human systems factors that influence the curriculum. These factors can be organized into two major categories: external and internal frame factors (Johnson, 1977). *External frame factors are defined as those factors that influence curriculum development in the environment and outside the parent institution. Internal frame factors are those factors that influence curriculum development and that are within the parent institution and the program itself.* Figure 5.1 depicts the external frame factors of a curriculum to consider when conducting a needs assessment.

▲ DESCRIPTION OF THE COMMUNITY

The first step in developing or revising a curriculum is to provide a description of the community in which the program exists (or will exist). A needs assessment ensures the relevance of the program to a community need and its eventual financial viability. Existing programs often identify the need for revision of their curricula based on recommendations from their consumers or an accreditation report. Whether developing a new program or revising an old one, an examination of the external frame factors is essential to study their impact on the program and its future needs. The program under development or revision is considered in light of its fit to the community that it serves. For the purposes of curriculum development, *community is defined as "people and the relationships that emerge among them as they develop and use in common some agencies and institutions and a physical environment; a locality-based entity composed of systems of formal organizations reflecting society's institutions, information groups, and aggregates"* (Stanhope and Lancaster, 2000, p. G-5).

Depending upon the nature of the educational program, the community can be as wide as an international focus to as narrow as a region within a state. Large universities or colleges with research notoriety often attract international scholars while some state-supported programs attract students who live nearby and who intend to spend their professional lives in their home community. *Sectarian (associated with or supported by a religious organization) and nonsectarian (not associated with a religious organization),* independent or private colleges and universities, state or other government sponsored institutions, and large or small schools face the same

Community

Financial Support

External

Demographics

Internal

Regulations and
Accreditation

The Curriculum

Political Climate
and Body Politic

Nursing Profession

Frame Factors

Health Care System
and Health Needs
of the Populace

Frame Factors

Need for the Program

Characteristics of the
Academic Setting

F I G U R E   5 . 1 External frame factors for a needs assessment for curriculum development. Adapted with permission from Johnson (1977).

challenges when assessing their external environment for program or curriculum development purposes. Therefore, it is important to identify if the community in which the program is situated is urban, suburban, or rural. Such factors as accessibility to students, faculty, learning resources, and financial support are influenced by the geographic location of the community.

The major industries and education systems in the community are identified as possible sources for students in the program and for potential partnerships for program support and learning experiences. Industry has resources for scholarship and financial aid programs and experts in the field who can serve as faculty or adjunct faculty. Health care industries in particular should be participants in the needs assessment and curriculum planning to bring the reality of the practice setting into the program. The major religious affiliations, political parties, and systems such as transportation, communications, government, community services, and utilities in the community are additional external frame factors. These factors have an effect on the curriculum as to its relevance in the community and the support it needs to meet its goal. For example, state supported schools are very dependent upon government funding while private schools must rely on tuition and endowments. There are many models in the literature that discuss the major components of a community assessment (e.g., Clemen-Stone, McGuire, & Eigsti, D.G., 2002; Stanhope and Lancaster, 2000).

Demographics of the Population

When considering a new program or revising a curriculum, it is useful to have knowledge of the people who live in the home community of the institution and the broader populace that it will serve. *Demographics are the data that describe the characteristics of a population, (e.g., age, gender, socioeconomic status, ethnicity, education levels, etc.).* The demographic information that is vital to program planners includes the age ranges and preponderance of age groups in the population; predicted population changes including immigrant and emigrant statistics; ethnic and cultural groups including major languages; education levels; and socioeconomic groups. This information identifies potential students and their characteristics and to some extent, the needs of the population that the students and graduates will serve.

Educational programs and curricula must be geared toward the needs of the learners. If the student body draws from the region surrounding the institution, the characteristics of the students should be analyzed for special learning needs. For example, if there are nurses seeking to advance their careers, then the curriculum needs to focus on adult learning theories and modalities. Younger students about to embark on their first professional degree will need curricula that focus on their developmental needs as young adults as well as the content necessary for gaining nursing knowledge, clinical skills, and socialization into the professional role. It is of interest to learn from students who come from greater distances what drew them to the program and if those factors are useful in curriculum planning. Faculty should identify potential students with needs for learning resources beyond the usual, for example, assistance for students whose primary language is not English. It is useful to learn of the financial resources for the potential student body and if there is a need for major financial aid programs. In light of the need for increased diversity in the nursing workforce, ethnicity and cultural values in the community particularly have an impact on recruitment strategies for higher education.

Another consideration related to demographics is the existence of potential faculty and identification of people who have the credentials to teach. Seeking potential sources of faculty through partnerships with industry and the community to supply adjunct teachers is helpful if the program needs to recruit new faculty. Resources for finding demographic information are plentiful. The U.S. Census Bureau (2002) has national and regional statistical and demographic information that is helpful in assessing the populations. Its website is located at http://www.census.gov.

▲ CHARACTERISTICS OF THE ACADEMIC SETTING

Other institutions of higher learning in the nearby community or region have an influence on the program and its curriculum. Identifying these institutions, their levels of higher education (technical schools, associate degree and/or baccalaureate and higher degree), financial base (private or public), and affiliations (sectarian or nonsectarian) gives the assessors an idea of the existing competition for recruiting students, faculty, and staff. Information about the types of programs in nursing that are available from other institutions and their intentions for the future enables developers to understand the gaps in the types of programs and the nature of the competition from other educational programs. For example, if the institution's curriculum offers a nurse practitioner program and two other programs in the region offer similar programs, perhaps the curriculum should be revised to a specialty primary care program such as a pediatric nurse practitioner or geriatric nurse practitioner track; discontinued; or, possibly, entered into a joint venture with the other schools. A private institution that is dependent upon tuition and endowments may question whether a particular track in its curriculum that is redundant with a state-supported school in the nearby vicinity should continue to offer the program. Other data to consider are the demands for nurses in the area and the success rates of graduates finding employment in the region.

Benchmarks that the faculty can use to compare its own curriculum with those of its competitors should be identified, for example, the pass rate on NCLEX. Other examples include costs of the program, admission and retention rates, accreditation status, and so forth. It is important to know how the nearby community agencies and health care systems view the graduates of the program. Yet another important factor is the productivity of the faculty members and how their educational credentials, track records in securing grants, publication histories, and research records compare to others.

A suggested resource for collecting data on other academic institutions is the regional accreditation agency. There are six regional accrediting associations in the United Sates. The umbrella organization that lists the agencies with addresses and contact information may be found at http://www.chea.org (Council for Higher Education Accreditation [CHEA], 2004). National databases may also be found at the National Center for Education Statistics website (2002), http://nces.ed.gov. Once the list of other academic institutions is developed, faculty can find descriptions for selected schools at their individual websites or in the library. Libraries or admission departments in most institutions of higher education have current copies of other college and university catalogs.

▲ POLITICAL CLIMATE AND BODY POLITIC

When assessing the community, part of the data describes the governmental structure. For example, if it is urban, it is useful to know if there is a mayor, a chief executive, and a city governing board. Likewise, if it is rural or suburban, vital information includes the type of county or subdivision of government, who the chief executive is, if the officials are elected or appointed, and what is the major political party.

Equally, if not more, important is information about the body politic. A simple definition for the body politic is: *the people power(s) behind the official government within a community. It is composed of the major political forces and the people who exert influence within the community.* The assessor should identify the major players and their visibility, that is, the high profiles or low profiles who are the powers behind the scenes. Additional information that reveals the body politic is how those in power influence decisions in the community and how they exert their power by using financial, personal, political, appointed, or elected positions. Specific information that is useful to educators is how the key politicians view the college or university and whether, during elections and other crucial times, they recognize the power of its people, that is, the students, faculty, and staff.

Relative to nursing, the politicians' and the body politic's specific interests in the profession are helpful. For example, if they have family members who are nurses or if they have been recipients of nursing care, they are more apt to support nursing education programs. All educational programs need the support of the community and its power structure. Therefore, the information learned from assessing the political climate is vital to planning for the future and seeking assistance when the call comes for additional resources or political pressure to maintain or increase the program.

▲ THE HEALTH CARE SYSTEM AND HEALTH NEEDS OF THE POPULACE

Providing nurses to care for the health care needs of the populace is of critical interest to the health care system and the consumers of care. It is obvious that information about these two factors is essential to education program planning and curriculum development. Schools of nursing expect that the majority of their graduates will remain in the region. However, nursing is a mobile profession and its members move to other geographic locations far from their alma maters. For example, in California, with one of the largest populations of nurses (247,138 in 1999), more than half of the nursing workforce immigrate into the state from other states and countries (Coffman, J. et al., 2001). Most state boards of nursing keep current data on the nursing workforce. Information about specific states can be obtained at the National Council of State Boards of Nursing website: http://www.ncsbn.org.

To assess the health care system, it is necessary to identify the major health care providers, types of organizations and health care agencies, and major health care financing resources. Box 5.1 presents a list of some of the major factors to assess in the health care system.

Information about regional health care systems is available through the following United States websites that contain lists of national, regional, and state health care agencies:

1. American Health Care Association: http://www.ahca.org (2004)
2. American Hospital Association: http://www.aha.org (2004)
3. American Public Health Association: http://www.apha.org (2004)
4. National Human Services Assembly: http://www.nassembly.org/nassembly (2004)
5. National Association for Home Care: http://www.nahc.org (2004)

Last but not least, the yellow pages of telephone directories have listings of regional and local health care agencies and facilities.

The assembled list provides an overview of the health care system within which the program is located. It describes the health care resources that are available or not available to the population, including the nursing school's aggregate. It points out the gaps of services in

▲ **BOX 5.1**   **Major Factors to Assess in the Health Care System**

- ▲ Major health care systems (i.e., private, public)
- ▲ Penetration rate of managed care* systems
- ▲ In the case of other countries, the nature of the health care system (i.e., a national system or predominantly private)
- ▲ Major health insurance programs
- ▲ Nonprofit or for-profit health care agencies and eligibility for services
- ▲ Sectarian and nonsectarian health-related agencies and eligibility for services
- ▲ Public health services
- ▲ Services for the underserved or unserved population groups
- ▲ Major primary health care agencies and providers
- ▲ Voluntary health care agencies and their services
- ▲ Other community-based health-related services staffed by nurses (e.g., schools, industry, state institutions, forensic facilities, etc.)
- ▲ Roles of nurses in the health care agencies
- ▲ Plans to increase or decrease health-related services in the future
- ▲ Influence of health care agencies on the curriculum, students' clinical experiences, and graduates' future careers

* Managed care is defined as "a system that integrates the financing and delivery of appropriate medical care by means of the following features: contract with selected physicians and hospitals that furnish a comprehensive set of health care services to enrolled members, usually for a pre-determined monthly premium; utilization and quality controls that contracting providers agree to accept; financial incentives for patients to use the providers and facilities associated with the plan; and the assumption of some financial risk by doctors, thus fundamentally altering their role from serving as agent for the patient's welfare to balancing their patient's needs against the need for cost control" (Lee and Estes, 1994, p. 231).

the community and the possibilities for community partnerships, including school-based services for the underserved and unserved populations. It identifies trends in health care services and anticipated changes for the future that can influence curriculum development.

It is useful to know if resources within the system, such as health care libraries, are available to students and faculty during clinical experiences or as resources for students enrolled in distance education programs. A review of the health care agencies & facilities list pinpoints existing clinical experience sites and the potential for new ones. Personnel in the agencies with qualifications as preceptors, mentors, and adjunct faculty are additional resources for possible collaboration opportunities. Research opportunities for students and faculty may emerge from the review and can influence curriculum development as well as foster faculty and student development.

An overview of the major health problems in the region contributes to curriculum development as exemplars for health care interventions. The National Center for Health Statistics' (2004) website, http://www.cdc.gov/nchs, provides general information on leading causes of death and morbidity. Vital statistics and other health statistics are located at the Healthy People website (2004), http://www.health.gov/healthypeople, which also describes leading health indicators.

▲ THE NEED FOR THE PROGRAM

An examination of the external environment informs the faculty about the increased or continued need for nurses. The following data points act as guides to document the need for the program:

▲ Characteristics of the nursing shortage and the extent of nursing shortage if it exists
▲ Predictions for the future nursing workforce needs
▲ Adequate numbers of eligible applicants to the program, currently and in the future
▲ Specific areas of nursing practice experiencing a shortage
▲ Employers' projections for the numbers of nurses needed in the future
▲ Employers' views on the types of graduates needed

A brief survey of health care administrators can provide this information, although it is sometimes difficult to expect a good return rate in light of the current pressures on administrators. Another strategy is to conduct focus groups that take no more than 15 minutes in the health agencies. Instructors who use the facilities for students or clinical coordinators are excellent people for collecting the information. There are several resources to identify the need for nurses, including the state nurses' associations that can be located through the American Nurses' Association (2004) website, http://www.nursingworld.org/about/index.htm; the Bureau of Health Professions (2004), http://bhpr.hrsa.gov; and the Colleagues in Caring Project (2004), http://www.aacn.nche.edu/CaringProject/index.htm.

As described previously in the characteristics of the academic setting, knowledge of other nursing programs in the region is useful to avoid curriculum redundancies. The data on the need for the program demonstrate to curriculum developers how many of its graduates are needed now and in the future, the level of education necessary to provide the level of care required, and short- and long-term needs in the health care system. A current demand indicates the possibility for accelerated programs. Shortages in specialties indicate advanced-practice curricula and increased opportunities for registered nurses to continue their education.

▲ THE NURSING PROFESSION

In addition to the need for nurses, it is important to learn about the nursing profession in the region. Professional organizations are rich resources for identifying leaders, mentors, and financial support such as scholarship aid. Curriculum developers should survey faculty and colleagues for a list of the nursing professions in the region. Such organizations include local or regional affiliates of the American Nurses' Association (ANA); the National League for Nursing (NLN); Sigma Theta Tau International; educator organizations such as the American Association of Colleges of Nursing (AACN) and the National Organization of Associate Degree Nursing (NOADN); and the plethora of specialty organizations. Questions to gather information about the profession are: Who are the nurses in the area? Are there professional organizations with which the program can link? What is the level of education for the majority of the nurses in practice? Are there nurses prepared with advanced degrees who could serve as educators or preceptors? Are research activities underway that present opportunities for students and faculty?

▲ REGULATIONS AND ACCREDITATION REQUIREMENTS

Whether the program is new or under revision, state regulations regarding schools of nursing should be reviewed for their requirements and any recent or anticipated changes in them that affect the curriculum. Information on regulations is available through the state boards of nursing. For a listing of specific state boards of nursing, consult the National Council of State Boards of Nursing (NCSBN) (2004) website at http://www.ncsbn.org.

National accreditation is not required of schools of nursing; however, it provides the standards for nursing curricula and demonstrates program quality. Sophisticated applicants to the school will look for accreditation. Alumni find it advantageous to graduate from an accredited institution when applying for positions in the job market, for future advanced education, and for positions in the military.

Nursing has two major accrediting agencies and a few specialty-accrediting bodies. The National League for Nursing Accrediting Commission (NLNAC) (2004) Inc. accredits licensed practical/vocational nursing, associate degree, and baccalaureate and higher degree nursing programs. Detailed information on its accrediting process and standards may be found on its website, http://www.nlnac.org. The Commission on Collegiate Nursing Education (CCNE) accredits baccalaureate and higher degree programs. Information on its accrediting process may be found at the American Association of Colleges of Nursing (AACN) (2004) Accreditation Standards, Accreditation Procedures, and Program Review Guidelines website, http://www.aacn.nche.edu/Accreditation/pubsguides.htm. An example of a specialty-accrediting body is that of the American Association of Nurse Anesthetists (AANA) (2004). Its website is http://www.aana.com/accreditation.

In addition to accreditation, there are standards set by professional organizations that can serve as guidelines or conceptual frameworks for curricula. Several examples for prelicensure and graduate-level programs are those developed by AACN (1995, 1998); Council of Associate Degree Nursing Competencies Task Force (2000), and the National Organization of Nurse Practitioner Faculty (NONPF) (2004).

Another external frame factor that influences the nursing curriculum is regional accreditation. The parent institution of a nursing program undergoes periodic review by its regional accrediting body. All programs within the institution are examined, although for some professional programs such as nursing, the most recent professional accreditation report is accepted by the regional organization. Nevertheless, members of the nursing faculty are involved in the regional accreditation process and should be mindful of the standards set by that organization. Information about regional accrediting bodies can be found at http://www.chea.org (Council for Higher Education Accreditation [CHEA], 2004). Detailed descriptions of accreditation processes and standards for educational programs are described in Section 5 under Evaluation. However, it is useful to review the processes for the standards and limitations they impose during the curriculum development process.

▲ FINANCIAL SUPPORT SYSTEMS

An analysis of the finances of the program provides curriculum developers with vital information on the economic health of the program. Indicators of financial health influence how the curriculum will be delivered, and faculty should recognize signs that demonstrate the program's financial viability. If new sources of income for the program are indicated, possible resources need to be identified. The proposed revisions in the curriculum must be realistic in terms of cost. If it is a new program, adequate resources including start-up funds for its implementation must be available. If it is an existing program, faculty and administration should consider whether to continue it at its present level of financial support or increase or decrease the level of support.

Other items of study include how the program is financed and the major sources of revenues such as fees, tuition, state support, private contributions, grants, scholarships, or endowments. Knowing if there are adequate resources to support the program to be self-sufficient is a critical element in the analysis of the financial viability. Although this type of information falls within the responsibility of administration, curriculum developers must have a basic understanding of the financial support systems that impact curriculum development.

▲ SUMMARY

Chapter 5 introduced the first step, a needs assessment, in curriculum development and revision. Prior to revising or developing new curricula, an assessment of the factors that influence the education program is necessary. In examining the environment that surrounds the program, curriculum developers look at external frame factors. Table 5.1 serves as a guideline for identifying the external frame factors, collecting the data for an assessment, and analyzing the factors to determine if there is a need for a new program or if changes are necessary for an existing program.

Analyzing external frame factors in light of proposed new programs or curriculum revisions helps faculty and their administrators to determine the type of new program needed, or in the case of an existing program, the extent to which changes in the curriculum are indicated. A review of the external frame factors provides a check with reality, including the community in which the program is located, the industry for which the program prepares graduates, and the economic viability of the program.

▲ TABLE 5.1	Guidelines for Assessing External Frame Factors

Frame Factor	Questions for Data Collection	Desired Outcomes
Description of the community	Is the community setting conducive to academic programs? Describe its major characteristics (i.e. urban, suburban, or rural)	The institution's campus is located in a safe and supportive environment for its students, faculty, and staff.
	What are the major industries, and do they financially support the institution as well as employ graduates?	Industries are stable and have a history of financial support of the institution and employ its graduates.
	Who are the major education systems in the community, and what is the quality of their programs? How do they feed into the parent institution?	The public and private school systems, kindergarten through 12th grade, provide graduates for the institution and are of high quality. The school counselors have a strong relationship with the institution's admission department.
		Community college and higher degree institutions collaborate with the parent institution and have articulation agreements for ease of transfer.
	What are the community services that provide an infrastructure for the institution (e.g., transportation and communications services)?	Students have easy access at reasonable cost to public transportation to and from home (for commuter students) and to stores and other community services.
		The community has multiple media communication networks of high quality for marketing, public relations, and education purposes. Postal service and other delivery systems are reliable.
	What are the community services that provide an infrastructure for the institution (e.g., recreation, housing, utilities, and human and health services)?	There are varied and multiple recreation sites for students' leisure activities.
		If there are no student health services, the community has quality health and human services for which students are eligible.
	What type of government is in place in the community, and what are its politics? Is the government supportive of the institution in its midst, and does it recognize its contributions to the community?	The government structure is supportive of the parent institution in its community. Key members of the parent institution serve on advisory boards for the local government.
Demographics of the population	What are the characteristics of the general population?	The population reflects multicultural and ethnic characteristics with a wide range of

(*table continues on page 118*)

▲ **TABLE 5.1**   **Guidelines for Assessing External Frame Factors** (*continued*)

Frame Factor	Questions for Data Collection	Desired Outcomes
		age groups. The average income level is at or above the average for the region. Poverty levels are low, or there are dedicated programs of assistance for the poor.
	What indications are there that the population supports higher education?	A majority of the population completed high school or higher levels of education and/or there is growing interest in and need for these levels of education.
	Within the population, what is the potential for student, faculty, and staff for the program?	There is an adequate applicant pool for the program(s). There are potential qualified faculty and staff in the locale.
Characteristics of the academic setting	Identify other institutions of higher learning in the region. Within those institutions, what types of nursing programs are offered, if any? Are there potential or existing competitors?	Other institutions of higher learning in the region have programs that are not in direct competition with the curriculum and can serve as feeder schools to the program. There are no known future plans that could conflict with the program.
Political climate and body politic	Identify the type of government and its structure. Who are the political power brokers in the community? What are the relationships of the parent institution to the political power brokers?	Key politicians and community leaders support the institution and have working relationships with the people within the educational institution.
The health care system and health needs of the populace	Identify the major types of health care systems and the predominant health care delivery patterns.	There are ample spaces currently and for the future for student nursing placements in the various health care systems and settings.
	Describe the major health care problems and needs of the populace in the education program's region.	The major health care problems and needs match those foci in the curriculum.
	Describe the role of nursing in the health care system.	Nursing, as the largest health care workforce, has a strong representation within the health care system.
The need for the program	Describe the nursing workforce in the region as well as in the state and nation.	There is a demonstrated need for nurses in the region, state, and nation currently and in the future.

▲ TABLE 5.1	Guidelines for Assessing External Frame Factors (*continued*)	
Frame Factor	**Questions for Data Collection**	**Desired Outcomes**
	Describe the numbers and types of nurses needed in the region, state, and the nation for the future.	The numbers and types of nurses needed meet the goals and type(s) of preparation available in the education program for the future.
The nursing profession	List the major professional nursing organizations in the region.	There are at least two major nursing organizations in the region that can support the program and provide collegial relationships for students and faculty.
	Describe the characteristics of nurses in the region.	The types of nurses in the region match the potential applicant pool for continued education or faculty and mentor positions.
Regulations and accreditation requirements	Identify the State Board of Registered Nursing regulations for education programs.	The nursing education program meets the state board regulations and has been approved or is eligible for approval.
	List accreditation agencies that impact the parent institution and the nursing education program.	The parent institution is accredited by its regional agency and the nursing program meets the standards of a national professional accrediting body.
Financial support	Review an analysis of the present financial health of the parent institution and the nursing program.	The institution and the nursing program are in solid financial condition and there is either guaranteed state support or substantial endowment funds for the future.
	Develop a list of existing and potential economic resources.	There are adequate economic resources for the present and the future of the program.
Analysis of the data and decision making	Summarize the findings by generating a list of positive, neutral, and negative external frame factors that influence the curriculum.	Make a final decision statement as to the feasibility of the program as it is affected by the external frame factors.

C A S E   S T U D Y

▼

A case study fictionalized from an actual feasibility study is presented in this chapter and the next to illustrate a needs assessment for curriculum development and evaluation purposes. It includes the collection of external and internal frame factors data, their analyses, and a curriculum decision based on the findings. Chapter 7 presents the proposed curriculum based on the needs assessment.

Description of the Community

An existing baccalaureate and higher degree nursing program is aware of the nursing workforce shortage in the nation and its region. It has anecdotal information that employers of nurses prefer baccalaureate or higher degree nurses owing to the complexity of the acute care setting and the shortages of nurses prepared to practice in community settings.

The School of Nursing program has a basic undergraduate program, a registered nurse (RN) Bachelor of Science (BSN) to Master of Science (MSN) accelerated program, an entry-level master's program, and the master's level specialties of nurse practitioner, clinical specialist, and case manager. It is a private sectarian program within a multi-purpose independent college with a strong liberal arts history. The nursing program affiliates with a religious-based health care organization of the same denomination as its parent organization. The health care organization structure is that of a health maintenance organization (HMO) and it has facilities located throughout the nation and the institution's region. The HMO indicated to the nursing program administration and its parent institution's administrators that it would support an outreach program to increase the numbers of nurses for its workforce. With this information in hand, the nursing administrator (or dean) asks the faculty to conduct a needs assessment for a possible outreach program located about 150 miles from the main campus in a large metropolitan area with at least four large HMO facilities located within the city's surrounding area.

Using the guidelines for assessing external frame factors, the faculty initiates a needs assessment. They divide the work into teams of two or three, each to collect information on one of the nine external frame factors. Once the data are collected, the teams present them to the faculty group, which organizes and refines the data for analysis according to the need for an outreach program.

The team assigned to community assessment identifies the city as a metropolitan area for the locale of the outreach program. They learn that their parent institution has several existing outreach programs in the city. The director of extended education consents to an interview to provide information for the community assessment. He is a willing partner in sharing classrooms, computers, staff, and student services facilities. (Sharing rental expenses for the facilities will result in cost savings to both the extended education and nursing programs.)

In addition to the interview, the team visits the city to conduct a windshield survey (Stanhope & Lancaster, 2000), look through the business and yellow pages of the telephone directory,

(continued)

and tour the extended education facilities. The team finds the city's website that describes the community and lists much of the information they seek. The major industries in the area include:

▲ Two large technology manufacturers
▲ Several food-processing plants
▲ A large inland port
▲ A railroad center that serves the region in the transportation of goods
▲ An airplane parts manufacturer
▲ A rocket engineering and manufacturing plant
▲ Several large health maintenance organizations that serve the city and its rural neighbors

All of the industries have a long history in the area and are financially stable, and the technology manufacturers plan to expand and employ at least 2,000 additional workers over the next 5 years. The non–health-related industries support the extended education program of the parent institution and send many of their workers to the programs for advanced preparation. In the past, two of the manufacturers gave grants to the parent institution for computer engineering scholarships and one manufacturer gave a $20 million grant toward a new science building on the home campus.

A state-supported baccalaureate and higher degree program with a nursing program is located in the city. Additionally, there are three state-supported community colleges in or near the city, there is one large university-based medical center that does not have a nursing program, and the closest private college (without a nursing program) is 300 miles away. Results from statewide achievement tests reveals that the city's kindergarten through 12th grade system ranked in the 60th percentile. Most of its students prefer to remain in the local area and the majority of those who continue schooling after high school (40%) go to the local community colleges. The extended education director collaborates with industry, the community colleges, and the state-supported university when marketing its program and recruiting students. Since, it is an extended education program, there is minimal contact with the kindergarten through 12th grade counselors. However, the parent institution has existing articulation agreements with all of the community colleges and the state school.

The public transportation system within the city includes buses and a light rail system. Three major highways intersect with the city, providing easy access for automobile travel. There is a middle-sized airport with commuter planes and some major airlines serving other major cities within the state, and AMTRAK services are available. Fares are reasonable and there are discounts for students. There is one major daily paper, several suburban papers, at least 15 radio stations, four television stations, TV cable service, and telecommunication services for computer access. There are many mailing services such as UPS, FedEx, and Pak Mail located throughout the area. The extended education director reports that mail service is speedy and reliable.

The city is located on a major river and there are several state and city recreation parks for picnicking, swimming, boating, and hiking. The city lies between the ocean and mountains; thus, winter, summer, and beach sports are no more than 2 to 3 hours away. Low-rent housing facilities are scarce and new home construction is barely able to keep up with the demand owing to the growth of industry in the region. Utilities are fairly reasonable in cost; however, as mentioned previously, low-rent housing including utilities is hard to come by. There is a municipal system for the delivery of utilities that is reliable.

(case study continues on page 122)

There are four major health maintenance organizations that serve their enrolled members, and students who have their coverage are eligible for care. With the projected population growth, two of the HMOs have plans for expansion. There are public health clinic services for students who do not have health coverage and who are eligible for state-supported health care programs.

The city has a board of supervisors with a mayor. At the present time, the Democratic party has the most representatives in the government. Although the parent institution has no representatives in the government, the director of extended education meets periodically with an ad hoc committee of the board of supervisors to discuss higher education issues that affect the city's populace. This activity on his part contributes to the presence and image of the parent institution in the city.

Preliminary Conclusions:

The location and size of the community indicate feasibility for the proposed outreach program. Collaboration possibilities with the existing extended education program are very positive. The infrastructure of the community provides support for the program and its students. Housing for students appears to be a major problem. There is only one baccalaureate and higher degree competitor for the nursing program. These issues will be examined in the "Characteristics of the Academic Setting Frame Factors" section.

Demographics of the Population

The faculty team assigned to gathering data on the demographics of the city's population in which the proposed outreach program will take place seeks information from the city's website. The team learns that the city's total population is 350,000. The racial breakdown by percentage is as follows: White: 48.3; Native American: 1.3; African American/Black: 15.6; Asian: 16.6; two or more races: 6.3; and other race: 15.0. The age distribution is as follows: 19 years and under: 30.2%; 20 to 34: 23.0%; 35 to 44: 15.0%; 45 to 59: 15.9%; 60 to 74: 10%; and 75 and over: 5.9%. The major languages spoken at home are English, 67.4%, and languages other than English, 32.6%. (The other major spoken languages are Spanish and several Asian languages.) Forty-two percent of the population have at least one vehicle per household. Of the population, 77.3% hold a high school diploma and 23.7% have a baccalaureate or higher degree. The following lists the major occupations for the working population and their percentage distribution: management or professional: 36.2; services: 16.2; sales or office work: 28.6; fishing, forestry, or farming: 0.4; construction: 7.6; and production: 11.0%. The unemployment rate is 4.2% (well below the state average) and the median household income is $37,000. There are 11.9% of households earning less than $10,000 per year. Indications are that the population is growing and that the demographics will remain stable as to ethnicity and occupations.

Preliminary Conclusions:

Overall, this population is growing and thriving economically. Its diverse ethnic population meets the program's goal to increase cultural diversity in its student population, while at the same time, there may be a need for programs to assist students whose primary language is not English. A large percentage of highly educated individuals in the population are potential faculty and staff for the

(continued)

program and might be interested in second career opportunities. Age breakdowns in the population indicate a large percentage of potential students between the ages of 20 to 44.

Characteristics of the Academic Setting

The team members assigned to identify other institutions of higher learning go to the regional accrediting body. There they find a listing of accredited colleges and universities in the region. They decide to identify those institutions within the selected city and 75 miles outside the radius of the city line. They also look at the city's website, which lists all of the institutions. Once the team members identify all schools and learn which schools have nursing programs, they divide the work among the members to interview the administrators of the schools of nursing. The information the team members seek includes types of nursing programs offered, the applicant pool, admission date(s), enrollments, graduation rates, licensure examination (NCLEX) pass rates, where the majority of graduates work, and impressions of the administrators for the need for an additional program in the area. The purpose for these interviews is twofold; that is, they give basic information about other nursing programs in the region, and they also inform the team of the potential for another program. The team members are aware that the interviews must be handled delicately with sincere reassurance to the administrators that the proposed program is meant to complement existing programs. This sets the pathway for collaborative relationships in the future should the program begin.

The academic setting team learns that the three community colleges offer associate degree in nursing (ADN) programs and the state-supported school offers a generic Bachelor of Science in Nursing (BSN) program as well as an accelerated RN-to-BSN program. It has four master's specialty tracks, one in education, one in nursing administration, one in community health nursing, and a nurse practitioner program. Additionally, the faculty learns that the program recently developed an online RN-to-BSN track that is proving to be very popular. The faculty also notes that there is one statewide online RN-to-BSN program and multiple nationwide programs for RNs to earn higher degrees.

The three community colleges are about equal in size, and their administrators report that their total enrollments approximate 150, with 50 graduates each year. Their qualified applicant pool numbers 350 each, although they believe they may be drawing from the same applicant pool. Their admission rates to fill slots average 93% to 95%, leaving a waiting list each year of about 50 qualified applicants. There are no plans to increase enrollments in the near future owing to the lack of state support for program expansion. The administrators report pass rates on NCLEX ranging from 82% to 100%. Most of their graduates remain in the local area to practice and are either in acute care, nursing home, or home health agencies.

The state-supported BSN and higher degree school administrator reports that they have a total enrollment of 300 students in the basic BSN program, 100 RNs in the RN-to-BSN program, and 150 in the graduate programs. The Master of Science in Nursing (MSN) nurse practitioner program is the most popular, with the community health nursing and education tracks each enrolling approximately 20 students each year. About 75% of the basic BSN students transfer in from the community college, having completed their nursing prerequisites. The remainder enters as freshmen. The basic BSN program graduates approximately 65 students each year, with an average NCLEX pass

(case study continues on page 124)

rate of 87% for the past 5 years. About 80% of its graduates remain in the area to practice. The qualified applicant pool for the basic BSN program is 350, and again, the administrator believes some of the applicants may be in the same pool as the ADN programs. Owing to constraints on state-supported funds, there are no plans to expand enrollments in the near future.

The RN students come from regional health care agencies, and based on the response to the online version of the program, the school may discontinue its traditional RN-to-BSN program. Most master's degree students come from the region as well and are seeking additional education for career mobility purposes. Although the MSN applicant pool is small compared to the capacity of the program (200 for 150 slots), the program remains viable. The administrator notes that there have been requests recently from people who have baccalaureates or higher degrees for a master's or second degree program. Upon further investigation with the ADN administrators, the faculty learns that they too have experienced these requests and, in fact, have students enrolled in their programs that have bachelor's or higher degrees other than nursing.

Preliminary Conclusions:

The region has four nursing programs—three ADN programs and one baccalaureate and master's degree in nursing program. There appears to be an adequate qualified applicant pool for these programs, and there are waiting lists for the generic programs (ADN and BSN). The RN pool seems satisfied with the new online program offered by the state-supported school, and there are multiple other options for them to complete a baccalaureate in nursing. All of the clinical specialties at the master's level are viable. One tantalizing fact is the interest on the part of college graduates in nursing. There are no fast-track baccalaureate or entry-level master's programs in the region. The faculty team advises the collection of additional data about this possibility.

Political Climate and Body Politic

The initial description of the community identified the city's government as consisting of a board of supervisors and a mayor. At the present, the Democrats are the political party in control. The team members assigned to investigate the political climate and body politic decides to attend a board of supervisors meeting. They also read the local newspaper metro section and the editorial pages. They interview the director of extended education for their home campus to seek his opinions on the political climate in the city as it relates to the parent institution.

The meeting of the board of supervisors that the team attended happened to have health care issues on its agenda. Citizens were concerned about the pending proposal to close two of the city's public health clinics owing to a shortfall in the state budget and a trickling-down effect of fewer public funds for the clinics. The faculty noted several political action groups in attendance that were vocal in their protests about the closures. It being an election year, the mayor and supervisors listened carefully to their pleas and by the end of the meeting, assured them that the clinics would remain open. The team observed that the mayor was a strong leader with little dissension among the board members on the various issues.

The survey team members were quite interested in learning that the mayor was an RN and quite knowledgeable about health cares issues. They decided to seek an interview with the mayor and

(continued)

were successful in meeting with her for a half-hour. At the meeting, they gained the mayor's support for the possible outreach program as long as the other nursing programs in the area supported it. She was well aware of the nursing shortage and the need for preparing additional nurses, preferably as fast as possible.

The city's newspaper had several articles on the closure of the public health clinics, and the editorial opinion page had a glowing account of the mayor's support for the groups who opposed the closures. The articles discussed the nursing shortage as well; thus, it was concluded that information about the increasing demand for nurses was reaching the public.

The director of extended education felt that most of the city's population was aware of the parent institution from the college's media campaign. The School of Extended Education runs spot announcements on the radio and even gained some free public service announcement on television, because one of its students is the manager of one of the major stations. The director also runs advertisements in the local newspaper, usually a month before the semesters start. The director described his role on the ad hoc committee on higher education for the board of supervisors. This role gives him the opportunity to meet other key educators and helps raise the visibility of the institution in the community. It was his overall impression that the awareness of the institution was increasing in the community.

Preliminary Conclusions:

The faculty team members concluded that although the parent institution's educational programs are relatively new in the community, the institution is recognized by some key members of the body politic and the public. They felt they had the initial support of the mayor, who is a leader in the community, but felt that the nursing program will need to nurture a relationship with her to gain further support. Depending upon other findings in the needs assessment, the team felt that there would at the very least be no opposition to the program, and at the most moderate support. One caution was issued and that was the need to work with the administrators and faculty of the existing nursing programs as colleagues. It would be advantageous to develop a program that would complement existing programs and not create a threat to them.

The Health Care System and Health Needs of the Populace

As identified in the community assessment, there are four major health care systems serving the city and its surrounding region. The team assigned to assess this frame factor gathers data from the websites of the American Hospital Association and the National Association for Home Care, as well as from looking in the yellow pages of the telephone directory. One health care system is a not-for-profit, large health maintenance organization that has a nationwide network. There are two nonprofit regional health care systems providing enrollees with a wide array of services. One is sponsored by the same religious-based organization as that of the nursing program's parent institution. The other is a federation of former independent nonprofit community hospitals that merged to share resources for cost savings. There is one moderately sized university-based medical center. There is no public hospital except for the state-supported university medical center; however, there are public health clinics that provide primary care for the medically indigent. The medically indigent receive Medicaid services through the

(*case study continues on page 126*)

existing health care systems and the county reimburses the agencies for services provided. There are no for-profit agencies except for three for-profit home care agencies that, in addition to home care, supply medical equipment. There is one nonprofit visiting nurse association, and that agency is under contract with several of the health care systems for home and hospice care. Most school districts have one school nurse, there is a nurse practitioner assigned to the city jail, and three of the major industries have occupational health nurses. The predominant pattern of health care is managed care. There are only a few *preferred provider organizations*—"loose networks of hospitals and physicians that provide services on a discounted fee-for-service basis" (Lee & Estes, 2000, p. 414)—and they contract for hospital and other services with one or more of the health care systems.

The major health care problems of the populace match those of the morbidity and mortality statistics of the state and the nation. Except for the lack of system-wide health care services for the poor, the systems meet the acute care needs of the populace. For those enrolled in health maintenance organizations, health promotion services seem adequate. The local Women, Infants and Children (WIC) program has public health nurses who provide health education and follow-up home visits. The public health clinics do not have a system-wide health education program, providing only immunizations and primary care services in their clinics.

The team members interviewed either the chief administrator of nursing or the associate administrator in the major health care systems. They learned that the majority of staff nurses are associate degree graduates while some of the older nurses are graduates of diploma programs. All of the large health care systems employ clinical specialists, and those with health maintenance services employ nurse practitioners. A few have staff educators, though those nurses also serve as risk managers. The university-based medical center has an all-RN staff and employs more clinical specialists than the other systems. The public health clinics use public health nurses prepared at the baccalaureate level for follow-up visits, and nurse practitioners staff the primary care clinics. The visiting nurse organization uses both public health nurses and RNs for home visiting and hospice services. All of the organizations use licensed practical nurses (LPNs), and the administrators report that they have seen an increase in the numbers of LPNs hired to fill the gap created by the RN shortage.

The administrators reported that they welcome nursing students and have existing articulation agreements with the regional nursing schools. The team decided to collect additional information in their interviews to share with the faculty team assigned to the "The Need for the Program" frame factor. The administrators said they could accommodate additional students for learning experiences, particularly if the program were to hold experiences on evening shifts or weekends. The religious-based system was especially open to having additional students in their agencies and indicated that the program's students would receive priority placements. All nursing specialties were represented in the agencies, though some had larger specialty units than others. A list was made of the agencies, their specialty units, and numbers of potential advanced-practice and experienced nurses who could serve as preceptors, mentors, clinical instructors, or faculty.

Preliminary Conclusions:

The faculty concluded that there is a wide variety of health care agencies with a plethora of potential clinical experiences available for students in an outreach program. Nursing administrators welcomed

(*continued*)

the idea of a new program in the region. This information would be passed on to the team investigating "The Need for the Program" The health care problems and needs of the populace are not unique and match the existing content of the curriculum. There is a need for health promotion activities, especially for the poor, which presents opportunities for faculty and student practice.

The Need for the Program

The faculty assigned to the frame factor that describes the need for the program goes to the state's Board of Registered Nursing website, the National Colleagues in Caring project, and the state nurses association for information on the nursing workforce in the region. The team members learn that there are 1,450 RNs, of whom 1,250 are employed. The four major health care systems report a vacancy rate of 15% and the schools, public health clinics, and home care agency report a total of 50 vacant positions. The team members did not include skilled nursing facilities in the survey; however, they learned from a few directors of nursing that they too are experiencing shortages of nurses with a rapid turnover of staff who move to acute care facilities. Calculating the needs for nurses in numbers of vacant positions, the team members estimated that there are at least 200-plus available positions. They note that the existing nursing programs plan to graduate only 125 entry-level nurses. The number of vacancies does not account for the numbers of nurses in the workforce who plan to retire within the next 5 years, especially in light of the fact that the average age of the nurse in the region is 48 years.

In addition to entry-level positions, 100% of the administrators of the nursing services programs told the team surveying the health care system that they anticipated increasing their staff, owing to the growing demand and complexity of health care. They reported shortages for staff nurses and those in advanced practice, especially clinical specialists. The administrators indicated a preference for baccalaureate-prepared nurses, and when informed about entry-level master's programs, their interest increased, especially if the programs are accelerated. They voiced a sense of urgency related to the increased need for nurses. The team's review of state and national studies demonstrated a similar need for nurses and an ever-increasing shortage of nurses.

Preliminary Conclusions:

There is a documented need for entry-level nurses in the city under study, region, state, and nation. In addition, nursing administrators report an increased need for baccalaureate-prepared graduates and advanced-practice nurses. The needs thus far match the types of options in the nursing program, that is, basic BSN, entry-level MSN, and the advanced-practice roles, especially clinical specialists.

The Nursing Profession

The team members to describe the nursing profession in the region go to the websites of the major nursing organizations in the nation. They discover that the state-supported baccalaureate and higher degree program sponsors a local Sigma Theta Tau chapter, the state nurses association has a regional affiliate, and there is a coalition of specialty organizations in the city. The nurse executive group meets periodically and is loosely affiliated with the American Organization of Nurse Executives. The

(case study continues on page 128)

administrators of the nursing schools belong to this group, and their faculty clinical coordinators have a group of educators who meet twice a year with staff educators in the four major health care systems to plan students' clinical experiences. There is one health care providers union, which represents nurses in two of the health care systems.

About 60% of the employed nurses work in acute care; the remainder are in community-based agencies. About 75% of the working nurses have an ADN or diploma, 18% have a BSN, 6% have a master's degree, and less than 1% have a doctorate degree. It was difficult to match the educational preparation of the nurses to the type of position they held, although anecdotal information demonstrated that the majority of master's-prepared nurses were either top administrators (vice presidents) or clinical specialists and nurse practitioners. The BSN nurses were employed in public health, schools, and home care, or as case managers or administrators. Only two nurses with doctorates were found in practice, and they were researchers at the university-based medical center. The faculty did not survey faculty of schools of nursing; however, it was acknowledged that there are additional master's- and doctorate-prepared nurses in the community, some of whom are faculty in other schools of nursing.

Preliminary Conclusions:

There are several nursing organizations whose members can serve as preceptors and mentors. There are two known doctorate-prepared nurse researchers who could serve as research mentors and, perhaps, faculty. There are master's-prepared nurse practitioners, administrators, and clinical specialists who are potential clinical faculty, preceptors, or mentors.

There is a shortage of nurses in the region, state, and nation. The existing workforce does not meet the preferred need for baccalaureate-prepared nurses and for clinical specialists. The existing schools of nursing cannot meet the current regional demand for nurses, and employers of nurses forecast an increasing need in the future. There is a need for another entry-level program as well as programs for RNs to complete the BSN and for advanced-practice roles, specifically clinical specialization.

Regulations and Accreditation Requirements

The dean of the nursing program and the coordinators of the undergraduate and graduate programs act as the team to investigate regulations and accreditation requirements. The program is due for a Commission for Collegiate Nursing Education (CCNE) reaccreditation visit in 2 years. The nursing program has approval of the State Board of Nursing. A phone call to the executive director of the state board by the dean verifies that the board must approve any proposed outreach program before starting the program. A proposal for the outreach program must be presented to the board at least 6 months in advance of the first class. The board has guidelines for the proposal and will send it to the administrator of the program. Included in the guidelines are congruency with existing approved programs; qualified faculty; adequate student services, including library facilities; approved clinical facilities; and adequate classroom and learning laboratories. Approval comes through the education committee of the board and can be reviewed within 3 months of receipt of the proposal.

The parent institution has regional accreditation. A call to that agency and a review of its standards indicate that proposed outreach programs must be preapproved by the agency at least 6 months prior to the enrollment of the first class. The criteria for approval are much the same as the

(continued)

State Board of Nursing. An ad hoc committee of the agency reviews and recommends approval for proposed outreach programs. In addition to the requirements of the State Board of Nursing, the regional agency looks for financial feasibility statements. The usual turnaround time for a response to a proposal is 2 months.

The nursing program has national accreditation through CCNE. A call to a consultant at that agency indicates that education programs are advised to submit an updated report of the addition to the program and show how it continues to meet the criteria of CCNE.

Preliminary Conclusions:

If the faculty and administrators of the nursing program develop an outreach program, the proposal for the program must be completed and submitted to the Board of Nursing and the regional accrediting agency at least 6 months prior to the start-up of the program. A description of the program as a point of information can be submitted to CCNE once the board and the regional accrediting agency approve the program and it is underway.

Financial Support

The dean and coordinators of the undergraduate and graduate nursing programs prepare a report on the financial resources of the parent institution and the nursing program. They consult with the comptroller of the institution as well as the director of human resources. The parent institution has an endowment fund of over $120 million. It has an active alumni association and raises at least $2 million each year for scholarships. Its capital operating costs match that of the tuition and fees each year. It has several million-dollar grants from private and federal sources for research in science and for program development in education. The nursing program has one federal grant ($300,000) for the nurse practitioner program, one managed care system grant ($50,000) for preparing case managers through online courses, and several scholarship funds totaling $11 million in endowments. The financial aid programs include a statewide tuition assistance program for needy students, the federally sponsored work-study program, PELL grants, nursing loan programs, and a forgivable loan program from a health care agency for students who agree to work for that agency for 2 years upon graduation. In addition, numerous private scholarships are available to nursing students from external sources.

The comptroller assures the team that the institution will provide a business plan for the nursing program to calculate start-up costs and the economic feasibility of an outreach program. If the program appears to be economically sound, the parent institution will provide the start-up costs. The director of extended education reiterates his interest in sharing classroom, staff, and computer facilities with the nursing program.

In addition to an analysis of the institution's financial health, the team members examine possible income sources for the outreach program. They contact the nursing administrators of the four major health care systems in the proposed site to discuss possible program development support, physical sites for student classrooms and laboratories, and scholarships or loans for nursing students. The religious-based system has some labs that students could use for clinical skills practice, and the students are quite interested in scholarship programs or forgivable loans for students who commit to a 2-year contract with that agency upon graduation.

(*case study continues on page 130*)

Preliminary Conclusions:

The parent institution and the nursing program are financially stable. There is the promise of start-up funds and professional consultation for a business plan if the decision to develop an outreach program is realized. In addition to the traditional economic resources, there are potential sources of income and support in the proposed site for the outreach program.

Conclusion

A needs assessment of nine external frame factors revealed a positive external environment for a potential outreach program when compared to the desired outcomes of the "Guidelines for Assessing External Frame Factors." The faculty organized their findings into a table for analyzing the factors and coming to a decision regarding the external frame factors (see Table 5.2).

▲ **TABLE 5.2**   **Case Study Analysis and Decision Making Based on an Assessment of External Frame Factors**

Frame Factor	Findings			Conclusions
	Positive	Negative	Neutral	
Community description	Size and location Infrastructure support through extended education	Student housing One major competitor (BSN+)		*Positive:* The community location and support systems are compatible with an outreach program.
Demographics	Thriving economically Diverse Some more educated	Possible language barriers	Possible emphasis on health promotion activities	*Positive:* Population has many positive attributes for an outreach program.
Academic settings	Adequate applicant pool Clinical specialties viable Interest in entry-level MSN	Four existing nursing programs RN pool satisfied with the RN-to-BSN state-supported program		*Neutral:* While there is an adequate applicant pool and there is interest in entry-level programs including the entry-level MSN, there are four existing nursing programs. The RNs are satisfied with the RN to BSN option in one of the programs.

(continued)

▲ **TABLE 5.2**	**Case Study Analysis and Decision Making Based on an Assessment of External Frame Factors (*continued*)**

| Frame Factor | Findings | | | Conclusions |
	Positive	Negative	Neutral	
Political climate	Parent institution recognized in the community Mayor is an RN and a strong leader	Need to work with existing nursing programs to avoid conflict	No opposition to new program	*Neutral:* The outreach program has a strong potential of success if it works with existing nursing programs and builds positive relationships with the body politic.
Health care system and health needs	Wide variety of health care agencies for learning experiences Nursing administrators in favor and support BSN or higher program Health care needs match curriculum content.		Possible opportunities for student and faculty practice in health promotion activities	*Positive:* The health care system is supportive and offers many learning opportunities for students. Health care needs match curriculum content and there is potential for health promotion practice.
Need for program	There is a need for additional entry-level nurses. There is a demand for BSN+ prepared nurses. Existing program tracks match the demand.			*Positive:* The proposed outreach program could meet the regional demand for additional nurses at the entry-level and advanced practice.

(*case study continues on page 132*)

▲ **TABLE 5.2** **Case Study Analysis and Decision Making Based on an Assessment of External Frame Factors (*continued*)**

| Frame Factor | Findings | | | Conclusions |
	Positive	Negative	Neutral	
Nursing profession	There are several nursing organizations with nurse leaders that support the program.			*Positive:* Professional nursing organizations and their members are potential supporters, mentors, and faculty for the program.
Regulations and accreditation			A proposal for the outreach program must be submitted to the regional accrediting body and the State Board of Nursing. After approval of the above agencies, a report can be sent to CCNE.	*Neutral:* Although proposals must be submitted to the accrediting and regulating bodies, this is not a major problem because a proposal is necessary for the parent institution if the assessment of external and internal frame factors is favorable toward an outreach program.
Financial support	Financial reports indicate economic health and stability. The parent institution will provide start-up funds. At least one health care system offered financial assistance.		There are other potential financial resources.	*Positive:* The financial picture is excellent and there are future potential resources that need to be explored further.
Overall decision	20 positive entries	5 negative entries	5 neutral entries	5 positive conclusions 3 neutral conclusions

(*continued*)

The faculty recommended that the potential for the program continue to be studied by conducting a needs assessment of the internal frame factors impacting the curriculum. Thus far, findings indicate a demonstrated need to increase the numbers of nurses in the proposed metropolitan area both at the entry level and advanced-practice level. Nursing administrators in the region and the community body politic are supportive, and there is strong support from one of the key health care systems. The parent institution indicates support through its extended education program in the area and offers to develop business plans and start-up funds should the faculty recommend an outreach program. Several recommendations were made:

▲ Consider an entry-level MSN program and possibly offer the clinical specialist track.
▲ Conduct focus groups of potential entry-level and advanced-practice students to determine community interest in the proposed program.
▲ Plan meetings with existing nursing program administrators and the mayor to nurture relationships.
▲ As the work continues, keep records that can eventually be the basis of a proposal, both as an internal document and as a report to regulating and accrediting bodies.

DISCUSSION QUESTIONS

1. Conducting a needs assessment is time consuming. Debate the value of conducting the assessment by paid consultants rather than by faculty members.
2. How does the process of a needs assessment apply to both curriculum development and curriculum evaluation?

LEARNING ACTIVITIES

Student Activities

1. As a student group, examine the community around you for its potential for a nursing program. Use Table 5.1, "Guidelines for Assessing External Frame Factors," to collect data on the external frame factors that you need to consider. After you collect the data, summarize your findings and compare them to the "Desired Outcomes" listed in the table. Based on the findings, justify why or why not a new nursing program is needed.

Faculty Activities

1. Using Table 5.1, "Guidelines for Assessing External Frame Factors," examine your existing nursing curriculum. Collect data for each external frame factor as it applies to the curriculum. Summarize your findings and compare them to the "Desired Outcomes" listed in the table. In light of your summary, is a program or curriculum revision indicated? Do you need additional information? Explain your rationale for your responses.

REFERENCES

American Association of Colleges of Nursing. (2003). *Accreditation standards, academic procedures, and program review guidelines.* Retrieved from May 30, 2004, http://www.aacn.nche.edu/Accreditation/pubsguides.htm

American Association of Colleges of Nursing. (1998). *Essentials of baccalaureate education for professional nursing practice.* Washington, DC: Author.

American Association of Colleges of Nursing. (1995). *Essentials of master's education for advanced practice nursing.* Washington, DC: Author.

American Association of Nurse Anesthetists. Council on accreditation of Nurse Anesthesia Educational Programs (2004). Retrieved May 30, 2004, http://www.aana.com/accreditation

American Health Care Association. (2004). *Home Page* Retrieved May 30, 2004, from http://www.ahca.org/

American Hospital Association. (2002). *Home Page* Retrieved May 21, 2002, from http://www.aha.org/aha/index.jsp

American Nurses' Association. (2002). *Home Page* Retrieved May 21, 2002, from http://www.nursingworld.org/about/index.htm

American Public Health Association. (2004). Retrieved May 30, 2004, from http://www.apha.org.html

Bureau of Health Profession. (2004). *Home Page* Retrieved May 30, 2004, from http://bhpr.hrsa.gov

Clemen-Stone, S., McGuire, S. L., & Eigsti, D. G. (2002): *Comprehensive community health nursing: Family, aggregate and community practice* (6th ed.). St. Louis, MO: Mosby.

Coffman, J., Spetz, J., Seago, J. A., Rosenoff, E, & O'Neil, E. (2001). Nursing in California: A workforce crisis. San Franciso, CA: California Workforce Initiative and the UCSF Center for Health Profession.

Colleagues in Caring Project. (2002). *Home Page* Retrieved May 21, 2002, from http://www.aacn.nche.edu/Caring-Project/index.htm

Council of Associate Degree Nursing Competencies Task Force, National League for Nursing (with support from the National Organization of Associate Degree Nursing). (2000). In G. Coxwell & H. Gleeman (Eds.), *Educational competencies for graduates of associate degree programs.* Sudbury, MA: Jones and Bartlett Publishers.

Council for Higher Education Accreditation (CHEA). (2004). *Home Page 2002–2003.* Retrieved May 30, 2004, from http://www.chea.org

Healthy People. (2004). *Home Page* Retrieved May 30, 2004, from http://www.health.gov/healthypeople

Johnson, M. (1977). *Intentionality in education.* Troy, NY: Walter Snyder, Printer, Inc. (distributed by the Center for Curriculum Research and Services, Albany, NY).

Lee, P. R., & Estes, C. L. (2001). The nation's health. Sixth Edition Sudbury, MA: Jones & Barilett Publisher.

National Human Services Assembly. (2004). Retrieved October 11, 2004, from http://www.nassembly.org/nassembly

National Association for Home Care. (2004). *Home Page* Retrieved May 30, 2004, from http://www .nahc.org

National Center for Education Statistics. (2004). *Home Page* Retrieved May 30, 2004, from http://nces.ed.gov

National Center for Health Statistics. (2004). *Home Page* Retrieved May 30, 2004, from http://www.cdc.gov/nchs

National Council of State Boards of Nursing. (2004). *Home Page* Retrieved May 30, 2004, from http://www.ncsbn.org

National League for Nursing Accrediting Commission. (2004). *Home Page* Retrieved May 20, 2004, from http://www.nlnac.org

National Organization of Nurse Practitioner Faculty. (2004). *Home Page* Retrieved May 30, 2004, from http://www.nonpf.com/ criteria.htm

Stanhope, M., & Lancaster, J. (2000). *Community and public health nursing* (5th ed.). St. Louis, MO: Mosby.

United States Census Bureau. (2004). *Home Page* Retrieved May 30, 2004, from http://www.census.gov

Internal Frame Factors:
Influence and Assessment

Sarah B. Keating, EdD, RN, FAAN

OBJECTIVES

Upon completion of Chapter 6, the reader will be able to:

1. Evaluate the essential internal frame factors that impact a nursing educational program for the need to either develop a new program or revise an existing one.
2. Compile resources for the collection of data related to internal frame factors for comparing the data to desired outcomes.
3. Examine a case study that illustrates a needs assessment of internal frame factors for a curriculum development project.
4. Apply the guidelines for Assessing Internal Frame Factors in a simulated or real curriculum development situation.

6

▲ OVERVIEW

Section 3 introduced the reader to the Frame Factors Model and Chapter 5 discussed the external frame factors that nurse educators should review when conducting a needs assessment for program planning and curriculum development purposes. The data collected from a review of the external frame factors provide information that leads to an assessment of the internal frame factors that influence the educational program and curriculum. These factors can have a major impact on the program's existence and decisions regarding changes. See Figure 6.1 for a conceptual model of the internal frame factors that impact the curriculum.

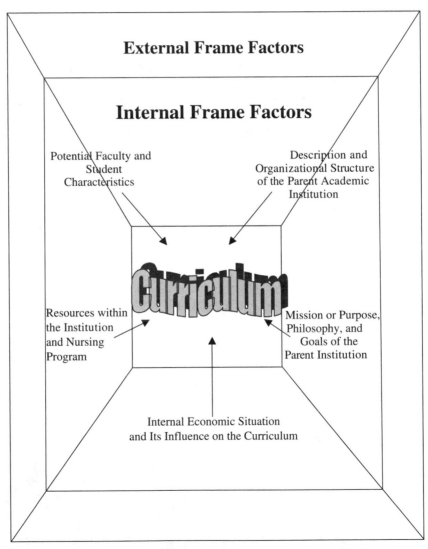

FIGURE 6.1 Internal frame factors for a needs assessment for curriculum development. Adapted with permission from Johnson (1977).

Faculty members continue to be responsible for curriculum development and evaluation and are part of the process for collecting information about the internal frame factors that impact the educational program. The internal frame factors include a description of the organizational structure of the parent academic institution; mission and purpose, philosophy, and goals; internal economic situation and its influence on the curriculum; resources within the institution (laboratories, classrooms, library, academic services, student services, etc.); and potential faculty and student characteristics. The information related to these factors is analyzed for its relevance to the program and the findings are weighed as to their importance to the quality of the program, its existence, and possible changes.

Chapter 6 provides detailed information about each of these internal frame factors, and there is a table with guidelines for collecting information about the factors and assessing the need according to the desired outcomes. The chapter ends by continuing the case study of a fictional nursing school based on an actual feasibility study for an outreach program.

▲ DESCRIPTION AND ORGANIZATIONAL STRUCTURE OF THE PARENT ACADEMIC INSTITUTION

When looking at the microenvironment that surrounds a nursing education program, the parent institution in which it resides is examined in light of the scenario it sets for the program. The physical campus and its buildings create the milieu in which the program exists, with the nursing program a reflection of its place within the institution. The nature of the institution influences the structure of the total campus and for nursing education programs, can be located in health care agencies, academic health sciences centers, liberal arts colleges, large research universities, land grant universities, multi-purpose state-supported or private universities, or community colleges. The history of the institution is important to know, such as its growth or change over the years and the role the nursing program had in its political fortunes or misfortunes. In small private institutions, the school of nursing can be one of the largest and most influential constituents, while in statewide university systems, nursing can be a small department within a health-related college that is within the greater university. To appreciate the vast number of different institutions within the United States, go to the University of Utah website (2004), which provides links to various U.S. higher education systems such as boards of regents, boards of governors, coordinating boards, and university system-wide administrations: http://www.utahsbr.edu/boards.htm.

All educational institutions and health care agencies have organizational structures, usually of a hierarchal nature. Faculty should analyze the structure of the parent institution as well as that of the nursing program to describe the hierarchal and formal lines of communication that guide the faculty in developing and revising programs. For example, as described in Chapter 2 on the roles and responsibilities of faculty, curriculum proposals and changes must be approved first on the local level (the nursing curriculum committee and faculty), then on the next level of organization (such as a college curriculum committee and dean), and finally, to an all-college or university- wide curriculum committee, with its recommendations going to the faculty senate (or its like) for final approval. There can be administrative approval along the way from department heads, deans, and perhaps academic vice presidents or provosts, especially with regard to economic and administrative feasibility.

Nevertheless, the major approval bodies are those that are composed of faculty and within faculty governance prerogatives.

At the same time, it is useful to know whom the major players are within the faculty and administrative structures to discuss with them the plans and rationale for proposed new programs or curriculum revisions. Prior consultation with these key people can help to smooth the way when the proposals are ready to enter the formal arena. Also, they can give advice related to changes that might enhance approval or advice on the best presentation formats that facilitate an understanding of the proposal. These contacts can be of a formal or informal nature; however, to avoid disastrous results, never blindside an administrator or decision-maker. It is wise to keep them informed of new proposals or possible changes that place them in the advocate role as the approval process winds its way through the system.

▲ MISSION, PHILOSOPHY, AND GOALS OF THE PARENT INSTITUTION

The mission and purpose in some institutions (this may be labeled as the "vision"), philosophy (or "value statement" or "beliefs"), and goals of the parent institution determine the character of the nursing program. Most institutions of higher education focus their missions and philosophies on three endeavors: education, service, and scholarship/research. Nursing must examine the mission and philosophy of the institution to determine its place within these three basic endeavors. For example, a state-supported university may have as part of its mission and philosophy the education of the people of the state for professional, leadership, and service roles. Thus, the nursing program could focus its mission and philosophy on the preparation of nurses for leadership roles and provision of health care services for the people of the state. If the statewide system is the predominant preparer of nurses within the state as compared to independent colleges, then the additional mission or purpose might be to provide an adequate nursing workforce for the state. For example, as nursing experienced its workforce shortages during the mid-1980s and into the early 21st century, there is evidence of federal and statewide programs for increased nursing scholarship support, and in some cases, a mandate for state-supported schools to admit more students to nursing programs (Health Resources and Services Administration, 2004; Keating & Sechrist, 2001; Rapson & Rice, 2002).

In contrast, independent or private colleges and universities may have missions and philosophies that have a sectarian flavor, such as preparing individuals with strong liberal arts foundations for public service or roles in the helping professions. Again, a nursing program's mission is compatible with this mission. Academic health science centers are yet another example of nursing's match to health disciplines housed in one institution whose mission is to prepare individuals for the health professions. Community college or junior college missions usually focus on technical education or on prerequisite preparation for entering into upper division level colleges and universities. Although the debate still rages about the role of nursing programs in these institutions, there is no question that they fit the mission of the 2-year college as most expect that their graduates will function as registered nurses (RNs) and continue with their education at the baccalaureate and higher degree levels (Joel, 2002; Mahaffrey, 2002).

▲ INTERNAL ECONOMIC SITUATION AND INFLUENCE ON THE CURRICULUM

As stated in Chapter 5, the economic health of the institution has a significant impact on the nursing program and curriculum. How much of the share of resources, income, and expenditures that the nursing program has can affect program stability and room for expansion. For example, nurse-managed clinics must be self-supporting or economic recessions can cause their demise. For state-sponsored programs, the parent institution is subject to the state economy during periods of recession and prosperity. Independent colleges, unless heavily endowed, depend on tuition, student fees, or other income-generating operations.

All institutions depend on endowments, financial aid programs for students including scholarships and loans, and grants. Nursing programs are eligible for many federal grants and have a history of securing other types of grants from private foundations, state-supported programs, and private contributions including those from alumni associations. These income-generating programs illustrate to the parent institution that the nursing program is viable, and at the same time, the institution's reputation and ability to garner external financial resources help the nursing program to secure funding.

Institutions usually have support systems for assisting faculty to write grants and seek outside financial support. Nursing programs should have close relationships with these support systems and have a plan in place for securing additional funds. Faculty plays a major role in writing grants, with the perks related to them, if funded, of released time for program development or research activities. Two sources of funding to support program development on the national level are the Health Resources and Services Administration (2004) and the National Institutes of Health (2004). The latter focuses on research; however, it is possible that faculty may wish to conduct curriculum and educational program research. A list of private foundations with funding opportunities for program development is located at http://www.research.ucla.edu/si2/Private.htm (University of California – Los Angeles, 2004).

Assessment of the economic status of the parent institution and the nursing program provides a realistic picture of the potential for program expansion and curriculum revision. When developing curricula, the first demand for financial support comes with the need for resources to conduct a needs assessment such as the costs of released time for those who are conducting the assessment, review of the literature, and surveys of key stakeholders. A cost analysis for revising a curriculum or initiating a new one requires a business plan to justify the costs and to forecast its financial viability. Unless there is a nursing program financial officer, the nursing program administrator and faculty should work closely with the parent institution's business office or chief financial officer in developing the business plan.

▲ RESOURCES WITHIN THE INSTITUTION AND NURSING PROGRAM

An analysis of the existing resources within the institution and the nursing program supplies information related to possible program expansion and curriculum revisions. First, there should be adequate classrooms, learning laboratories, computer facilities, clinical practice simulations, and distance education support systems for the current program. When planning for revisions of the curriculum or for new programs, the need for expansion of these facilities should be identified. If expansion is not possible, then creative approaches to scheduling for the maximum use of these facilities can be examined (e.g., evening classes, weekend learning experiences, or online courses).

Academic support services such as the library, academic advisement, teaching–learning resources, and instructional technology contribute to the maintenance of a quality education program and are internal frame factors that should be assessed when developing new programs or revising existing ones. If there are to be new programs or expansion of current curricula, the library resources must be adequate. Library resources include not only those resources on campus, but also services for off-campus programs and students. There should be Internet and web-based library resources for students and faculty; this is especially true when the campus has a large commuter student population or distance education programs, or proposes new programs. Library support staff must be large enough and knowledgeable about nursing education needs. Thus, faculty should have collaborative relationships with librarians and their staff to build the resources needed to revise the curriculum or develop new programs.

Academic advisement services play an important role in program planning because new programs entail additional staffing for those purposes. If the curriculum is revised, updates for academic advising are necessary so that the faculty and its support staff who provide the services have current information to impart to the students. Teaching–learning resources need to be available to keep faculty current in instructional strategies, particularly if the revisions to the curriculum have an effect on instructional design. For example, a baccalaureate program may decide to convert its RN program to a web-based delivery system. In this case, the faculty needs training in preparing and implementing web-based courses.

Instructional support systems are also part of planning because the nature of the proposed program or the revised curriculum may call for additional resources. These resources include programmed instruction units, audio-visual aids, hardware and software, computer technologies, simulated clinical situations, and so forth. They can generate large costs to the program and should be calculated into the business plan and the costs associated with their maintenance and replacement over time. Some instructional support systems include monthly or annual fees as well. For new programs or revisions, these costs are often included in requests for external funding, and because many times they are one-time-only costs, they are funded more easily.

Student support services are equally important to nursing education programs and are an integral part of the curriculum development process. Major student services include enrollment (recruitment, admissions, registrar activities, and graduation records), maintenance of student records, advising and counseling, disciplinary matters, remediation and study skills, work-study programs, career counseling, job placement, and financial aid. Depending on the size of the university or college, these services can be congregated into one department or subdivided into several. Their role in curriculum development is important because expanding or changing educational programs require their support. For example, if a new program is proposed, then the recruitment and admissions staff will need to be apprised of the program to best serve the needs of the new program in recruitment and admission activities.

Financial aid programs are crucial to the recruitment, admission, and retention of students. If the proposal brings in new revenues through grants or other financial support structures, financial aid staff members must be cognizant of the proposal. They can provide useful information to program planners and thus, a partnership between the student services staff and the nursing program staff is beneficial.

Work-study programs and job placement information can supplement the curriculum if these programs are in concert with the educational plan and not in conflict with the program of study. An example is a revised curriculum that calls for accelerated study and clinical experiences that disallow student employment and therefore prohibits enrollment in the program. Another aspect is the potential influence of students' part-time employment on the curriculum and its role in intended and unintended outcomes on the educational experience.

The informal curriculum often takes place through the planned activities of the student services department. Again, partnerships between that staff and nursing faculty can increase the effectiveness of the formal curriculum. Students who can benefit from remediation or learning skills workshops can be referred to student services. Faculty can help the student services staff identify the learning needs of nursing students; this is especially relevant when curriculum changes are taking place. In return, the student services staff can educate faculty about the special needs of students with learning disabilities and the special accommodations they require without sacrificing the privacy of the clients for whom the students provide care. Bourke, Strehorn, and Silver (2000) found that assistance from the support services staff for faculty who had students with learning disabilities resulted in increased provision of accommodations for the students.

▲ POTENTIAL FACULTY AND STUDENT CHARACTERISTICS

When proposing new educational programs or revising existing curricula, thought needs to go into the characteristics of the existing faculty and the student body who will participate in the educational program. If a new program is proposed, the faculty composition should be reviewed. There should be enough faculty members to reach the desired faculty-to-student ratio. Depending on the nature of the program, clinical supervision of students requires a low faculty-to-student ratio but can differ according to program. For example, master's and doctoral students are usually RNs, and therefore may not need the close clinical supervision required of entry-level students. Although for some advanced-practice roles there is a need for closer faculty supervision, preceptorships or internships are the usual format and a faculty member can supervise more students. In entry-level programs, there are usually eight to 10 students to one faculty member; however, in the senior year, it is possible to have preceptorships with approximately 12 to 15 students, depending on the nature of the clinical experiences. While lecture can accommodate many students to one teacher, seminars and learning laboratories demand fewer numbers of students and additional faculty. These are very practical issues that must be addressed owing to the quality perspectives and cost factors that they present when developing curricula. Another consideration related to faculty is the match of their knowledge to the subject matter, clinical expertise, and pedagogical skills. Numbers and types of faculty members are pieces of information that feed into decisions about curriculum development because they are critical to the delivery of the curriculum and instructional design.

As with faculty considerations, the characteristics of the student body and types of students the faculty hopes to attract to the new program or the revised curriculum are important. If it is a new program, the potential applicant pool should be identified according to interest, numbers, availability, and competition with other nursing programs. If a new program is contemplated, its type dictates the kind of applicant pool that the program and the admission department need to target. If it is a curriculum revision to update the program and plan for future demands, the applicant pool might be the same as the current one. The characteristics of the students in the program help to tailor the curriculum according to their learning needs. For example, if it is an entry-level associate degree or baccalaureate program, the applicants may be a mix of new high school graduates, transfer students with some college preparation, and adult learners with some work experience. The curriculum is then planned to meet a diversity of learning needs from traditional pedagogical learning theories to andragogical adult learning theories. Diversity of racial, ethnic, and cultural characteristics is another factor to consider, and the educational program must plan to be culturally responsive, including preparing professionals with cultural competence in the curriculum.

▲ SUMMARY

Chapter 6 reviewed the internal frame factors to consider when conducting a needs assessment for developing new educational programs or revising curricula. These factors follow the assessment of external frame factors that influence the educational program and are equally important to the decision for changing a curriculum or developing a new program. While the external frame factors examined the macro environment surrounding the program, the internal frame factors looked at the factors that are closer to the program and include the parent institution as well as the nursing program itself.

Factors that were examined include the characteristics of the parent institution and its organizational structure. How the nursing program fits into this structure can determine the economic, political, and resource support for program changes, as well as set the stage for the processes that the nursing faculty must undergo to gain approval for the proposed changes. The mission and purpose, philosophy, and goals of the parent institution influence the nature of the nursing program and to ensure success, they must be congruent with those of the parent institution. The internal economic status and the available resources of both the parent institution and the nursing program are assessed for the financial viability, as are the necessary additional resources and support services for any proposed revisions to the curriculum or proposed new programs. Finally, the characteristics of the faculty and the potential student body are reviewed to determine their match to the proposed change. See Table 6.1 for guidelines to assess the internal frame factors when conducting a needs assessment for curriculum revision or new program proposals.

▲ **TABLE 6.1**	**Guidelines for Assessing Internal Frame Factors**	
Frame Factor	**Questions for Data Collection**	**Desired Outcomes**
Description and organizational structure of the parent academic institution	In what type of educational institution is the nursing program located? What is the milieu of the parent institution in regard to the nursing program? What is the organizational structure of the parent institution? What place in the institution does the nursing program hold? What influence does it have?	A supportive organizational system for program planning and curriculum revision
	What are the layers of approval processes for program approval and curriculum revisions? In what order must a program go through for the approval process? Who are the major players in the various levels of approval processes?	A fair and comprehensive review process that results in economically sound and high-quality educational programs
Mission and purpose, philosophy, and goals of the parent institution	What are the mission, purpose, philosophy, and goals of the parent institution? Are they congruent with and supportive of the nursing program?	The mission and purpose, philosophy, and goals of the parent institution are congruent with and supportive of the nursing program.
Internal economic situation and its influence on the curriculum	What is the operating budget of the nursing program? Is it adequate for the support of the existing program?	The nursing program has adequate resources for supporting its educational program from the parent institution.
	Are there resources for program or curriculum development activities?	The nursing program has the resources for program or curriculum development activities.
	Does the program have a financial officer or administrative assistant who can develop a business plan for the proposed program or curriculum revision? If not, are there resources available from the parent institution for this activity?	The nursing program has a business plan for initiating a new program or revising the existing curriculum.
Resources within the institution and nursing program	How many classrooms, laboratories, and computer laboratories does the nursing program have, and are they under the control of the nursing program? Can they accommodate additional students and newer technologies in the proposed	The current physical facilities are adequate and can accommodate a new program or revised curriculum, there are plans for expansion that are part of the business plan and have the support of the financial bodies of the institution.

(table continues on page 144)

▲ **TABLE 6.1** **Guidelines for Assessing Internal Frame Factors** (*continued*)

Frame Factor	Questions for Data Collection	Desired Outcomes
	program or for the revised curriculum? Are the plans for these facilities included in the proposal and are their costs calculated in the business plan?	
	What are the available resources for program planning and curriculum revision? Is there released time available for those people involved? Is there support staff available? Are there teaching/learning continuing education programs available for faculty?	There are teaching and learning support systems for faculty that facilitate program planning and curriculum revisions.
	What instructional support systems are in place in the institution and the nursing program? Are they adequate, and what plans are there for increasing and updating them according to the revised or new program needs?	There are adequate instructional support systems available for the current program and for proposed future programs.
	How many texts and journal holdings does the library have, and will they meet the needs of student and faculty in the future, especially in light of new program or revised curricula? Is there access to the library and other electronic resources and communications for commuter students and faculty and for distance education programs?	The current and proposed library holdings are adequate to meet the needs of the nursing program and proposed curriculum revisions. There is access to the library and other electronic resources for commuter students and faculty and for distance education programs.
	Is the current academic advising system working to students' and faculty's satisfaction? Is there appropriate faculty-to-student ratios for academic advising? Will a revised curriculum or new program require additional faculty and staff for academic advising purposes?	The academic advising system can accommodate appropriate faculty-to-student ratios and there are support systems within it to ensure the quality of advisement. There are adequate faculty and staff for the academic advising system.
	What are the current relationships of the nursing program's administration, faculty, and staff with those of student services? Is the student services department aware of the proposed revision or new program, and have they been consulted regarding future student services needs that may occur owing to the changes?	The student services system (recruitment, enrollment, registrar, financial aid, remediation support, student counseling, and other related services) works in partnership with nursing administration and faculty to enhance the formal curriculum.

▲ **TABLE 6.1**	Guidelines for Assessing Internal Frame Factors (*continued*)

Frame Factor	Questions for Data Collection	Desired Outcomes
Faculty and student characteristics	Describe the current faculty compositions. Is it adequate in number and qualifications for meeting program needs?	The faculty is adequate in number and meets the qualifications for delivering a quality nursing education program.
	Describe the characteristics of the current student body and the history of the applicant pool to the nursing program. Has the program been able to meet its enrollment targets in the past 5 years? If not, what strategies have taken place to meet the target?	The parent institution and the nursing program have the resources to recruit, educate, and graduate the type of student body that the new program or curriculum revision requires.
	What are the characteristics of the student body for the proposed program or revised curriculum? Is there an adequate applicant pool to fulfill enrollment targets? Are there plans in place for their recruitment? Does the nursing program have a partnership with the admissions department for recruiting and retaining students?	
Analysis of the data and decision making	Summarize the conclusions by generating a list of positive, negative, and neutral findings that can influence the curriculum and program planning.	A final decision statement as to the feasibility for developing a new program or revising the curriculum based on the needs assessment of the external and internal frame factors is developed.

C A S E   S T U D Y

▼

The case study initiated in Chapter 5 presented a fictional baccalaureate and higher degree School of Nursing seeking to develop an outreach program to meet the region's increasing nursing shortage. The faculty was divided into teams, and each team gathered data related to the external frame factors that influence program and curriculum development. Thus far, the information the team members gathered indicates a positive milieu for developing an outreach program for either entry-level baccalaureate or master's degree students and the possibility for a clinical specialty track in the graduate program. The next step is to assess the internal frame factors that can further inform the decision for offering or not offering an outreach program.

Description and Organizational Structure of the Parent Academic Institution

The School of Nursing dean and the coordinators of the undergraduate and graduate programs put together a description of the parent institution (college) and the School of Nursing. The most recent accreditation reports for the Commission on Collegiate Nursing Education (CCNE) and the State Board of Nursing provide the description, including the organizational structure of both. With a few minor edits of the documents to update them, they have the report ready to analyze for information related to the proposed outreach program.

The home campus of the college is located in the outskirts of a large metropolitan area, with the campus a self-contained unit within a pleasant pastoral atmosphere. The School of Nursing shares offices, classrooms, and several laboratories with the School of Arts and Sciences. However, it has two clinical skills laboratories that are under its control. There is easy access to public transportation to travel into the metropolitan area, where many learning and leisure time experiences for the students take place.

The School of Nursing represents about 11% (350 undergraduates and 200 master's students) of the student body and was founded within the 100-year-old institution almost 60 years ago, being the first professional school in the college. The institution averages 4,500 undergraduate students each year, with the graduate enrollment at 500. It has six schools: arts and sciences (40% of the enrollment), business administration and economics (30% of the enrollment), computer science (6% of the enrollment), education (5% of the enrollment), extended education (8% of the enrollment) and nursing. All but the arts and sciences school have graduate programs, and the education school is graduate-level only. The highest degree that the institution awards is the master's degree and it awards both bachelor of arts and bachelor of science degrees. It has an excellent reputation in the community for its dedication to community service and high-quality programs, all of which hold regional and national accreditation.

Although the college originally had a strong liberal arts focus, it has become multipurpose with the addition of the professional schools including business, education, and nursing; computer

(continued)

sciences still is a relatively young school, having started 10 years ago. The School of Extended Education offers distance education programs in business administration, computer sciences, and education from the home campus and its outreach program in the metropolitan area that is under study by nursing for the needs assessment. Each school has a dean and the School of Nursing dean has been in his position for 9 years, and therefore has a strong voice in the council of deans. There is a provost to whom the deans report, and the president, who is an ordained minister within the religious sect that sponsors the college, administers the college. There is a comptroller, a dean of student affairs, a dean of enrollment services, a director of human resources, and a director of library and instructional support services.

The faculty full time equivalent (FTE) totals about 210, with almost 100 part-time lecturers. There is an academic senate composed of two representatives from each school's faculty, three members-at-large, undergraduate and graduate student representatives, a presidential appointee, and the academic provost. There are three major committees of the senate: the curriculum, graduate, and faculty affairs committees. The faculty elects the chair of the senate, chair-elect, and secretary. The faculty also votes for members of the three committees from the senate membership. The committees then select their chairs. There is one nursing faculty member on the graduate committee, one nursing member is chair of the faculty affairs committee, and another is a member-at-large of the senate. The School of Nursing faculty and the senate curriculum committee must approve new academic programs and curriculum revisions. If the proposals are for graduate programs, then the graduate committee, which recommends approval of those curricula, must review them and send them to the senate with recommendations.

The School of Nursing faculty numbers 29 full-time tenured or tenure-track faculty and 25 part-time clinical faculty, not including the dean and three administrative support staff. There are two coordinators, one for the graduate program and one for the undergraduate program. The coordinators have 30% released time for coordination duties. The part-time faculty's teaching role occurs primarily in supervising students during their clinical experiences. The faculty members teach in both undergraduate and graduate programs, although some are predominantly assigned to one or the other depending on their clinical expertise and academic preparation. Sixty-five percent of the full-time tenured or tenure-track faculty members have doctorates, and there are currently three enrolled in doctoral programs. The School of Nursing faculty meets once a month during the academic year, and there are three major committees, the curriculum, graduate, and peer evaluation. Ad hoc task forces or committees are assembled as needed (e.g., search committee, faculty affairs, etc.). All program and curriculum revisions must be approved through the appropriate nursing committee structure and then approved by the faculty as a whole, with final administrative review and approval by the dean. Proposals are then forwarded to the appropriate senate committee, which makes recommendations to the senate, which votes for approval or disapproval. Upon approval of the senate, the provost completes a final review and makes a recommendation to the president.

Preliminary Conclusions:

The college has a strong reputation for high-quality liberal arts and professional education programs within the region, and the School of Nursing has a significant role within the college. The dean of

(*case study continues on page 148*)

nursing is an active and respected member of the college's administrative structure and has a sense of the history of the college and School of Nursing.

There are clear hierarchal lines of communication for administrative decisions and for gaining curriculum and program approval. The school had three senators with two on senate committees but none on the curriculum or graduate committees; thus, some political maneuvering will be necessary to educate the senate about the proposed program and solicit their support. The president, provost, and comptroller have been aware of the proposal and they are supportive owing to community demand for more nurses in the health care system.

Mission and Purpose, Philosophy, and Goals of the Parent Institution

Owing to the institution's religious base, nursing's mission is congruent with the institution's mission and goals, which focus on the preparation of compassionate and responsible citizens for society and professionals who provide services to the community. While the School of Nursing sometimes finds itself in conflict with the large School of Arts and Sciences, which emphasizes strong liberal arts and science foundations for all undergraduate students, nursing often allies itself with the other professional schools, and thus can forestall additional prerequisites by arts and sciences that can overburden the student load for the undergraduate degree in nursing.

Preliminary Conclusions:

The School of Nursing is in congruence with the mission and purpose, philosophy, and goals of the college. It recognizes the need to educate other schools in the college about the nursing shortage and the need to increase enrollments through a possible outreach program. At the same time, it must collaborate with them in regard to the impact the new program might have on the other schools.

Internal Economic Situation and Its Influence on the Curriculum

The same team who examined the organizational structure of the college meets with the comptroller of the college to discuss some additional issues related to the economic situation and its effect on the proposed new outreach program. When they conducted the assessment of the external frame factors, faculty members found that both the college and School of Nursing were financially stable, the comptroller was willing to help develop a business plan for the proposed program, and there were potential external funding resources for the program should it start up. Recently, the nursing faculty identified several state and federal programs that might fund a new program, especially if it included strategies to reduce the current nursing shortage. However, this requires released time for faculty to write the grants. It is calculated that two faculty members each need at least 5% released time for the next semester to write these grants. The comptroller refers the dean and faculty to the provost, who may have some faculty development funds that could cover the costs for this released time. The provost agrees to provide a total of $2,000 as released time for the next semester for faculty to write grant proposals for program development.

(continued)

Thus far, there has been no financial support for the needs assessment, and as it progresses, the dean and faculty feel the need for some support to continue to develop the proposal. Of special concern is the need to provide released time for curriculum development when and if the outreach program is approved. This would involve at least three faculty members and would take about 10% of their workload in assigned time activities to develop or revise the existing curriculum to fit the outreach program. This released time needs to be built into the next year's budget for the School of Nursing. The comptroller suggests that the dean of nursing bring up this need when the council of deans and the provost develop next year's proposed budgets. The dean discussed this with the provost, who is willing to place the item in next year's budget request.

Preliminary Conclusions:

The college and the School of Nursing are economically stable. The college administration has indicated support for developing a business plan for the proposed program. This plan will calculate estimated start-up costs and program maintenance funds for 3 years, by when the program should become self-sufficient. The provost will provide $2,000 next semester for faculty-released time to write grants for program development funds. The dean will write in the cost for faculty-released time for curriculum development for the next year's budget with the approval of the provost.

Resources Within the Institution and Nursing Program

A team of faculty members, including two representatives who teach in the nursing laboratory, the liaison from the library and instructional support, the school's curriculum committee chair, and the undergraduate and graduate coordinators, assess the resources within the college and the School of Nursing. Because the proposed outreach program must depend on the resources of the existing program and yet meet the needs of students at a distance from the school, the team assesses the existing resources that could have an effect on the proposed program and the additional resources needed at the outreach site.

The on-campus classrooms, learning laboratories, and computer classrooms, although not under the school's control, are adequate in size and number for the on-campus student enrollment. The library has one of the largest holdings in the region for nursing journals and texts as well as for other disciplines. Recently, the library upgraded its off-campus access so that students are able to log into databases with full-text journal articles including CINAHL, ERIC, and MEDLAR. The instructional support services department and the School of Extended Education have distance education programs including videoconferencing with a dedicated broadcasting suite and classroom, and there is a contract with a web-based delivery system for online courses. These facilities were developed for the Schools of Business Administration and Education graduate programs, the extended education program, and the RN-to-BSN program. The director of library and instructional support services meets with the team and indicates that nursing has access to these technologies, although videoconferencing dictates scheduling of classes

(case study continues on page 150)

to avoid conflict with the School of Extended Eeducation programs. She also indicates that monthly in-service workshops are held for faculty to improve teaching effectiveness as well as to learn new technologies such as developing web-based courses and designing videoconference classes. Many nursing faculty members attend these workshops and are always welcome as new programs and technologies are developed.

As for off-campus facilities, the team knows from the assessment of external frame factors that the dean of extended education indicated that the classrooms he rents in the proposed off-campus outreach program site are available for rental by the nursing program. These rooms include an office space for faculty, one office for the coordinator of the program, a traditional classroom, and a dedicated high-technology computer and videoconferencing room that can be shared with other extended education students. Special clinical learning laboratories are available to the program, rent free, from the religious-based health maintenance organization in the proposed outreach site.

The academic advisement system in the School of Nursing requires that each faculty member carry an average of 20 advisees. Advisees are matched to faculty members' expertise and interests. In the graduate program, advisors are usually the students' thesis or research project chairs and therefore have fewer student advisees.

The team assesses student services needs for the outreach program. They meet with the director of enrollment services and discuss recruitment, student records, counseling services, financial aid programs, and work-study options for nursing students. The proposed outreach program would call for at least one additional staff member in enrollment services for all of the services mentioned above, although it is possible that such a person could work with the extended education program staff located in the proposed site for the program. This would have to be included in the business plan and is duly noted for bringing to the attention of the comptroller.

Preliminary Conclusions:

Current facilities and services for the School of Nursing are adequate for the on-campus program. However, the following is a list of the needs for an outreach program with possible resources to fill the needs:

Classrooms	One room shared with extended education. There is a rental fee.
Office space	Two rooms in the extended education facility. There is a rental fee.
Computer and video-conferencing classroom	One room shared with the School of Extended Education. There is a rental fee.
Skills labs	One room with equipment. Donated by the health care lab facilities system.
Library and instructional support systems	Current facilities are adequate and accessible.
Academic counseling	Additional faculty and staff
Student services	Services are in place; however, one additional staff member may be necessary.

(continued)

Potential Faculty and Student Characteristics

Four faculty members representing the undergraduate and graduate programs are charged with identifying potential faculty and student characteristics and needs for the proposed program. They agree that a full-time coordinator for the outreach program is necessary during the planning stages as well as for managing the program when it commences. At that time, depending on the size of the student enrollment, that person could assume some teaching responsibilities in addition to coordinating the program. Faculty characteristics and needs must match those of the current faculty with tenure track and clinical positions available to the program. The size of the faculty will be determined by the choice of program, the specialty if it is not a prelicensure program, and the delivery mode of the program. For example, some lecture courses might be developed and delivered through videoconferencing or web-based courses that are already part of the on-campus program and the faculty's repertoire, while new faculty will be needed for clinical supervision of students and some theory and skills laboratory courses. Although precise numbers of teachers needed cannot be calculated until the final decision is made to offer the program and what kind of program it will be, the faculty sets the parameters for the characteristics of the faculty and its size.

Like the faculty, the characteristics and size of the student body depends on the decision to offer the program and the type of program it will be. Based on the needs assessment of the external frame factors, the decision appears to be going toward the initiation of an entry-level program, either at the baccalaureate or master's degree level. If it is an undergraduate program, the numbers of students are likely to be larger than for a graduate program. However, because both programs are prelicensure programs, the faculty-to-student ratio for clinical supervision must be calculated into the costs for starting the program. A critical mass for the number of students needed to meet the cost of initiating the program must be calculated as well. The same prerequisites and other admission criteria for students on the home campus program must be applied to the outreach program.

With these factors in mind, the faculty team members look at the enrollment and retention patterns of the School of Nursing's home campus. The undergraduate program enrollments have been stable for the past 5 years; however, the applicant pool decreased in the past 4 years by 8%, with a slight increase this past year. The team attributed the slight increase in the applicant pool to the lay public's increasing awareness of the nursing shortage. Although enrollment targets were met for the past 5 years, the result was that students admitted to the program had lower overall high school GPAs and scores on the SATs. They met the prerequisites and admission criteria, but the average overall GPA and SAT scores fell by 3 percentage points. Thus, the students required more academic counseling and remediation programs than in the past for retention purposes and the attrition rate increased slightly from 6% to 8%. The NCLEX passing score for first-time takers averaged 85% over the past 5 years.

The entry-level master's program began 3 years ago with the first graduations occurring this past May. All students passed the NCLEX and are gainfully employed in beginning-level staff positions. Although formal follow-up studies have not been conducted, anecdotal information indicates high satisfaction with the graduates on the part of their employers, and the graduates are equally satisfied with the program. The majority of faculty members enjoy working with these students and find them challenging owing to their adult-learner needs, previous work experience, and new perspectives on nursing as a profession. The graduates have not assumed advanced-practice roles as yet.

(case study continues on page 152)

The nursing faculty works closely with the admissions department in recruiting the entry-level master's students into the home campus program, and the applicant pool is increasing with word-of-mouth information about the program spreading and news of the nursing shortage increasing in the public's mind. The assessment team meets with the admissions department staff, whose major responsibility is the recruitment of these types of students. They learn from the staff that the applicant pool is more than adequate, all met the admission criteria, and the enrollment target was realized every year of its existence.

Based on their experiences, the admissions staff believes that recruitment for both types of students should be fairly easy for the outreach program; although owing to the other existing nursing programs, the entry-level master's program is more attractive because there is no competition for those types of students. However, it requires meetings of the staff with regional college and university advising centers' staff, public media advertisements and spot announcements, and on-site information meetings. These activities would have to be included in the business plan.

Preliminary Conclusions:

The current nursing faculty-to-student ratio is 1 to 13 (average of theory and clinical ratios with the clinical ratio at 1 to 8), which is lower than the other schools in the college; thus, a new program will require a coordinator, additional faculty, and staff. A full-time coordinator is necessary to build relationships with extended education and the community and to help the admissions staff recruit students. Eventually, the coordinator role could include some teaching activities. Current faculty may be able to deliver their lecture and theory-type courses via distance education; however, skills labs and clinical experiences must take place on-site, requiring part-time clinical faculty services at the very least.

The coordinator and faculty will need to work closely with enrollment services in the recruitment of students into the program. A marketing and recruitment plan, including a timetable, needs to be developed with that staff.

Analysis of the Internal Frame Factors Needs Assessment Data and Decision Making

Table 6.2 provides a summary and analysis of the internal frame factors data collected for the needs assessment. Included are the decisions or recommendations based on the analysis.

Conclusion

The needs assessment of the internal frame factors clarified some of the issues raised by the assessment of the external frame factors. Overall, the college and School of Nursing have the experience and knowledge to develop an outreach program. Other schools in the college, particularly the professional schools and extended education, are supportive of nursing. The nursing faculty is well prepared and the library and instructional support systems of the college can facilitate the development of distance learning courses. Some released time for faculty to write grants for external funding for program development is available. However, released time for program planning and curriculum development is

(*case study continues on page 155*)

▲ **TABLE 6.2**	**Analysis of the Internal Frame Factors Needs Assessment Data and Decision Making**			
	Findings			
Frame Factor	**Positive**	**Negative**	**Neutral**	**Conclusion**
Description and organizational structure of the parent academic institution	The college and school of nursing have positive reputations. Organization and hierarchal communication lines are clear for program and curriculum development processes and approvals. The dean has influence in the college. The college administrators are aware of the proposed program and supportive thus far.	There are no nursing senators on the senate curriculum or graduate committees.	The school has three senators on the academic senate.	*Positive:* The college organizational structure and administrators are supportive. The dean has influence. *Neutral:* There is a need to educate key members of the Senate about the program.
Mission and purpose, philosophy, and goals of the parent institution	The school of nursing matches the college mission, purpose, philosophy, and goals. It has good relationships with the professional education schools.	A few of the other schools may present roadblocks to the development of an outreach program if it impacts their programs.		*Positive:* Nursing is congruent with the college mission, etc. It has the support of the professional schools. *Neutral:* A campus-wide education effort regarding the nursing shortage and nursing's role in responding to the shortage is indicated.
Internal economic situation and its influence on the curriculum	The college and school of nursing are financially secure.	There is no support for the needs assessment and program or	The costs for released time to develop the curriculum will be	*Positive:* The college and school of nursing are financially secure.

(table continues on page 154)

▲ **TABLE 6.2**　　**Analysis of the Internal Frame Factors Needs Assessment Data and Decision Making** *(continued)*

Frame Factor	Findings			Conclusions
	Positive	**Negative**	**Neutral**	
	The college administrators favor the proposed program and will develop a business plan for it. There is a $2,000 grant for faculty released time to write grant proposal next-semester.	curriculum development.	included in next year's proposed budget.	The comptroller will develop a business plan for the proposal. There is money for faculty to write grants. *Negative:* Plans for released time for curriculum development must be included in next year's budget.
Resources within the institution and nursing program	The current on-campus program has adequate resources and services. The costs for some facilities may be offset by donated space.	An outreach program will require rental fees for classrooms, labs, offices, a coordinator, support staff, and faculty. Student services may need to increase staff for marketing and recruitment purposes.	Some support staff and instructional support services can be covered by existing services.	*Positive:* The college and school of nursing have adequate resources for the on-campus program, some of which can be shared with the outreach program. *Negative:* The business plan must include the costs for a coordinator and increases to faculty and support staff, physical facilities, and student services.
Potential faculty and student characteristics	The current faculty is well qualified.	A coordinator for the program and support staff for the position for start-up is necessary.		*Positive:* The school's existing faculty is well qualified. *Negative:* Selecting a coordinator for the program is of priority to coordinate the outreach program.

(continued)

▲ **TABLE 6.2** **Analysis of the Internal Frame Factors Needs Assessment Data and Decision Making** (*continued*)

| Frame Factor | Findings | | | Conclusions |
	Positive	Negative	Neutral	
		Part-time faculty at the very least will be necessary for learning lab and clinical supervision purposes.		*Neutral:* Faculty and staff needs can be identified when the decision is reached to start the program.
	The entry-level master's program applicant pool has been increasing. Entry-level master's graduates and their employers are satisfied with the program. One hundred percent of the graduates passed NCLEX.	Recently, the quality of the undergraduate applicant pool decreased. Additional marketing and recruitment services are indicated for recruiting students.	The applicant pool to the baccalaureate had a slight increase in the past year.	*Positive:* There is an increased interest in the entry-level master's program. One hundred percent of the graduates passed NCLEX and they and employers are satisfied with the program. *Negative:* Support for marketing and recruitment purposes are of highest priority.
Overall decision internal frame factors	16 positive entries	9 negative entries	4 neutral entries	12 positive conclusions 3 negative conclusions 3 neutral conclusions with recommendations

of the highest priority. The dean and provost plan to place a request to support these activities into next year's budget. Student services works closely with the school and with a small increase in staffing can provide marketing and recruitment support. Applications and enrollment patterns have been stable for the School of Nursing, though the entry-level master's program has been more stable than the undergraduate program. Employers of the entry-level master's graduates and the graduates are very satisfied with the program.

Specific items for the business plan have been iterated. The recommendations from the needs assessment of the external factors and the conclusions reached from the assessment of the internal factors led to the decision to initiate an entry-level master's degree outreach program.

(*case study continues on page 156*)

It was determined by the faculty and administrators that there is an adequate applicant pool for graduates of the program, there is no other program like it in the region, and it meets the demand for preparing additional nurses for the workforce. When the curriculum is developed, the option for students to continue their education in a clinical specialty after completing prelicensure requirements will be considered. A program coordinator and the marketing and recruitment of students have been identified as the first order of business. The following are the recommendations for initiation of the program and plans for their follow-up.

1. Expand the entry-level Master of Science in Nursing curriculum to an outreach program in the designated metropolitan area.
   1.1 Initiate information meetings about the program to the college community and the outreach site.
   1.2 Select two faculty members to write grants for program development funds.
   1.3 Appoint faculty members to revise the existing entry-level master's curriculum to fit an outreach program.

2. Appoint an on-site coordinator for the program and support staff.
   2.1 Work with the dean of nursing and faculty to recruit and appoint a coordinator and support staff for the program.
   2.2 Work with the dean of extended education to set up an office for the coordinator and support staff.

3. Develop a business plan for an entry-level Master of Science in Nursing outreach program in the designated metropolitan area studied.
   3.1 Work with the comptroller to develop a business plan for the start-up year and implementation of the program for the following 3 years leading to self-sufficiency.
   3.2 Identify all costs for management and planning for the program, support staff, faculty, facilities, resources, and services.
   3.3 Balance the costs with income from start-up grants, tuition, and fees.

4. The coordinator of the program will initiate start-up activities for the program including the following plans:
   4.1 Meet on-site with key stakeholders about the program (e.g., the director of extended education, the body politic, other nursing program directors and faculty, focus groups of potential students, health care facilities administrators and educators, potential funding agencies, and feeder educational institutions).
   4.2 Hold information and planning meetings on-campus with the dean and other deans of schools within the college, the provost and the president, the director of the library and instructional support services, the dean of enrollment services, nursing faculty, the nursing graduate committee, current enrolled entry-level master's students and graduates of that program, and members of the senate.
   4.3 Begin a written record for the program that can be incorporated into grant proposals, accreditation reports, and proposals for approval by the School of Nursing and the academic senate.

DISCUSSION QUESTIONS

1. To what extent do you believe an assessment of the internal frame factors that affect a nursing education program influences a decision to revise a program or propose a new one?
2. Of the five major internal frame factors, how would you prioritize findings from their assessment in terms of the potential success for a proposed education program or revision of the curriculum?

LEARNING ACTIVITIES

Student Activity

1. As a student group, continue your needs assessment for a potential nursing program that you started in Chapter 5. Use Table 6.1, "Guidelines for Assessing Internal Frame Factors," to collect data on the frame factors that you need to consider. After you collect the data, summarize your findings and compare them to the "Desired Outcomes" listed in the table. Based on the findings, justify why or why not a new nursing program is needed.

Faculty Activity

1. Using Table 6.1, "Guidelines for Assessing Internal Frame Factors," continue your work on the existing nursing curriculum that you identified in Chapter 5. Collect data for each internal frame factor as it applies to the curriculum. Summarize your findings and compare them to the "Desired Outcomes" listed in the table. In light of your summary, is a curriculum revision indicated? Explain your reasons for the decision to revise or not to revise.

REFERENCES

Bourke, A. B., Strehorn, K. C., & Silver, P. (2000). Faculty members: Provision of instructional accommodations to students with LD. *Journal of Learning Disabilities, 33*(1), 26–32.

Health Resources and Services Administration, Bureau of Health Professions, Nursing. (2004). *Nurse education and practice grant programs.* Retrieved May 31, 2004, from http://bhpr.hrsa.gov/nursing/

Joel, L. A. (2002). Education for entry into practice: Revisited for the 21st century. *Online Journal of Issues in Nursing, 7*(2),.8.

Johnson, M. (1977). *Intentionality in education.* Troy, NY: Walter Snyder, Printer, Inc. (distributed by the Center for Curriculum Research and Services, Albany, NY).

Keating, S. B., & Sechrist, K. R. (2001). The nursing shortage in California: The public policy role of the California Strategic Planning committee for Nursing. *Online Journal of Issues in Nursing. 6*(1), 14.

Mahaffrey, E. H. (2002). The relevance of associate degree nursing education: Past, present, future. *Online Journal of Issues in Nursing, 7*(2), 8.

National Institutes of Health. *National Institute of Nursing Research.* Retrieved May 31, 2004, from http://www.nih.gov/ninr

Rapson, M. F., & Rice, R. B. (2002). Regions' spadework helps speed caring solutions to challenges of rapid changes in nursing. *Patient Care Management, 17*(12), 2–7.

University of California – Los Angeles (UCLA). Office of Contract and Grant Administration. (2004). *Private foundations and organizations.* Retrieved May 31, 2004, from http://www.research.ucla.edu/ocga/sr2/Private.htm

University of Utah. (2004). U.S. higher education systems. Retrieved May 31, 2004, from http://www.utahsbr.edu/boards.htm

Curriculum Development

▼

Sarah B. Keating, EdD, RN, FAAN

▲ OVERVIEW

Prior to discussing curriculum development, it is useful to review the definition of curriculum. According to this text, *a curriculum is the formal plan of study that provides the philosophical underpinnings, goals, and guidelines for the delivery of a specific educational program.* Chapter 7 of this section introduces the components of the curriculum and the process for its development followed by two chapters devoted to undergraduate and graduate nursing education curricula.

Experienced educators will testify to the fact that as a curriculum ages, changes occur that were unintended in the original curriculum plan. These changes occur in response to feedback from students, faculty, and consumers; faculty's individual interpretations of the objectives and course content; changes in faculty personnel who are not familiar with the curriculum; changes in the practice setting; and expansion of nursing knowledge. Unless there is continuous evaluation of the curriculum, the plan will eventually become so corrupted that it is barely recognizable.

Section 5 describes in detail the value of evaluation activities as they apply to the curriculum and for approval and accreditation of the nursing program. However, it is wise in this section to recognize the need for continually monitoring the curriculum plan at least annually to ensure that it is meeting the original mission, framework, goals, and objectives. The data collected for evaluation reports and the recommendations issuing from them indicate to faculty the need for revising the curriculum, discontinuing certain programs within it, or initiating new tracks. If this exercise is conducted every year, maintaining the integrity of the curriculum becomes easy and there are fewer hoops to go through in seeking approval for minor or major changes. Annual reviews contribute to a curriculum that is a living, vibrant organism that prepares nursing professionals for current and future markets or, in the practice setting, educates staff and the public on current practice and health care matters.

▲ PURPOSE OF CURRICULUM DEVELOPMENT

The purpose of curriculum development in nursing is to meet learners' needs by ensuring that the curriculum meets educational and professional standards and is responsive to the current and future demands of the health care system. Curriculum development cannot occur in a vacuum, and though it is the responsibility of the faculty or nurse educators, consumers of the program also need to be involved in its processes. Consumers include students, families, communities, the health care system that utilizes graduates of schools of nursing programs, and nurse educators and staff in the practice setting.

▲ LEVELS OF NURSING EDUCATION

Chapter 1 reviewed the history of nursing education in the United States and described the evolution of various levels of nursing education beginning with diploma programs and ending with doctoral programs. For clarification, throughout this section's discussion and the remainder of the text, the usual types of undergraduate nursing education programs are defined in the following paragraphs.

A licensed practical nurse or licensed vocational nurse (LPN or LVN) is a graduate of an education program that prepares students to sit for licensure to practice as LPNs or LVNs. (The terms LPN and LVN are interchangeable.) Each state defines the title, scope of practice, and requirements for eligibility to sit for the licensure examination. Most programs take place in technical schools or community colleges and are usually 12 to 18 months in length. Credits for the work that took place in a community college can be transferred directly into an associate degree or undergraduate program as lower-division credit. In the case of technical schools, credit is awarded through a variety of methods. These methods include challenge exams to demonstrate knowledge and skills equivalent to specified content in the associate degree or undergraduate program, portfolios to demonstrate knowledge and clinical skills, or standardized examinations that measure knowledge and competency.

A diploma program is a hospital-based nursing program usually 3 years in length. Though these programs are gradually being phased out, it should be noted that many convert to associate degree or baccalaureate programs in recognition of the need for nursing programs to take place in institutions of higher learning rather than apprentice-type programs sponsored by hospitals. Much like the LPN/LVN programs, credits earned are usually not transferable into associate degree or baccalaureate programs unless they were earned in institutions of higher learning. Thus, community colleges and baccalaureate nursing programs have a variety of ways for diploma graduates to earn credit for previous learning, much the same as those listed for LPN/LVN programs.

Associate degree programs are based in community or junior colleges that usually offer 2-year lower-division programs. (Lower-division units are equivalent to undergraduate freshman and sophomore levels and include introductory courses, courses that provide broad knowledge from the disciplines, or technical level training.) Nursing programs may award the Associate of Arts (AA) or Associate of Science (AS) degree in nursing; thus, this text refers to them as Associate Degree in Nursing programs (ADN). These programs vary from 2 years to 3 or 4 years in length depending on the number of prerequisite courses required and the number of credits in the nursing program. Nevertheless, the credits earned are in lower-division units. Prelicensure nursing content in the United States is regulated by State Boards of Nursing, thus some of the nursing courses in these programs may contain content similar to upper-division level courses in undergraduate and higher degree programs. The same strategies for awarding upper-division level credit for LPN/LVN and diploma graduates can be used to recognize previous knowledge and skills. This results in less time spent in earning the bachelor's degree, ranging from 1 to 2 calendar years.

Baccalaureate (undergraduate) nursing programs have many versions of degree titles including Bachelor of Arts (BA), Bachelor of Science (BS), and Bachelor of Nursing Science (BNSc). Depending on the school of nursing and its parent institution, these degrees reflect curricula that may have emphases in the sciences or liberal arts; however, all prepare graduates for licensure as registered nurses (RNs) and contain the required prelicensure content as prescribed by the State Board of Nursing or, in the case of other countries, national regulating agencies. This text recognizes all of these degree titles, but for the sake of simplicity refers to them as baccalaureate programs or as the Bachelor of Science in Nursing (BSN).

▲ COMPONENTS OF THE CURRICULUM

The classic components of a school of nursing curriculum include statements on the mission or vision of the program and the philosophy of the faculty, which usually includes beliefs and values about teaching and learning processes, diversity, and the metaparadigm of nursing (i.e., nursing, person, health, and environment). Following these statements are the purpose or overall goal of the program; a conceptual framework around which to organize the curriculum plan; the end-of-program objectives; and an overall implementation plan. These same components apply to the practice setting when developing staff and patient education programs. The components should be congruent with the parent institution's mission and philosophy for both the academic and the practice settings. Chapter 7 discusses these components in detail and the pros and cons of conceptual frameworks, including the use of nursing and other disciplines' theories as organizing themes for the curriculum plan. While a review of all of the components may seem cumbersome at times, in the long run, it results in a logical order for planning and evaluating the curriculum.

Chapter 8 discusses the three major curricula for entry into practice (i.e., the diploma, associate degree [ADN], and the baccalaureate in nursing). The latter two programs have been in existence since the mid-20th century, replacing the hospital-based diploma programs, which continue to exist but are decreasing in numbers. The old issue of entry into practice rears its ugly head as the ADN and baccalaureate are examined; however, with the need to produce more nurses as rapidly as possible to meet health care demands and the need for additional education beyond the ADN, the authors of Chapter 8 offer alternative curricula that embrace both programs and foster career ladder opportunities.

Chapter 9 examines graduate education at the master's and doctorate levels, including entry-level master's and doctoral programs. Graduate programs are particularly hard-hit by the looming shortage of doctorally prepared teachers as the faculty workforce ages and retires and the numbers of new graduates from doctoral programs do not meet the demand. This situation provides the impetus for accelerating access to graduate education for both new entrants into the discipline and practicing nurses and educators who have an interest in teaching. Other issues facing graduate education are discussed in the chapter, including differentiation of research activities at the master's and doctorate levels, faculty-to-student ratios in graduate education, and the necessity for available research opportunities and resources for both faculty and students in graduate programs.

Components of the Curriculum

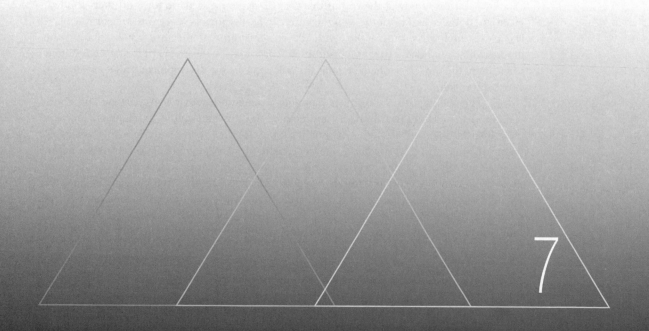

Sarah B. Keating, EdD, RN, FAAN

OBJECTIVES

Upon completion of Chapter 7, the reader will be able to:

1. Compare curriculum development activities among various types of educational institutions.
2. Distinguish the formal curriculum from the informal curriculum.
3. Review classic philosophies and trends in nursing education that influence curriculum development and evaluation.
4. Analyze the components of the curriculum according to their place in producing a curriculum plan.
5. Analyze a case study that illustrates the adaptation of an existing curriculum to a distance education program.
6. Assess an existing curriculum or educational program by using the "Guidelines for Assessing the Key Components of a Curriculum or Educational Program."

▲ OVERVIEW

Faculty members continually examine the curriculum and make minor revisions based on its relevance to the preparation of nurses for today and the future. The curriculum must also undergo complete periodic reviews based on feedback from its stakeholders and external demands such as program review and accreditation. Chapter 7 discusses the classic components of the curriculum, which include the mission and/or vision; philosophy, including beliefs about teaching and learning, critical thinking, diversity, optional conceptual or theoretical framework, and overall goal and purpose; and the implementation plan. It discusses the components in detail and the pros and cons of conceptual frameworks including the use of nursing and other disciplines' theories as organizing themes for the curriculum plan. Based on the overall purpose or goal, end-of-program and intermediate or level objectives are developed that provide the basis for the curriculum plan (i.e., the prerequisites and the courses with their respective descriptions, objectives, and content outlines). Table 7.1, "Guidelines for Assessing the Key Components of a Curriculum or Educational Program," summarizes methods for assessing each curriculum component. A case study is presented at the end of the chapter to illustrate the adaptation of an existing curriculum to a distance education program. It is a continuation of the case study found in Chapters 5 and 6 that is based on an actual feasibility study.

Curriculum Development Applied to Various Levels of Institutions

The principles and components of curriculum development are quite similar for private and public institutions as well as community colleges, small liberal arts colleges, large multi-purpose or comprehensive colleges and universities, research universities, and academic health sciences centers. The differences arise when examining the overall purpose of the institution and the financial and human resources that are available for revising or initiating new programs.

The case study at the end of this chapter depicts a scenario for a privately funded, sectarian, middle-sized institution. In this case, the faculty members act as the major role players in developing the curriculum, with the administrator of the program facilitating the process. In larger, heavily endowed institutions, there may be the luxury of hiring a consultant to facilitate the process. Nonetheless, faculty still controls the development processes (i.e., the curriculum plan).

Depending on the regional economy, academic health science centers and state-supported universities usually have funding available for curriculum development because these institutions must answer to the public and, as is true for all institutions, the quality of the institution must be maintained to meet accreditation and program approval criteria. Thus, there are usually funds provided by these parent institutions for periodic curriculum development. For example, when accreditation reports and visits are due, the budget for that year includes self-study activities, costs for preparing reports, released time for faculty and staff to coordinate activities, and consultant fees, if indicated. Smaller institutions should plan so that funds are available to them when curriculum development, evaluation, and accreditation activities are approaching.

For all types of programs, administrators and faculty should plan for the financial support of curriculum development activities and investigate external resources such as grants that support curriculum changes and program development. An example of a program that

| ▲ TABLE 7.1 | Guidelines for Assessing the Key Components of a Curriculum or Educational Program | |

Component	Questions for Data Collection	Desired Outcomes
Mission/vision	What are the major elements in the missions of the parent institution and subdivision (if applicable)? Are these same major elements in the nursing mission? If not, give a rationale as to why they are not.	The nursing mission is congruent with that of its parent institution and, if applicable, the academic subdivision in which it is located.
	How does the nursing mission speak to its teaching, service, and research/scholarship roles?	The mission reflects nursing's teaching, service, and research/scholarship role.
Philosophy	Is the nursing philosophy congruent with that of the parent institution philosophy and subdivision (if applicable)? If not, give the rationale as to why they are not.	The philosophy statement is congruent with that of the parent institution and academic subdivision (if applicable).
	What statements in the philosophy relate to the faculty's beliefs and values about teaching and learning, critical thinking, diversity, and nursing's metaparadigm?	The philosophy reflects the faculty's beliefs and values on teaching and learning, critical thinking, diversity, and nursing's metaparadigm.
Organizing framework	What is the organizing framework for the curriculum, and how does it reflect the mission and philosophy statements?	The curriculum has an organizing framework that reflects its mission and philosophy.
	To what extent does the framework appear throughout the implementation of the curriculum? Are its threads readily identified in all of the tracks of the programs?	The threads of the organizing framework are readily identified in all tracks of the nursing education program.
Overall purpose/goal of the program	To what extent does the overall goal or purpose statement reflect the mission, philosophy, and organizing framework?	The overall goal or purpose statement reflects that of the mission, philosophy, and organizing framework.
	Is the statement broad enough to encompass all tracks of the nursing program?	The overall goal or purpose includes all tracks of the nursing program.
	To what extent does the statement lead to the measurement of program outcomes?	The overall goal or purpose is stated in such a way that it is a guide for measuring outcomes of the program.
End-of-program, intermediate, and course objectives	To what extent are the mission, overall goal or purpose, and conceptual framework reflected in the objectives?	The objectives reflect the mission, overall purpose or goal, and organizing framework.
	Are the objectives arranged in logical and sequential order?	The objectives are sequential and logical.

has been available over the years for nursing program development or expansion is the Division of Nursing's Title VIII program for advanced nurse training grants, scholarships, diversifying the workforce through education programs, and scholarships (Health Resources and Service Administration, Bureau of Health Professions, Nursing, 2004). Detailed information is available at the following website: http://bhpr.hrsa.gov/nursing.

The Formal and Informal Curricula

Throughout curriculum development activities, the faculty should be aware of the influence of the informal curriculum on student learning. The informal curriculum is also termed the cocurriculum or extracurricular activities and can be planned or unplanned. Examples of informal curricula are athletic activities and events, special convocations such as invited speakers, student study groups, student organization activities, faculty and student interactions, and travel. Some specific examples for nursing are nursing convocations, pinning ceremonies, graduations, honor society meetings, study groups, student nursing association meetings, and invited attendance at faculty meetings.

Several studies in higher education looked at extracurricular or cocurricular activities and their influences on students' learning. Of special interest to nursing are the positive influence of out-of-class experiences on learning and the acquisition of critical thinking skills and cognitive development (Terenzini and others, 1995; Terenzini, Pascarella, & Blimling, 1999). Kuh (1995) discusses some of the specific out-of-class experiences that have a positive influence on students' learning. They include leadership activities, peer interactions, faculty contacts, work, and travel. Many schools of nursing schedule informal student–faculty meetings, holiday parties, and special events. They provide opportunities for student–faculty interchanges to enrich and supplement the formal classroom setting as well as facilitate leadership opportunities for the students.

Yet another influence on the formal curriculum with application to nursing is the experience students have when transferring into another college. Many nursing students transfer into upper division higher education institutions from community colleges where they fulfilled prerequisites for the major. Laanan (2000) studied the experiences of transfer students from community colleges into the University of California, Los Angeles (UCLA). His study found that students who were products of honors programs in the community colleges were more apt to have higher grade point averages (GPAs) in the baccalaureate program and more likely to engage in extracurricular activities than those students who did not participate in honors programs. However, both groups expressed similar satisfaction with UCLA and had similar levels of involvement in the university. Additionally, there were no statistically significant differences between the two groups in psychological or social adjustment.

There are no studies in nursing on the effects of the transfer process on students' learning. Since so many nursing students, including registered nurses (RNs), transfer into the major, it would be interesting to study if there are any differences between them and students who started in the program at the freshman level. Questions might be raised as to the need for mentoring programs for transfer students to ease transition or to the possibility of experienced learners providing peer support and study strategies for novice learners in the home institution.

Students in the RN program are a rather unique group of adult learners who, in essence, are transfer students. They require responsive educational programs that recognize their needs and their strengths as adult learners in both bachelor's completion and graduate programs. Some of the strategies for meeting the needs of RN students include distance education (especially attractive to working RNs), clinical experiences in which teachers respect the RNs' clinical competence, learning contracts, alternative validation approaches for previous learning, and classroom teaching tailored to the preferences of the adult learner. There is a plethora of studies that relate to educational programs for the RN returning to school and teaching strategies to meet their needs. Recent studies include those by Armstrong and Gessner (1999); Diaconis (2001); Reale (2001); Thompson and Scheckley (1997); Vivarais-Dressler and Kutschke (2001); and Waddell and Stephens (2000).

Kellogg (1999) cites findings from various organizations in higher education that urge the promotion of student learning through collaboration between academic programs and student services. Examples include orientation, faculty–student–staff activities, remediation activities, study skills workshops, and peer mentoring. When planning the formal curriculum, faculty may wish to identify those learning activities that take place outside of the formal curriculum and that have a positive influence on learning to enhance the planned curriculum.

The Mission and Vision Statements

Traditionally, higher education institutions in the United States have three major components in their mission statements—teaching, service, and research (scholarship). The mission statement for each institution depends on the nature of the institution, and the three major components are often divided into separate permutations of the components. In more recent times, some organizations either replace or supplement the mission statement with a vision statement. For the purposes of this discussion, the mission statement is the institution's beliefs about its responsibility for the delivery of programs through teaching, service, and scholarship. A vision statement is outlook oriented and reflects the institution's plans and dreams about its direction for the future. It is possible that a mission statement includes its vision and that a vision statement includes its mission. With this in mind, the following discussion emphasizes the development of the traditional mission statement, but also recognizes the more recent utilization of vision statements.

Chief administrators (presidents) of institutions of higher learning assume much of the responsibility for ensuring that the mission is current and reflects the purpose of the college or university. They provide the leadership for administrators, staff, faculty, and students to implement the mission, to maintain the mission's relevancy in the community, and to meet future education needs. Developing or revising a mission statement is usually a part of a strategic planning process that involves all of the constituents within the institution. The purpose of the institution is examined and then a vision statement is developed that looks into the future for the next decade or two. These activities foster creativity and a movement toward the future that provide the framework for planning. After consensus is reached, the mission statement evolves and guides the development of subsequent components of the curriculum, including the philosophy, organizing framework, long-range goals, and objectives for implementing them.

Another consideration related to the mission is the congruence of the statement with its actual implementation. Measures to determine if the mission is realized throughout the educational process and according to the expectations of graduates' performance in the real world give feedback as to how well the mission is met. For example, if the mission has a strong research emphasis, there should be adequate support and funding for faculty and students to write research grant proposals, released time, facilities to conduct research, and money to fund their activities.

Another aspect to the implementation of the mission is a cost analysis of the institution's budget to relate the amount of funds allocated to the various educational programs for carrying out the mission. Academic and infrastructure support systems are analyzed for congruency with the mission. An example from nursing's is a parent institution's support and commitment to a school of nursing's nurse-managed primary care clinic that serves the under- and unserved populations of the community. In this example, the clinic meets the institution's mission to serve the community.

Unless the school or department of nursing is a stand-alone academic entity, the mission of the major academic division (e.g. college or school) in which it resides is examined in addition to that of the parent institution. The missions of both the parent institution and its academic subdivision should be congruent with each other and provide guidelines for the mission statement of the nursing program. These statements depend on the nature of the institution and the nursing program. Smaller institutions may focus on liberal arts as a basis for all disciplines and professional programs to meet societal needs, while a large research-oriented university or academic health sciences center might emphasize graduate education and new knowledge breakthroughs by its faculty's and graduate students' research activities. In the case of the former, nursing's mission statement would reflect the graduation of well-prepared nurses to meet current and future health care demands; the latter would have an emphasis on nursing research and leadership in the profession. As mentioned previously, mission statements focus on the three elements of higher education—teaching, service, and research; thus, nursing's mission statement will reflect all three with emphasis on certain ones according to the nature of the parent institution and its divisions.

As with the presidents of universities and colleges, deans and directors of nursing education programs have a leadership role in developing nursing missions that not only are congruent with the parent institutions but also look to the future (Starck, Warner, & Kotarba, 1999). Additionally, the mission needs to be examined frequently for its relevance to the rapidly changing health care system and needs of society. In the recent past, nursing and other health care disciplines recognized the need for interprofessional education (Fitzpatrick, 1998) and with the complexity of the United States' health care system, this is an important consideration for nursing programs to include in their mission statements and philosophies.

▲ PHILOSOPHY

Developing a statement of philosophy that flows from the mission gives faculty members the opportunity to discuss their beliefs, values, and attitudes about nursing and the educational processes for imparting nursing's body of knowledge to the next generation of care providers. Faculty members discuss their beliefs about their school of nursing and its role in preparing nurses for the future, including statements on teaching and learning theories, the development of critical thinking, diversity, and the nursing metaparadigm (i.e., nursing, person, health, and the environment). Each individual member holds his or her own personal philosophy and thus, the development of a philosophical statement can become an arduous task for reaching consensus. Nevertheless, the resulting statement reflects the faculty's (as an entity) rationale for the school of nursing's existence and it serves to flavor the remainder of the curriculum components, its implementation, and its outcomes.

When developing or revising a statement of philosophy, it is useful to be familiar with common terms from philosophy to identify the basic underlying precepts in which faculty believe. The Encyclopedia Britannica (2003) defines philosophy as follows: *the critical examination of the grounds for fundamental beliefs and an analysis of the basic concepts employed in the expression of such beliefs. Philosophical inquiry is a central element in the intellectual history of many historical civilizations.* It outlines the many subdivisions of philosophy, such as logic, ethics, aesthetics, and metaphysics, and further classifies knowledge into epistemology, existentialism, axiology, realism, idealism, empiricism, pragmatism, phenomenology, and humanism.

Three basic components of philosophy are metaphysics, epistemology, and axiology. Csokasy (2002) defines them as such: "*Metaphysics seeks to answer the basic questions of reality and what is real and true; epistemology is the study of nature, the validity of knowledge, and how the truth differs from opinion; and axiology seeks to describe that which is ethical logical and of value*" (p. 32). Csokasy goes on to discuss the differences in philosophical approaches and the eclectic nature of nursing with its humanistic values and, at the same time, its need to fill behaviorist expectations to meet licensure and accreditation requirements. Csokasy discusses the use of philosophical frameworks in nursing curricula and the need for them to be congruent with the outcomes of the programs. If the philosophy is harmonious with what is valued currently and for the future, the philosophy remains intact; if it is not, it may be time for a change or revision.

As with the mission statement, the nursing philosophy is congruent with that of the parent institution and its subdivisions (if applicable). In instances of incongruity, a rationale as to why and how the nursing program meets other components of the philosophy statements should be discussed. Eventually, this rationale is documented so that members of the school and external reviewers understand the fit of the nursing program to its parent institution and subdivisions. The following discussion reviews common elements found in nursing statements of philosophy.

Beliefs About Teaching and Learning and the Roles of Faculty and Students

Chapters 3 and 4 of this text include in-depth discussions regarding teaching and learning theories and principles, critical thinking, and educational taxonomies. When developing or assessing a philosophy, these chapters provide useful information regarding the faculty's beliefs about teaching and learning and the development of critical thinking. Watson (2001) discusses postmodernism in terms of nursing and nursing education. She states that it is the process of critiquing and demystifying modern traditions and beliefs. Applied to curriculum development, it frees faculty from old, traditional ways of thinking and curricula to developing new, creative, and innovative curricula.

Espeland and Shanta (2001) discuss student–teacher interactions by a description of two concepts—empowering and enabling—as part of the role that faculty plays in the student learning process. Their observations of the interactions between students and their teachers are pertinent to nursing education techniques, which so often in the past focused on faculty control over students to transmit a large body of knowledge. It is their contention that this type of teaching does not foster critical thinking, the development of autonomy, or a professional identity.

Metcalfe (1998) discusses the mandate from the 21st century's changing health care system that includes a movement away from behaviorism concepts toward humanism. Multidisciplinary teaching and learning experiences are encouraged to enhance the development of students' critical thinking skills. Learning becomes problem-based and is a collaborative experience for the student, teacher, and others in the clinical experience. Mallow and Gilje (1999) raise some interesting questions related to the philosophy of nursing education and the utilization of technology-driven teaching and learning modalities. They point out that at that time (1999) there were few articles in the nursing literature related to the impact of technology-based instruction on outcomes valued by nursing such as caring, communication, moral and ethical behaviors, and other humanism and holism aspects of nursing. Since that time, technology has played a major role in nursing education, such as total programs that are web-based. The questions these authors raise persist and are ones that faculty need to reflect upon and incorporate into their beliefs about the teaching and learning process and critical thinking.

Beliefs About Critical Thinking

Chapter 4 of this text discusses critical thinking and its application to nursing education. The development of critical thinking is an essential element for preparing nurses for the professional role and their skills for clinical decision making and judgment. Most philosophies for nursing curricula contain some mention of critical thinking. Hicks (2001) discusses the myriad definitions of critical thinking utilized in nursing practice and education and the fact that many of these definitions come from disciplines other than nursing. In his review of the literature, he found that research on the attainment of critical thinking focused on outcomes and that more meaningful studies on the nature of critical thinking came from qualitative research that examined the process of acquiring these skills though interactions with clients in clinical experiences. His thesis is significant to the development of curricula philosophies as faculty consider the relationship of the place of critical thinking in the development of professionals and its contribution to nursing science.

Bowles (2000) conducted a study of critical thinking and its influence on the clinical judgment skills of graduates from two schools of nursing. Her findings demonstrated a relationship between critical thinking and clinical judgment that also confirmed previous research. Like Hicks, she recommends additional studies that show how the educational process has an impact on the development of critical thinking and, hence, clinical judgment. Both articles demonstrate the need for studies on processes and outcomes related to the development of critical thinking in nursing. After reviewing theories and concepts related to teaching and learning and critical thinking, faculty comes to a consensus for a statement in the philosophy that reflects their beliefs and values related to these themes.

Beliefs About Diversity and Cultural Competence

Diversity can be considered, in its broadest sense, not only in terms of race, ethnicity, culture, linguistics, religion, and gender, but also in terms of the diversity of opportunities in nursing. For example, while the majority of the nursing workforce remains in the acute care delivery system, there are many opportunities in community-based settings such as primary care, public health, industry, schools, home care, skilled nursing facilities, and rehabilitation hospitals. While the core of nursing knowledge and practice remains the same for all settings, community-based settings call for different interests, values, educational preparation, and skill sets. Thus, when faculty develops the curriculum philosophy, it must consider these factors and how the curriculum will meet the health care needs of a multicultural society through graduates who can function with cultural sensitivity and competence in all settings.

Diversity of the Nursing Workforce

Though many gains were realized in the latter part of the 20th century, the nursing profession and its education system must still commit itself to diversifying the workforce to more closely resemble that of the populace. According to the Bureau of Health Professions, Health Resources and Services Administration, Division of Nursing (2002), in March 2000 about 12% of the nursing workforce represented racial/ethnic minority backgrounds compared to about one-third of the general population. At the same time, the minority nurses were more likely to be employed in nursing and employed full time than nonminority nurses.

Bauerhaus and Auerbach (1999) discuss the slow growth of the number of minorities in the nursing workforce and the need to study the barriers that face ethnic and cultural minorities in gaining admission to nursing schools. California, whose minority population in 2000 was 52%, has one of the best records for increasing the diversity of the nursing workforce, with 27.5% of the RN population representing minorities and 8.2% men compared to the national averages of 12% and 5.4%, respectively (Sechrist, Lewis, Rutledge, Keating, & the Association of California Nurse Leaders, 2002; Bureau of Health Professions, Health Resources and Services Administration, Division of Nursing 2002).

These data illustrate the need to increase the diversity of the nursing workforce and to develop curricula that speak to diverse learning needs as well as to the health needs of the multicultural and ethnic population. Diversifying the health professions workforce is a goal at the national level to help eliminate health disparities in the population by increasing access to health care services and providing health professionals who can provide culturally competent care for underserved areas (HRSA, Bureau of Health Professions, Division of Nursing 2004a).

An understanding of cultural differences in the population and its health values and responses to illness has become increasingly important to global health. Language, as a major part of culture, is an important component in formulating value statements about graduates' communication skills. Many nursing programs are considering proficiency in a language other than the native language as a competency expected of their graduates. For English as a second language (ESL) students, Abriam-Yago, Yoder, and Kataoka-Yahiro (1999) offer a model of language proficiency as a framework for assisting faculty and ESL students in gaining proficiency in the predominant language. (p. 143).

While the discussion thus far involved increasing the diversity of the nursing workforce through the recruitment, retention, and graduation of a more representative student body, another major issue is the need to increase the diversity of nursing faculty who serve as role models for students. Although a review of the literature yielded only one article on the breakdown of cultural and ethnic diversity in faculty, it is widely accepted that nursing needs to increase the diversity of its faculty as well as its general workforce (Grossman et. al., 1998).

Overall in the United States, nursing faculty in all types of nursing schools is 90% to 92% Caucasian (Berlin, Stennett, & Bednash, 2002; Bureau of Health Professions, Health Resources and Services Administration, 2002).

Grossman et. al. (1998) surveyed deans and directors of Florida schools of nursing regarding the diversity of their faculties. They compared faculty and student demographics to the general population of Florida and found that nursing students and faculty under-represented the diversity of the general population. There were even fewer diverse faculty representatives than student representatives. The groups least represented in the faculty were: Hispanic (2.16%, compared to 12.2% of the general population) and Black/non-Hispanic (8.19%, compared to 13.6% of the general population). The article included the deans' and directors' opinions about barriers to recruitment of diverse faculty and some of their recruitment methods. While this is only one state, it is possible that similar findings could be found in other states, especially those with multicultural and ethnic population groups.

Cultural Competence

According to the Health Resources and Services Administration Bureau of Health Professions, Division of Nursing (2004b) the definition of cultural competence is: "a set of academic and interpersonal skills that allow an individual to increase their understanding and appreciation of cultural differences and similarities within, among and between groups. This requires a willingness and ability to draw on community-based values, traditions, and customs and to work with knowledgeable persons of both and from the community in developing targeted interventions, communications, and other supports." Additional definitions from the perspectives of other disciplines may be found at http://bhpr.hrsa.gov/diversity/cultcomp.htm.

Several authors discuss the importance of diversity to education, research, and practice. Leininger (2001) discusses the growth of transcultural nursing knowledge from the 1950s to the present and its application to practice. She urges nursing to continue integration of knowledge related to both Western and non-Western cultures into research, education, and practice. Sloand, Groves, and Brager (2004) discuss cultural competence and its place in the nursing curriculum. They describe its role in providing care for a diverse population in America where the predominant culture is Western but the need is for individualized care for other cultural groups. They also describe a specific nursing curriculum that integrates culturally competent care into the program.

Several authors studied diversity issues in the curriculum and cocurriculum that influenced the development of students' racial-policy beliefs and openness to diversity. Some of the positive influences include a nondiscriminatory racial environment, racial/ethnic composition of the classroom, diversity of student acquaintances, and exposure to political ideologies (DeAngelo, 2001; Terenzini, Cabrera, Colbeck, Bjorklund, and Parente, 2001; Terenzini et al., 1999). A specific teaching strategy in nursing as reported by Koening and Zorn (2002) is storytelling. These authors found that this method of instruction appealed to various types of learners and had special relevance to ethnically diverse students to empower them to share their culture and transform ideas and concepts into learning situations.

Nurse educators must build their curricula to support the diversification of the workforce and to graduate health professionals who not only represent the multicultural/ethnic general population, but also are sensitive to the varying health care needs of the people.

Integrating beliefs, values, and concepts about diversity is as important as the application of learning and teaching theories, critical thinking, and educational taxonomies when developing the curriculum. The recognition of the concepts of multiculturalism and ethnicity should appear in the mission, philosophy, and statements of beliefs and values of the curriculum. These concepts should be threaded throughout the curriculum plan and should address the health care needs of the people nurses serve and the learning needs of an increasingly diverse student population.

Nursing's Metaparadigm

While the debate continues about nursing as a discipline, in most nursing education circles, a metaparadigm for the nursing discipline is recognized and included in the philosophy and organizing framework of the curriculum. Though there are numerous terms for the four domains of the nursing metaparadigm, the most commonly accepted terms are nursing (practice), environment, health, and the client (Fawcett, 1984; Kim, 1998; Newman, Sime, & Corcoran-Perry, 1991; Paillé & Pilkington, 2002).

Smith (2000) gives arguments for and against nursing as a science and a profession. In her review of the literature, she found that disciplines base their scientific practice on a unified paradigm and that there are some who say there is no one unifying theory in nursing. Added to this is the problem of multiple entries of education into practice and the need to base practice and research on theory. However, counterarguments in favor of nursing as a profession are the commonly recognized four-domain nursing metaparadigm, increasing numbers of doctoral programs to prepare nurse scientists and researchers, and research studies that test nursing theories. Smith concludes by saying that nursing meets the definition of a profession and that it is a young, ever-evolving science. She urges members of the nursing profession to continue to build nursing science by testing theories and applying them to practice.

Theoretical and Conceptual Frameworks

The majority of nursing programs and curricula in the United States are organized around a nursing theoretical or conceptual framework. Most State Boards of Nursing require documentation of the basic elements in the curriculum, including a conceptual framework. The National League for Nursing Accrediting Commission's (2004) standards and criteria are explicit in asking for the philosophy/mission and organizing framework. For example, for all nursing programs from licensed practical/vocational through master's programs, Standard IV: Curriculum and Instruction states: "Curriculum developed by nursing faculty flows from the nursing education unit philosophy/mission through an organizing framework into a logical progression of course outcomes and learning activities to achieve desired program objectives/ outcomes."

The Commission on Collegiate Nursing Education does not specify an organizing framework, although its statement provides guidance for faculty in the development of the curriculum. Standard III, Program Quality Curriculum and Teaching-Learning Practices, states: "The curriculum is developed with clear statements of expected results derived from the mission, philosophy, and goals/objectives of the program with clear congruence between the teaching-learning experiences and expected results" (American Association of Colleges of Nursing, 2004).

Although accreditation is voluntary, most schools of nursing in the United States are accredited by a national organization. Therefore, depending on which accrediting organization grants the accreditation, the school may or may not elect to choose an organizing framework. However, because most state boards require a framework, the majority of programs in the United States choose a conceptual, theoretical, or organizing framework for their curricula.

Some programs may elect to use the metaparadigm; nursing theories or models; other disciplines' theories and models such as systems theory, human development, or the medical model; or several frameworks as an eclectic model. When developing or revising a nursing curriculum, faculty selects the framework that best fits its philosophy and the nature of the program and its students. The framework serves to logically organize the body of knowledge and provides a checklist of sorts that ensures that no parts are omitted.

McEwan and Brown (2002) surveyed National League for Nursing Accreditation Commission (NLNAC) undergraduate nursing programs for the use of conceptual frameworks in their curricula. One hundred sixty schools responded, which represented 12.8 % of the total schools accredited by NLNAC. Because part of the criteria for NLNAC accreditation includes the use of an organizing framework, all of the programs had conceptual frameworks. The authors found the most common curricular framework to be the nursing process. One-third of the programs used a simple-to-complex organization, biopsychosocial models, and nursing theorists. Orem was the most common of the nursing theorists, with other mentioned theorists including Parse, Levine, King, Newman, and Henderson.

There were some significant differences among types of programs and selection of conceptual frameworks. Associate Degree in Nursing (ADN) ($p = .003$) and diploma programs ($p = .024$) were more likely to use the nursing process as a component of the framework than baccalaureate programs. ADN programs were almost twice as likely to use a simple-to-complex framework than baccalaureate programs ($p = .024$). Diploma programs were more likely to use an integrated medical model ($p = .082$). The respondents were asked to what extent they used the metaparadigm (nursing, health, person, and environment) in the conceptual framework; nursing had the greatest emphasis, with the diploma and ADN programs spending significantly more time on nursing and the baccalaureate programs spending more time on the environment (McEwan & Brown, 2002).

Organizing frameworks serve to guide curriculum development and provide ways in which the faculty can continually evaluate the curriculum for its completeness and quality. Weaving threads from the theory or conceptual framework throughout the curriculum assists in ensuring that essential nursing content is there and helps to identify gaps or redundancies as the curriculum plan develops. Chinn and Kramer (1999) define conceptual frameworks and theoretic frameworks as follows:

> A logical grouping of related concepts or theories, usually created to draw
> together several different aspects that are relevant to a complex situation such as
> a practice setting or an educational program. Term used synonymously with
> theoretic framework. A knowledge from within the empirics pattern (p. 252).

One example from the literature that describes the use of a nursing theory in an associate degree curriculum is the use of Martha Rogers' (1970) model (Hellwig & Ferrante, 1993). Comley (1994) describes the process of comparing two nursing theories (Orem, 1985; Peplau, 1952) as they relate to the nursing metaparadigm, usefulness, generalizability, and testability in choosing one to match one's personal philosophy or, in the case of a nursing education program, to match the faculty's conceptual framework statement. Gulitz and King (1988) discuss the use of King's theory in organizing and implementing a curriculum utilizing definitions within that model's concepts as core components of the curriculum.

Several more recent models are described in the literature that pertain to partnerships between types of nursing programs, the use of an organization's recommended essentials of education, and standards of practice. In Arizona, a joint curriculum plan was developed to improve articulation between five associate degree programs and that of a baccalaureate program (Lusk & Decker, 2001). Called the "Healing Community," its purpose was to form a seamless articulation from associate degree programs to baccalaureate programs. Faculty from all of the schools developed a joint statement of philosophy and a conceptual framework for the curriculum. The major concepts in the organizing framework were competency, critical thinking, caring, culture, communication, learning/teaching, accountability, and management/leadership.

Daggett, Butts, and Smith (2002) describe the revision of a nursing curriculum in response to the current and future demands of the health care system and health care needs of the people. They argue that many nursing programs' curricula are based on "yesteryear's" premises that include the nursing process and are not equipped to meet the challenges of changing health care systems. Using the American Association of Colleges of Nursing's (1998a, 1998b) recommendations for essentials of baccalaureate and master's education, they developed a new conceptual framework. The model of their organizing framework for the curriculum has a compass in its center pointing to four core concepts—nursing knowledge, competencies, role development, and professional nursing values. Surrounding the model is an outer circle that defines the outcomes of the curriculum.

Nursing theories, the nursing metaparadigm, and other disciplines' frameworks traditionally served as conceptual frameworks for nursing education curricula; there are, however, several newer ideas that relate to changes in the health care system and the demographics of the population. Cloutterbuck and Cherry (1998) present a curricular and teaching–learning model that proposes to prepare nurses for interdisciplinary practice and the future. They contend that educational programs must respond to the rapid changes in the health care system as well as the health care demands and needs of the population. The Cloutterbuck model consists of the consumer's health status, behavior, and outcomes that are assessed across three dimensions, personal, situational, and structural. These dimensions are defined in detail with additional items for assessment and intervention. The model has a strong emphasis on preparing health professionals for working with diverse population groups and other disciplines. While the model has been tested with only two groups of senior-level baccalaureate students in a community health nursing course, it has possibilities as a model for a total curriculum plan.

Taybei, Moore-Jazayeri, and Maynard (1998) discuss another curriculum model that meets the needs of first-generation, low-income, and ethnically diverse students. This type of model has potential for integration into other curriculum conceptual or theoretical models to ensure relevancy to the current and future health care system and the needs of students and the population.

Webber (2002) briefly describes the history and development of conceptual frameworks of nursing curricula in the United States and then presents a new nursing framework, the KSVME model. KSVME signifies nursing Knowledge, Skills, Values, Meaning, and Experience. The model is designed in such a way that it can apply to all levels of education (associate degree, baccalaureate, and graduate education) and moves cumulatively and progressively. The author states that it is flexible and can be adapted to the individual school's mission and philosophy. It is used as an example in the case study at the end of this chapter.

▲ OVERALL PURPOSE AND GOAL OF THE PROGRAM

After the philosophy, mission, and organizing framework are chosen, the next logical step in curriculum development is to state the overall purpose or goal of the program. There are arguments against behavioral statements for goals as postmodernist and humanism philosophies take hold in the 21st century. The arguments against them relate to the lack of freedom they provide for the learner and for the teacher, whose role is to empower the learner. At the same time, there are accountability issues that relate to graduates' competencies in meeting the health care system's demands and the needs of the people they serve. Faculty must grapple with these issues as it develops statements on the purpose of the nursing program and the overall long-term goal for graduates. Whether the statement becomes global and idealistic or specific and stated in measurable terms depends on the faculty's philosophy, values, and beliefs.

In addition to the choice of the format for the goal statement, there are certain components belonging to nursing that faculty may wish to consider and include, if not explicitly, implicitly. Clinical competence is a factor, and Lenberg (1999) discusses this category in terms of outcomes and performance assessment. Depending on the conceptual framework, the purpose or overall goal may include statements on caring, health promotion, and other types of nursing interventions, client systems, professional behaviors, and so forth.

The type of nursing education program influences the overall program purpose or goal statement. For example, levels of clinical competence and knowledge acquisition will differ among licensed vocational nursing, associate degree, baccalaureate, master's, and doctoral programs. Programs with multiple layers of preparation have a global statement of purpose or goal and then each program, in symphony with that statement, adapts it to meet its own level of education.

Failla, Maher, and Duffy (1999) studied the clinical competencies of associate degree graduates in terms of that level of education's overall goal. They surveyed graduates, faculty, and employers at the time of graduation and 6 months following graduation. They found that graduates rated themselves higher than faculty and employers, who were in agreement about the graduates' competencies. Overall, employers rated the graduates as competent in practice as measured by interpersonal relations and communication, teaching and collaboration, professional development, planning and evaluation, clinical care, and leadership. Findings such as these reinforce the purpose and overall goals of the program in preparing clinically competent nurses.

Most baccalaureate programs speak to the contribution of the liberal arts to professional education; thus, the purpose or goal of a program might include mention of the liberal arts. Nursing and other professional programs continue to defend their place in higher education. Halter and Polet (2002) discuss this issue, the history of nursing in higher education, and the value of the liberal arts in preparing professionals. Griffiths and Tagliareni (1999) describe a collaborative program between an associate degree and baccalaureate nursing program in accelerating minority students into the bachelor's program to prepare them to address minority health issues as well as to develop research goals. At the graduate level, several authors give examples of overall goals for advanced-practice nurses and the role that society's health needs and political influences can play in developing goal statements (Gagan, Berg, & Root, 2002; Vezeau, Peterson, Nakao, & Ersek 1998).

Although the statement of purpose and overall goal can be succinct, they act as guides for end-of-program objectives. The statement must also reflect the curriculum's mission statement, philosophy, and conceptual framework.

End-of-Program, Intermediate, and Course Objectives

End-of-program objectives reflect the organizing framework and define the specific expectations of graduates upon completion of the nursing program. To reach these objectives, intermediate or level, semester, and course objectives are developed in sequential order. For example, in a two-year associate degree program there are end-of-first-year expectations and end-of-second-year expectations, all of which lead to the end-of-program objectives. In a baccalaureate program there may be freshman-, sophomore-, junior-, and senior-level objectives. Some programs prefer to divide the objectives into semesters and could be titled in that fashion (i.e., first semester, second semester, third semester, etc.). Graduate programs may indicate junior or senior levels, semester levels, doctorate candidate, and so forth. These intermediate objectives lead to course objectives though in some programs course objectives are directly linked to the end-of-program objectives instead of level or semester objectives.

Chapter 4 presents the classic educational taxonomies and assists in developing end-of-program, intermediate, and course objectives. To develop or assess end-of-program objectives, the first task is to look at the program mission, purpose, and overall goal. Faculty members discuss what they expect of their graduates at the end of the program to meet the overall goal. A list of these expectations is developed into end-of-program objectives, which are assessed for their specificity in meeting the overall goal or purpose and the selected organizing framework of the curriculum. For example, if Watson's theory (1979) on caring as the central core of nursing is the theoretical framework, the end-of-program objectives should include a statement(s) on knowledge and skills in caring.

Intermediate, level, or semester objectives follow the end-of-program objectives, and each of these steps may be viewed deductively or inductively to ensure that the total body of knowledge and skills expected at the end of the program are included in the curriculum plan. All levels of objectives provide information for planning and implementing the curriculum. Faculty reviews each level for the progression of objectives toward the end-of-program objectives. Some programs start from basic knowledge and skills at the first level or semester to the complex knowledge and skills expected at the senior level of the program. Other programs expect mastery of specific knowledge and skills earlier in the program at lower levels. Decisions on the patterns of progression will depend on the philosophy and conceptual framework, including the developmental stage of the learner. These decisions should be documented with rationales for their placement in the curriculum to aid in evaluation of the curriculum and total quality management of the program.

Implementation Plan

The overall goal, end-of-program objectives, level or intermediate objectives, and organizing framework serve as a master plan for placing content into the curriculum. Faculty is responsible for developing the curriculum plan and revising it periodically as needed. The prerequisites for the program are examined for their logical location in the curriculum. Prerequisites for prelicensure nursing programs include the liberal arts; social, physical, and biologic sciences; communications; mathematics; and other general education requirements specific to the institution.

Graduate nursing programs usually require a baccalaureate in nursing, although students with associate degrees in nursing and baccalaureates in other disciplines can sometimes be admitted conditionally, subject to completing prescribed courses in nursing that the faculty designates as meeting the equivalent of a baccalaureate in nursing. The same principles apply to nursing or other disciplines' doctorate programs. Each doctoral program will prescribe the courses or degree work necessary to meet the equivalent of their lower degree requirements.

Once the prerequisites are completed, the nursing curriculum plan has a progressive order for nursing courses. For example, a Nursing 101 Fundamentals of Nursing course is a prerequisite for Nursing 102 Nursing Care of the Older Adult; similarly, Nursing 501 Nursing Research is the prerequisite for Nursing 502 Master's Thesis. Corequisites are courses that can be taught simultaneously and are complementary, for example, Nursing 301 Health Promotion of Children and Adolescents and Nursing 303 Nursing Care of Children and Adolescents. Again, the placement of courses depends on the organizing or conceptual framework with the level objectives and the course content matching that of the level and/or end-of-program objectives.

The numbers of units or credits are assigned to each course factoring in the total allotted to the major. For associate degree in nursing programs, nursing units average 30 units with total degree requirements averaging 60 to 70 units. Baccalaureate programs average 60 nursing units with a total of 120 to 130 units for the degree. The master's in nursing program ranges from 30 to 60 or more total units depending on the nature of the program, with advanced-practice roles requiring the higher number of units. The majority of the master's degree units are in the nursing major, with only a few from other disciplines or electives.

Content experts serve as guides for nursing course placements, and once the courses are placed in logical sequence, the course descriptions are written, usually by the content expert or the person who will serve as "faculty of record" (in charge of the course). Course descriptions are brief paragraphs with several comprehensive statements that provide an overview of the content of the course.

Course objectives follow the description and are based on the content of the course, place in the curriculum plan, relationship to the level and end-of-program objectives, and relevance to the conceptual framework. Finally, an outline of the course content is listed and should be tied to the objectives of the course. All of these components are subject to approval by faculty as well as the parent institution and serve as the template for course syllabi. Once established, faculty members who are assigned to courses have the freedom to rearrange or update the content and to teach the courses in their preferred method. However, changes to the course title, units, pre- or corequisites, objectives, or descriptions must undergo the same approval processes as the original courses. While this may appear stifling to academic freedom, it ensures the integrity of the curriculum.

Usually these course descriptions, objectives, and content outlines are presented to the program's curriculum committee for recommendations and approval, submitted to the total faculty for approval, and continue through the appropriate channels of the parent institution for final formal approval. Owing to the many layers of approval, faculty must be mindful of the initial proposals so that they will not need frequent revising as any changes are subject to the same review processes.

▲ SUMMARY

Chapter 7 reviewed the components of the curriculum and the processes faculty undergo in developing or revising curricula. Assessing and revising (if necessary) each component of the curriculum in logical sequence helps to maintain its integrity and ensure its quality. Faculty members are experts in their discipline and are, therefore, responsible for ensuring that essential knowledge as well as the latest breakthroughs in science is in the curriculum. Curriculum development and revision processes must be based on information from evaluation activities; the latest changes in the profession, health care, and society; and forecasts for the future. Table 7.1 provides guidelines for assessing the key components of a curriculum or educational program.

C A S E   S T U D Y

▼

The case study from Chapters 5 and 6 continues with a description of the processes faculty used in a fictional school of nursing to develop a curriculum for an outreach program. If the same degree is to be offered from the same institution, the curriculum needs to be the same. The administration and faculty of the nursing school completed the recommendations from the needs assessment of the external and internal frame factors. The decision to initiate an entry-level Master of Science in Nursing (MSN) program was agreed upon, the accrediting agencies approved it, and the program is to start in the summer semester from the time the curriculum is developed. Because the School of Nursing has an entry-level MSN program on its home campus, the task is to take that same curriculum and adapt it to an outreach program. The process is based on the guidelines found in Table 7.1 and the components of the curriculum.

Mission

The faculty reviewed the existing college and School of Nursing mission statements in the most recent accreditation reports as well as the college catalogue and recruiting materials. The college mission states: "The mission of the College is to educate students in the traditions of the liberal arts, sciences, and spiritual beliefs of its founding fathers to become intellectually and socially responsible, compassionate citizens and leaders in their communities and society." The School of Nursing mission statement states: "The mission of the School of Nursing is to prepare intellectually and socially aware, competent, and compassionate nurses and nurse leaders to meet the health care needs of their communities and society."

(*case study continues on page 180*)

The faculty agrees that both missions are similar and contain elements of teaching, service, and research. Specifically, the School of Nursing mission implies teaching and learning by the verb "prepare" and all that it entails, including acquisition of knowledge and skills. The service element specifies that the graduates will provide competent and compassionate care to communities and society and the allusions to intellectual and social awareness imply research or in this case, scholarly activities. Because the outreach program is an adaptation of the existing entry-level master's track on campus and operates within the mission, it is determined that the outreach program is not in conflict with the current college and School of Nursing mission statements, which, in turn, are congruent.

Philosophy

The philosophy statement of the college is as follows: "The College fosters the liberal study of the arts and sciences, of humanity in its diverse historical and cultural forms, and of the insight derived from spiritual and religious study. Students and faculty interact in critical and creative thinking processes and effective communication to acquire the skills needed for active participation and leadership in transforming their communities and the world. Through faculty's research and scholarly activities and collaborative teaching and learning processes, students cultivate a global perspective that embodies the values of social justice and compassion and results in the responsible valuing and sharing of knowledge and skills as articulate and responsible citizens and leaders in their communities."

The School of Nursing philosophy states: "Students and faculty of the School of Nursing interact in teaching and learning processes that empower students to build upon a strong liberal arts and sciences foundation and assimilate the nursing knowledge and skills that lead to the provision of competent and compassionate nursing care and leadership for multicultural and ethnic persons, families, aggregates, and communities. The nursing paradigm guides the students and faculty in the teaching and learning processes to foster creative thought, critical thinking, clinical decision making, and ethical and professional judgments. The faculty defines the metaparadigm as:

Nursing: a science and profession that provides independent and interdependent nursing and health care for multicultural and ethnic clients in multiple health care settings. The profession has a major role in recognizing social justice issues and shaping public policy that affect the health of the local, regional, and world communities.

Client system: is composed of multicultural, racial, and ethnic individual persons, families, aggregates, or communities and is the focus of nursing care. The individual person is a spiritual, biopsychosocial being in need of nursing care and health services. The family is composed of persons with close biologic or psychosocial ties that bind them together as a subsystem of the community in which they are members. The aggregate is a group of persons with at-risk health needs within the community in which they are members. The community is composed of individuals, groups, and aggregates with social, geographic, functional, or political ties.

Health: the optimum state of well-being along a continuum of wellness and illness throughout the life span from conception to death.

Environment: the milieu and external factors that surround the care-giving phenomenon and the interactions of the client system and care provider with these factors."

(continued)

An analysis of the philosophies of the college and School of Nursing reveals that they are congruent. Although the nursing philosophy does not speak specifically to that of the college's statement on religious study, it incorporates the notion of spirituality and designates the study of liberal arts and sciences including religious studies as the foundation for nursing knowledge and skills. The nursing statement includes teaching and learning, ethnic diversity, critical thinking, clinical decision making, and professional and ethical judgments. It adapts its definitions of the client systems that relate to the four-domain nursing metaparadigm. The philosophy is broad enough to incorporate all of the programs within nursing including the outreach program.

Organizing Framework

The organizing framework for the curriculum that applies to all programs in the School of Nursing is that of Webber's (2002) Nursing Knowledge, Skills, Values, Meaning, and Experience (KSVME) model. Nursing knowledge is defined as "the cumulative, organized, and dynamic body of scientific and phenomenological information used to identify, relate, understand, explain, predict, influence and/or control nursing phenomena. Skills are deliberate acts or activities in the cognitive and psychomotor domain that operationalize nursing knowledge, meanings, and experience" (Johnson & Webber, 2001; Webber, 2002, pp 4-5, Webber, 2000). "Values are enduring beliefs, attributes, or ideals that establish moral boundaries of what is right and wrong in thought, judgment, character, attitude, and behavior that form a foundation for decision making throughout life" (Johnson & Webber, 2001; Kozier, Erb, & Blais, 1997; Webber, 2002, p 6). "Meanings define the context, purpose, and intent of language. Nursing Experience refers to the unique and active process of defining, refining, and changing" (Webber, 2002, p. 6).

Faculty members analyze the framework for its relationship to the mission and philosophy statements and find it to be congruent. The "knowledge and skills" portions of the framework apply to the statements on teaching and learning and scholarly activities. The "values" of the model relate to the philosophy's statements on ethical and professional judgments and preparation for competent and compassionate care. "Meanings" in the framework are directly applicable to the definitions of the nursing metaparadigm found in the philosophy, and "experience" is implied in the mission and philosophy when referring again to preparing nurses who provide competent and compassionate nursing and health care. All levels of nurse education preparation relate to this framework as well as the entry-level MSN outreach program. As the faculty prepares to adapt the entry-level curriculum to the outreach program it will look for evidence of the KSVME model in the program.

Overall Purpose and Goal of the Program

The School of Nursing's overall goal is: "The School of Nursing prepares highly competent and compassionate nurses and nurse leaders to deliver professional nursing care and interdisciplinary health care for multicultural and ethnic people, families, aggregates, and communities in all settings."

The faculty agrees that the goal is broad enough to encompass the undergraduate and graduate programs. Some members raise the question about the term *nurse leaders* as it applies to the baccalaureate program; however, they agree that leadership in its broadest terms apply to those graduates as well as the graduates of the master's program. They point to the baccalaureate senior-level nursing

(case study continues on page 182)

management course as well as the health policy course as foundations for preparing nurse leaders. The overall goal provides guidelines for the end-of-program objectives for all of the tracks and for evaluation of the outcomes of the program. By analyzing the mission and philosophy of the school, terms in the goal statement can be traced back to terms in those statements.

End-of-Program and Level Objectives

Because the outreach program is an adaptation of the entry-level master's program, its end-of-program objectives are examined for their flow from the overall goal, mission, and philosophy. The objectives are as follows:

At the end of the entry-level master's program the graduate will:

1. Synthesize knowledge from other disciplines to develop intellectual and social knowledge and skills that apply to nursing and responsibilities as citizens and leaders in the community and society.
2. Apply advanced nursing knowledge and skills to provide competent and compassionate nursing care for multicultural and ethnic people, families, aggregates, and communities across the lifespan in a variety of health care settings.
3. Value the professional role of nursing and interdisciplinary collaboration in the delivery of health care through community service and scholarly activities.
4. Contribute to the development of nursing as a science through the use of theory and scientific processes.
5. Using a broad understanding of social justice issues and participate in nursing and health policy actions to improve the health care delivery system.
6. Commit to lifelong learning through continuing education.
7. Gain the foundation for advanced-practice nursing and doctoral studies.

The analysis of the objectives demonstrates a congruency with the mission, philosophy, conceptual framework, and overall goal. Thus, the faculty moves on to the level or intermediate objectives.

Level Objectives

The entry-level master's program consists of two levels. The first level is the prelicensure content and is three semesters in length. The second level is at the graduate level and is another three semesters. The program begins in the summer and runs through another summer. Thus, the program is a total of 2 and 1/4 calendar years. The level objectives are as follows:

Level One: At the end of the Level One courses the student will be able to:

1. Apply knowledge from other disciplines to the nursing care of multicultural and ethnic individuals and families across the lifespan.
2. Apply nursing knowledge and skills with competency and compassion for multicultural and ethnic individuals and families in select health care settings.
3. Analyze the professional role of nursing and its collaborative role with other health care disciplines.

(continued)

4. Analyze the organization of the health care system and the role of nursing in health-related issues and public policy.
5. Apply current and relevant nursing research to the practice of nursing.

Level Two: At the end of the Level Two courses, the graduate will be able to:

1. Apply knowledge from other disciplines to the nursing care of multicultural and ethnic individuals, families, aggregates, and communities.
2. Apply advanced nursing knowledge and skills with competency and compassion for multicultural and ethnic individuals, families, aggregates, and communities in select health care settings.
3. Value the professional role of nursing and interdisciplinary collaboration in the delivery of health care through community service and scholarly activities.
4. Contribute to the development of nursing as a science through the use of theory and scientific processes.
5. Using a broad understanding of social justice issues, participate in nursing and health policy actions to improve the health care delivery system.
6. Commit to lifelong learning through continuing education
7. Gain the foundation for advanced-practice nursing and doctoral studies.

The faculty agrees that the level objectives come from the end-of-program objectives, are learner focused, and contain the content of what is to be learned, when, and to what extent. The level objectives imply mastery of the content and, because they must be met by the end of three semesters of course work for each level and are arranged in sequential order, it is assumed they are feasible. However, analysis of the courses in each level will provide further information as to their feasibility. The courses will also be analyzed for their relationship to the KSVME conceptual framework (Webber, 2000). The following is the implementation plan for the existing entry-level MSN track with course descriptions, objectives, and content outlines.

Curriculum Plan: Outreach Entry-Level Master of Science in Nursing

Prerequisites

A baccalaureate with a 3.0 or higher cumulative grade point average in the last 60 credits
One semester Anatomy with a lab
One semester Physiology with a lab (or two semesters of a combined Anatomy and Physiology course with labs)
One semester Microbiology with a lab
One semester Statistics
One semester Chemistry
Two semesters of Communications, written and oral
One semester of a Social Sciences course
One semester Human Development across the Lifespan

(case study continues on page 184)

Level 1

SEMESTER 1

Nursing and Health Care
3 units of theory (**KVM**)*

Prerequisite Courses
Human Development, Social Science, Written and Oral Communications

Description
Introduces the student to the nursing profession, its history, the science of nursing, current issues, and ethics. Discusses the role of the multidisciplinary health care team. Reviews the definitions of health and the health and illness continuum across the lifespan.

Objectives
At the end of the course the student will be able to:

1. Analyze the history of nursing and its impact on its status as a profession and a discipline.
2. Compare the definitions of a profession and an academic discipline to nursing.
3. Review the major health disciplines and their role in providing health care.
4. Formulate a definition of health and illness across a continuum and the lifespan for multicultural and ethnic people.
5. Examine selected issues in health care and nursing that have an impact on health care and the ethics for providing nursing care.

Content Outline
1. Nursing History
2. Nursing as a Profession
3. Nursing as a Science and an Academic Discipline
4. The Multi- or Interdisciplinary Health Care Team
5. Health and Illness Definitions
6. Diversity and the Delivery of Competent and Compassionate Nursing Care
7. Health Care Issues and the Ethics of Nursing Care

Pathophysiology
3 units theory (**KM**)*

Prerequisite Courses
Anatomy and Physiology, Chemistry, Human Development, Microbiology

Corequisites
Basic Skills I, Health Assessment, Nursing Care of Older Adults

Description
Focuses on alterations and responses of the human body to altered states of health, environmental stresses, and the aging process.

(continued)

* Signifies the components of the Nursing Knowledge, Skills, Values, Meanings, and Experiences (KSVME) conceptual framework.

Objectives

At the end of the course the student will be able to:

1. Analyze each body system for alterations and responses to disease, varying states of health, environmental stresses, and the aging process.
2. Analyze the body as a whole in its alterations and responses to disease, varying states of health, environmental stresses, and the aging process.
3. Discuss selected diagnoses of health problems, their pathophysiology, and common interventions for their resolution.

Content Outline

1. Review of Normal Anatomy and Physiology of the Human
2. Effects of Disease on Selected Body Systems
3. Effects of Environmental Stresses on Selected Body Systems
4. Effects of the Aging Process on the Human Body
5. Major Health Problems, Their Pathophysiology, Diagnosis, and Common Interventions for Their Treatment

Health Assessment

2 units: 1 unit theory, 1 unit lab (2-hour lab on campus) (**KSVME**)*

Prerequisite Courses

Anatomy and Physiology, Human Development, Oral and Written Communications, Social Science

Corequisites

Basic Skills I, Pathophysiology, Nursing and Health Care, Nursing Care of Older Adults

Description

Introduces the nursing process. Applies communication skills and knowledge from the biologic and social sciences to the subjective and objective assessment of multicultural and ethnic individuals across the lifespan to identify deviations from normal.

Objectives

At the end of the course the student will be able to:

1. Apply the nursing process to the health assessment of multicultural and ethnic individuals and families across the lifespan.
2. Apply oral and written communications skills in the assessment of multicultural and ethnic individuals and families across the lifespan.
3. Apply knowledge of sociology and human development to the health history of multicultural and ethnic individuals and families across the lifespan.
4. Apply knowledge of anatomy and physiology to the physical examination of multicultural and ethnic individuals and families across the lifespan.
5. Diagnose major deviations from normal in the health assessment of multicultural and ethnic individuals and families across the lifespan

(case study continues on page 186)

Content Outline
1. The Nursing Process and Practice
2. Interview Techniques and Lab Practice
3. Written Documentation and Lab Practice
4. Components of the Health History and Lab Practice
    a. Individuals
    b. Families
5. Components of the Physical Examination and Lab Practice
    a. Individuals
    b. Families
6. Diagnosis of Deviations from Normal and Lab Practice

Basic Skills I
1 unit (2-hour lab on campus) (**KSVME**)*

Prerequisite Courses
Anatomy and Physiology, Chemistry, Human Development, Microbiology, Oral and Written Communications, Social Science, Statistics

Corequisite
Care of the Older Adult, Health Assessment, Pathophysiology, Nursing, and Health Care

Description
Introduces fundamental nursing skills including oral administration of drugs, activities of daily living, transfer techniques, and documentation of nursing care.

Objectives
At the end of the course the student will be able to:

1. Demonstrate competent nursing skills in the provision of care for activities of daily living for multicultural and ethnic individuals across the lifespan.
2. Demonstrate safe transfer techniques for physically compromised individuals across the lifespan.
3. Demonstrate competence in the calculation and administration of oral medications.
4. Demonstrate competence in the documentation of nursing care.

Content Outline
1. Activities of Daily Living and Lab Practice
2. Transfer Techniques and Lab Practice
3. Oral Medications Calculations and Administration and Lab Practice
4. Documentation and Legal Issues With Lab Practice

Care of the Older Adult
3 units (1 unit theory and 2 units lab with 6 hours clinical experience in elder care settings) (**KSVME**)*

Prerequisite Courses
Anatomy and Physiology, Human Development, Microbiology, Oral and Written Communications, Social Science

(continued)

Corequisites
Basic Skills I, Health Assessment, Pathophysiology, Nursing and Health Care

Description
Provides theories and concepts in geriatric nursing and opportunities for students to practice nursing care for multicultural and ethnic elders in community settings, assisted-living, and skilled nursing facilities.

Objectives
At the end of the course the student will be able to:

1. Develop an awareness of the aging process and its impact on individuals and their families.
2. Analyze major health problems and the biopsychosocial and spiritual needs of the multicultural and ethnic elder population and their families.
3. Apply health assessment knowledge and skills to multicultural and ethnic elders in a variety of care settings.
4. Apply the theories and concepts of the aging process to the provision of competent and compassionate basic nursing care for multicultural and ethnic elders in a variety of care settings.
5. Demonstrate awareness of the role of other health care providers in the delivery of health care services to elders.

Content Outline
1. The Aging Process
   a. Individuals
   b. Families
2. Major Health Problems Related to Aging
   a. Individuals
   b. Families
3. Biopsychosocial Health Needs of the Older Population
   a. Individuals
   b. Families
4. Roles of Other Health Care Providers in Elder Health Care Services
5. Health Assessment and Nursing Care of Individual Elders and Clinical Practice
   a. At home
   b. In assisted-living facilities
   c. In skilled nursing facilities

Total Units: 12 Units

SEMESTER 2

Nursing Care of Reproductive Families
5 units (2 theory and 3 clinical hours for 9 clinical hours per week in reproductive health care settings) (**KSVME**)*

(*case study continues on page 188*)

Prerequisite Courses
Basic Skills I, Care of the Older Adult, Health Assessment, Pathophysiology, Nursing and Health Care

Corequisite Courses
Basic Skills II, Pharmacology, Nursing Care of Children and Adolescents

Description
Reviews theories and concepts related to health promotion strategies for multicultural and ethnic reproductive families. Introduces nursing care for well families and those who are experiencing deviations from normal or major health problems. Applies health assessment and nursing skills to the care of reproductive families in a variety of multidiscipline health care settings.

Objectives
At the end of the course the student will be able to:

1. Apply human development theories and concepts to the competent and compassionate care of multicultural and ethnic reproductive families.
2. Apply family theories and concepts to the competent and compassionate care of multicultural and ethnic reproductive families.
3. Analyze normal reproductive life processes as they apply to the care of multicultural and ethnic families.
4. Diagnose deviations from normal and major health problems in multicultural and ethnic reproductive families.
5. Provide knowledgeable, competent, and compassionate nursing care for multicultural and ethnic reproductive families in a variety of care settings.
6. Coordinate care with other health care providers.

Content Outline
1. Review of Human Development in Reproductive Families
   a. The reproductive systems
   b. Biopsychosocial and spiritual effects of reproduction on individuals and families
2. Family Theories and Concepts
   a. General theories
   b. The reproductive family
3. Nursing Care of Multicultural and Ethnic Reproductive Families
4. Deviations from Normal in the Reproductive Cycle
5. Major Health Problems and Complications Related to the Reproductive Process
6. The Nursing Process in the Care of Multicultural and Ethnic Reproductive Families and Clinical Practice in a Variety of Interdisciplinary Settings

Nursing Care of Children and Adolescents
5 units (2 theory and 3 clinical hours for 9 clinical hours per week in pediatric and well child/adolescent health care settings) (**KSMVE**)*

Prerequisite Courses
Basic Skills I, Care of the Older Adult, Health Assessment, Pathophysiology, Nursing and Health Care

(*continued*)

Corequisite Courses
Basic Skills II, Pharmacology, Nursing Care of Reproductive Families

Description
Reviews theories and concepts related to health promotion strategies for children and adolescents and nursing care for those who are experiencing deviations from normal and major health problems. Applies health assessment and nursing skills to the care of multicultural and ethnic children and adolescents in a variety of multidiscipline health care settings.

Objectives
At the end of the course the student will be able to:

1. Apply human growth and development theories and concepts to the competent and compassionate care of multicultural and ethnic children and adolescents and their families.
2. Apply family theories and concepts to the competent and compassionate care of multicultural children and adolescents and their families.
3. Interpret well-child guidelines to the care and health education of multicultural and ethnic children, adolescents, and their families.
4. Diagnose deviations from normal and major health problems in multicultural and ethnic children and adolescents.
5. Provide knowledgeable, competent, and compassionate nursing care for multicultural and ethnic children and adolescents and their families in a variety of care settings.
6. Coordinate care with other health care providers.

Content Outline
1. Review of Human Development in Children, Adolescents, and Their Families
2. Family Theories and Concepts as they apply to:
   a. Children and their families
   b. Adolescents and their families
3. Well-Child Care and Health Promotion of Multicultural and Ethnic Children, Adolescents, and Their Families and Clinical Practice
4. Deviations from Normal in Children, Adolescents, and Their Families
5. Major Health Problems in Children and Adolescents
6. The Role of Other Disciplines in the Care of Children and Adolescents
7. The Nursing Process in the Care of Multicultural and Ethnic Children and Adolescents and Clinical Practice in a Variety of Settings

Pharmacology
3 units theory (**KM**)*

Prerequisite Courses
Basic Skills I, Care of the Older Adult, Health Assessment, Pathophysiology, Nursing and Health Care

Corequisite Courses
Basic Skills II, Nursing Care of Reproductive Families, Nursing Care of Children and Adolescents

(*case study continues on page 190*)

Description
Introduces the student to pharmacology and its role in health care. Differentiates among prescribed drugs, over-the-counter drugs, and substance abuse. Reviews the pharmacology and the major classifications of drugs and their actions, interactions, and side effects.

Objectives
At the end of the course the student will be able to:

1. Describe the role of pharmacology and its practitioners and clinicians in health care.
2. Differentiate among the use of prescriptions, over-the-counter drugs, and substance abuse.
3. Analyze the actions, interactions, and side effects of the major classifications of drugs.

Content Outline
1. Pharmacology
   a. Discipline
   b. Practitioners and clinicians
2. Definitions
   a. Pharmacotherapeutics
   b. Over-the-counter drugs
   c. Substance abuse
3. Major Classifications of Drugs
   a. Actions
   b. Interactions
   c. Side effects

Basic Skills II
1 unit (2-hour lab on campus) (**KSME**)*

Prerequisite Courses
Basic Skills I, Care of the Older Adult, Health Assessment, Pathophysiology, Nursing and Health Care

Corequisite Courses
Nursing Care of Reproductive Families, Nursing Care of Children and Adolescents, Pharmacology

Description
Continues nursing skills including all routes of administration of medications, immunizations, treatments, and documentation.

Objectives
At the end of the course the student will be able to:

1. Apply nursing skills safely and competently for the care of multicultural and ethnic individuals experiencing episodes of illness and in need of immunizations, including:
   a. The components of a prescription
   b. Multiple routes of administration for medication interventions and immunizations

(*continued*)

    c. Review of prescribed orders for:
      i. Drug actions
      ii. Correct calculation of dosage
      iii. Possible side effects or interactions with other drugs
      iv. Medically and nursing prescribed treatment interventions
2. Document nursing care according to legal requirements, nursing responsibilities, accuracy, and accepted terminology.

Content Outline
1. Drug Administration and Immunizations and Lab Practice
    a. Routes of administration
    b. Dosage calculation
    c. Actions, interactions, and side effects
2. Treatments and Lab Practice
3. Documentation and Lab Practice
    a. Legal requirements and nursing responsibilities
    b. Accuracy
    c. Terminology

Total Units: 14 units

SEMESTER 3

Nursing Care of Adults
5 units (2 theory and 3 clinical hours for 9 clinical hours per week in acute care settings) **(KSVME)***

Prerequisite Courses
Basic Skills II, Nursing Care of Children and Adolescents, Nursing Care of Reproductive Families, Pharmacology

Corequisite Courses
Mental Health and Psychiatric Nursing Care, Nursing Management and Leadership

Description
Reviews theories and concepts of health promotion strategies for adults and nursing care for adults experiencing acute episodes of illness. Applies nursing management and leadership skills to the care of adults in acute care settings and coordinates care with other disciplines.

Objectives
At the end of the course the student will be able to:

1. Analyze health promotion and maintenance theories and concepts and their application to the nursing care of well, multicultural and ethnic adults.
2. Analyze the disease processes in major acute episodes of illness and their effects on multicultural and ethnic adults individuals and their families.

(*case study continues on page 192*)

3. Provide competent and compassionate health promotion nursing strategies for adults and their families.
4. Provide competent and compassionate nursing care to adults experiencing episodes of acute illness.
5. Apply leadership and management skills to the acute care setting in the care of adults and their families.
6. Coordinate care with other disciplines.

Content Outline
1. Health Promotion and Health Maintenance in the Care of Multicultural and Ethnic Adults
   a. Theories and concepts
   b. Competent and compassionate nursing strategies and clinical practice in a variety of community settings.
2. Major Illnesses and Health Problems in Multicultural and Ethnic Adults
   a. Diseases, diagnoses, and treatment
   b. Health problems, diagnoses, and interventions
   c. Competent and compassionate nursing interventions through clinical practice in a variety of acute care settings
3. The Role of Other Health Disciplines in the Health Care of Adults and Their Families
4. Application of Nursing Leadership and Management Skills in a Variety of Acute Care Settings

Mental Health and Psychiatric Nursing Care
5 units (2 theory and 3 clinical hours for 9 clinical hours per week in pediatric and well child/adolescent health care settings) (**KSMVE**)*

Prerequisite Courses
Basic Skills II, Nursing Care of Children and Adolescents, Nursing Care of Reproductive Families, Pharmacology

Corequisite Courses
Nursing Care of Adults, Nursing Management and Leadership

Description
Reviews theories and concepts of mental health promotion strategies across the lifespan. Provides opportunities for nursing care practice for multicultural and ethnic individuals and families who are experiencing episodes of psychiatric illness. Reviews coordination of care and provides opportunities for practice with other mental health and psychiatric care providers.

Objectives
At the end of the course the student will be able to:

1. Analyze mental health promotion and maintenance theories and concepts and their application to the nursing care of multicultural and ethnic individuals across the lifespan.
2. Analyze the disease processes related to major acute episodes of psychiatric illness and their effects on multicultural and ethnic individuals and their families.

(continued)

3. Provide competent and compassionate mental health promotion nursing strategies for multicultural and ethnic individuals and families across the lifespan.
4. Provide competent and compassionate nursing care to multicultural and ethnic individuals and families across the lifespan experiencing acute episodes of psychiatric illness.
5. Coordinate mental health and psychiatric nursing care with other disciplines.

Content Outline
1. Mental Health Promotion Maintenance in the Care of Multicultural and Ethnic Individuals and Families Across the Lifespan
  a. Theories and concepts
  b. Competent and compassionate nursing strategies and clinical practice in a variety of interdisciplinary mental health community settings
2. Major Psychiatric Illnesses in Multicultural and Ethnic Individuals and Families
  a. Disease processes, diagnoses, and treatment
  b. Competent and compassionate nursing interventions through clinical practice in a variety of acute psychiatric care settings
3. Other Health Disciplines in the Mental Health and Psychiatric Care of Individuals and Their Families
  a. Roles and coordination of care
  b. Clinical practice opportunities to coordinate care

Nursing Management and Leadership
3 units theory (**KSMV**)*

Prerequisites
Basic Skills II, Nursing Care of Children and Adolescents, Nursing Care of Reproductive Families, Pharmacology

Corequisite Courses
Nursing Care of Adults, Nursing Management and Leadership

Description
Introduces organizational behavior in health care settings. Provides the theory and concepts for nursing management and leadership including the supervision of nursing staff and collaboration with other health care providers. Analyzes the role of nursing in leadership and management in health care settings.

Objectives
At the end of the course the student will be able to:

1. Analyze health care organizational behavior and its influence on nursing.
2. Analyze theories, models, and principles of nursing leadership and management.
3. Apply team and supervisory processes in nursing to health care settings.
4. Participate in the collaborative role of nursing with other health care providers.

(case study continues on page 194)

Content
1. Health Care Organizational Behavior and Nursing
2. Theories, Models, and Principles of:
    a. Nursing management
    b. Nursing leadership
3. Team Management
4. Supervisory Roles and Processes in Nursing
5. Composition of the Nursing Staff
    a. Education and qualifications
6. Collaboration and Roles of Other Health Care Providers

Introduction to Nursing Research
2 units theory (**KSMV**)*

Prerequisite Courses
Basic Skills I, Care of the Older Adult, Health Assessment, Pathophysiology, Nursing and Health Care

Description
Introduces nursing research and theories and their application to practice. Includes the research process and how to critique research studies.

Objectives
At the end of the course the student will be able to:

1. Differentiate between research, surveys, studies, and program evaluation.
2. Analyze the steps in the research process.
3. Demonstrate knowledge of the various types of nursing research.
4. Critique several nursing research studies from the literature.
5. Describe the application of a research study to nursing practice.

Content Outline
1. Studies, Program Evaluation, and Surveys Versus Research
2. Types of Research
3. The Research Process
4. Nursing Research in the Literature and Its Critique
5. Application of Research Findings to Nursing Practice

Total Units: 15 units

Level 2

SEMESTER 4

Community Health Nursing
5 units (2 theory and 3 clinical hours for 9 clinical hours per week in community health settings) (**KSVME**)*

(continued)

Prerequisite Courses
Introduction to Nursing Research, Nursing Care of Adults, Mental Health and Psychiatric Nursing, Nursing Management and Leadership

Corequisite Courses
Epidemiology, Health Care Policy and Social Justice, Theoretical Foundations of Nursing Science

Description
Reviews theories and concepts of public health and community health nursing. Examines the roles of health care team members in community settings. Applies disease prevention and health promotion strategies for multicultural and ethnic families, aggregates, and communities in community health care settings.

Objectives
At the end of the course the student will be able to:

1. Analyze the discipline of public health and its role in the health care system.
2. Analyze the role of the multidisciplinary health care team in public and community health.
3. Compare and contrast community health and public health.
4. Analyze the classic levels of prevention.
5. Apply health promotion and disease prevention strategies for multicultural and ethnic individuals, families, aggregates, and the community in community health settings.

Content Outline
1. Public Health
   a. Organization
   b. Services
   c. Nursing role
2. Community Health
   a. Definitions
   b. Services
   c. Nursing role
3. The Multidisciplinary Health Care Team in Public Health and Community Health
4. The Target Systems in Public Health and Community Health
   a. Families
   b. Aggregates
   c. Communities
5. Levels of Prevention
   a. Disease prevention
   b. Health promotion
   c. Health maintenance
6. Health Promotion and Disease Strategies in the Care of Individuals, Families, Aggregates, and the Community and Practice in a Variety of Public Health and Community Health Settings

(*case study continues on page 196*)

Epidemiology
3 units of theory (**KM**)*

Prerequisite Courses
Introduction to Nursing Research, Nursing Care of Adults, Mental Health and Psychiatric Nursing, Nursing Management and Leadership

Corequisite Courses
Community Health Nursing, Health Care Policy and Social Justice, Theoretical Foundations of Nursing Science

Description
Presents theories and models of epidemiology and their application to nursing and health care interventions. Reviews environmental health and ecology and their contributions to epidemiology. Utilizes biostatistics as it applies to the analysis of health data and epidemiology models.

Objectives
At the end of the course the student will be able to:

1. Define the science of epidemiology and the role of the epidemiologist.
2. Analyze common theories and models in epidemiology and their application to the public health and community health practices.
3. Discuss environmental health and ecology and their role in epidemiology.
4. Analyze epidemiologic methods and the application of biostatistics in the diagnosis of health problems in aggregates and communities.
5. Relate the role of epidemiology in nursing.

Content Outline
1. Epidemiology
   a. Definition
   b. Common terms
   c. The role of the epidemiologist in health care
2. Common Theories and Models in Epidemiology
   a. Application to public health and community health
   b. Methodology
3. Environmental Health and Ecology and Their Role in Epidemiology
4. Biostatistics
   a. Common rates
   b. Application to epidemiologic studies
5. Role of Epidemiology in Nursing

Health Care Policy and Social Justice
3 units theory (**KMV**)*

Prerequisites
Introduction to Nursing Research, Nursing Care of Adults, Mental Health and Psychiatric Nursing, Nursing Management and Leadership

(*continued*)

Corequisite Courses
Community Health Nursing, Epidemiology, Theoretical Foundations of Nursing Science

Description
Examines local, regional, national, and international health care systems and the social policy issues related to them. Describes strategies for shaping public policy in the health and social political arenas.

Objectives
At the end of the course the student will be able to:

1. Compare local, regional, national, and international health care systems.
2. Identify major social policy issues related to the various health systems.
3. Debate the public policy issues that affect aggregates, communities, or health care systems in terms of social justice and the delivery of health care.
4. Discuss the nursing profession's responsibilities in responding to injustices in the health care of multicultural and ethnic aggregates and communities.
5. Formulate nursing strategies for shaping public policy in health care.

Content Outline
1. Local Regional, National, and International Health Care Systems
2. Social Policy Issues in Health Care Systems
3. Social Justice and the Delivery of Health Care
4. The Nursing Profession's Responsibilities
5. Nursing Strategies for Shaping Public Policy in Health Care

Theoretical Foundations of Nursing Science
3 units theory (**KMV**)*

Prerequisite Courses
Introduction to Nursing Research, Nursing Care of Adults, Mental Health and Psychiatric Nursing, Nursing Management and Leadership

Corequisite Courses
Community Health Nursing, Epidemiology, Health Care Policy and Social Justice

Description
Discusses concepts, theories, and models for building bodies of knowledge, disciplines, and professions. Reviews the nursing metaparadigm and leading nurse theorists as they apply to the science and practice of nursing.

Objectives
At the end of the course the student will be able to:

1. Differentiate among theories, concepts, models, and constructs in the process of theory building.
2. Analyze the nursing metaparadigm and its application to the development of the discipline and profession.
3. Compare major nursing theories for their relevance to the nursing metaparadigm.
4. Evaluate major nursing theories and their application to nursing as a science and practice.

(*case study continues on page 198*)

Content Outline
1. Theory Building
    a. Theories
    b. Concepts
    c. Models
2. Constructs
3. The Nursing Metaparadigm
4. Major Nursing Theories
5. The Application of Nursing Theory to the Body of Knowledge and Practice

Total Units: 14 units

SEMESTER 5

Nursing Management of Acute Disease With Internship in a Clinical Specialty
6 units: 2 theory units and 4 clinical units for 12 clinical hours per week in select health care settings
(KSVME)*

Prerequisite Courses
Community Health Nursing, Epidemiology, Health Policy and Social Justice, Theoretical
Foundations of Nursing Science

Corequisite Courses
Advanced Health Assessment, Advanced Pharmacology, Research Methods

Description
Reviews the diagnosis and treatment of major acute diseases and traumatic injuries and their impact
on multicultural and ethnic client systems in a clinical specialty. In collaboration with other disciplines, applies the nursing process to the care of select client systems in acute, emergency, and/or
intensive care settings.

Objectives
At the end of the course the student will be able to:

1. Analyze major acute illnesses and traumatic injuries and their diagnoses, causes, pathophysiology,
    effects, and interventions in the care of multicultural and ethnic clients in a selected clinical
    specialty.
2. Evaluate the health care system's effectiveness in caring for the acutely ill or injured.
3. Collaborate with other health care providers in the acute care setting.
4. Provide skillful, competent, and compassionate advanced nursing care for acutely ill or injured
    multicultural and ethnic clients in select acute, emergency, and/or intensive care settings.

Content Outline
1. Major Acute Illnesses and Traumatic Injuries
    a. Diagnosis

(continued)

    b. Cause and effects

    c. Interventions

2. Acute Health Care Systems

3. Collaborative Role With Other Health Care Providers

4. Advanced Nursing Care for Acutely Ill or Injured Multicultural and Ethnic Clients and Practice in Acute, Emergency and/or Intensive Care Specialty Settings

Advanced Health Assessment

2 units: 1 unit theory and 1 hour lab for 3 hours in the clinical setting(**KSVME**)*

Prerequisite Courses

Community Health Nursing, Epidemiology, Health Policy and Social Justice, Theoretical Foundations of Nursing Science

Corequisite Courses

Advanced Pharmacology, Nursing Management of Acute Disease with Internship in a Clinical Specialty, Research Methods

Description

Reviews theories and skills for the advanced health assessment of multicultural and ethnic individuals and families with acute health problems and major traumatic injuries and interventions for their management. Applies advanced health assessment skills and interventions for major acute health problems or major traumatic injuries in the specialty clinical setting.

Objectives

At the end of the course the student will be able to:

1. Systematically assess the acutely ill client for common health problems related to disease processes or major traumatic injuries.

2. Review interventions for the treatment of major acute illnesses or major traumatic injuries.

3. Apply advanced health assessment skills to the care of multicultural and ethnic clients experiencing acute episodes of illness or major traumatic injuries in acute care, emergency, and/or intensive care specialty settings.

Content Outline

1. Systematic Assessment of Body Systems Experiencing Acute Illness or Major Traumatic Injury

2. Interventions for Major Acute Illnesses and Traumatic Injuries

3. Advanced Health Assessment Skills in the Care of Acutely Ill Multicultural and Ethnic Clients

4. Advanced Health Assessment Skills in the Care of Clients With Major Traumatic Injuries

Advanced Pharmacology

3 units theory (**KSVM**)*

Prerequisite Courses

Community Health Nursing, Epidemiology, Health Policy and Social Justice, Theoretical Foundations of Nursing Science

(*case study continues on page 200*)

Corequisite Courses

Advanced Health Assessment, Nursing Management of Acute Disease with Internship in a Clinical Specialty, Research Methods

Description

Builds upon previous knowledge of drug classifications, effects, interactions, and side effects for the pharmacologic therapeutics for the management of chronic and acute illnesses.

Objectives

At the end of the course the student will be able to:

1. Review the major classification of drugs and their actions, interactions, and side effects.
2. Examine the role of the advanced-practice nurse in pharmacotherapeutics.
3. Analyze the clinical and therapeutic use of drugs in the treatment of illnesses in acute care, pain control, and management of chronic disease.

Content Outline:

1. Major Classifications of Drugs
   a. Actions
   b. Interactions
   c. Side effects
2. The Role of the Advanced-Practice Nurse in Pharmacotherapeutics
3. Clinical and Therapeutic Use of Drugs
   a. Management of acute illnesses
   b. Pain control
   c. Management of chronic disease

Research Methods

3 units theory (**KSVM**)*

Prerequisite Courses

Introduction to Nursing Research, Nursing Care of Adults, Mental Health and Psychiatric Nursing, Nursing Management and Leadership

Corequisite Courses

Advanced Health Assessment, Advanced Pharmacology Nursing Management of Acute Disease with Internship in a Clinical Specialty

Description

Reviews quantitative and qualitative research and the methodology for various types of research inquiries. Includes review of the literature and research processes and leads to a research (thesis) or special project proposal.

Objectives

At the end of the course the student will be able to:

1. Compare quantitative and qualitative research.

(continued)

2. Analyze research methodologies and their application to researchable questions.
3. Analyze each step of the research process for a variety of types of research studies.
4. Develop a research (thesis) or special project proposal, including an initial review of the literature pertaining to the topic.

Content Outline
1. Quantitative and Qualitative Research
2. Research Methodologies and Application to Research Inquiries
3. Steps of the Research Process and Application to Various Types of Research Studies
4. The Literature Review
5. Formulating a Research Question
  a. Thesis project
  b. Special project

Total Units: 14 units

SEMESTER 6

Nursing Management of Chronic Disease with Internship in A Clinical Specialty
6 units: 2 theory units and 4 clinical units for 12 clinical hours per week in select health care settings.
(KSVME)*

Prerequisite Courses
Advanced Health Assessment, Advanced Pharmacology, and Nursing Management of Acute Disease with Internship in a Clinical Specialty, Research Methods

Corequisite Courses
Leadership and Role Development in Nursing, Research Project or Thesis

Description
Reviews major chronic diseases, their diagnosis and treatment, and their impact on client systems in a selected clinical specialty. Reviews the effectiveness of the health care system in providing chronic disease services. In collaboration with other disciplines, applies the nursing process to the care of client systems in select health care settings.

Objectives
1. Analyze major chronic diseases and their diagnoses, causes, effects on the body, and interventions for care for selected multicultural and ethnic clients in a selected clinical specialty area.
2. Evaluate the effectiveness of the health care system in providing chronic disease services.
3. Collaborate with other health care providers in chronic care settings in providing health maintenance and health promotion services.
4. Provide skillful, competent, and compassionate advanced nursing care for the chronically ill in a selected clinical specialty.

(*case study continues on page 202*)

Content Outline
1. Major Chronic Diseases
   a. Diagnosis
   b. Cause and effects
   c. Interventions
2. Chronic Disease Health Care Systems
3. Collaborative Role with Other Health Care Providers and Practice in a Variety of Health Care Settings
4. Advanced Nursing Care of the Chronically Ill Multicultural and Ethnic Clients and Practice in a Selected Clinical Specialty

Leadership and Role Development in Nursing
3 units theory (**KSVM**)*

Prerequisite Courses
Advanced Health Assessment, Advanced Pharmacology, Nursing Management of Acute Disease with Internship in a Clinical Specialty, Research Methods

Corequisite Courses
Nursing Management of Chronic Disease with Internship in a Clinical Specialty, Research Project or Thesis

Description
Discusses theories, concepts, and models of health care economics, organization, and quality assurance as they apply to nurse leader, manager, educator, and consultant roles. Reviews teaching and learning theories for application to staff development and patient education.

Objectives
At the end of the course the student will be able to:

1. Apply advanced nursing knowledge to the leadership and management role of nursing.
2. Analyze health care economic systems and their impact on the delivery of health care services and the role of nursing.
3. Analyze quality assurance methodologies and their impact on the delivery of health care services and the role of nursing.
4. Apply teaching and learning theories to staff development and patient education situations.
5. Offer consultation as a community service according to one's expertise in health care for individuals, families, aggregates, and communities.

Content Outline
1. Leadership and Management in Nursing
   a. Theories and models
   b. Processes
   c. Roles as experts, clinicians, leaders, managers, and administrators

(*continued*)

2. Theories and Models in Health Care Economics
   a. Organizational systems
   b. Budgeting
   c. The role of nursing
3. Quality Assurance
   a. Theories and models
   b. Accreditation
   c. Program evaluation
   d. The role of nursing
4. Education
   a. Theories and concepts in teaching and learning
   b. Staff development and patient education
   c. The role of nursing
5. Consultation
   a. The role of consultant
   b. The nursing role

Research Project or Thesis
3 units theory (**KSVM**)*

Prerequisite Courses
Advanced Health Assessment, Advanced Pharmacology, Nursing Management of Acute Disease with Internship in a clinical Specialty, Research Methods

Corequisite Courses
Leadership and Role Development in Nursing, Nursing Management of Chronic Disease with Internship in a Clinical Specialty

Description
This is the capstone experience for the master's graduate program. The student completes a research project based on a literature review and an original proposal that applies to nursing practice or health care innovation, OR the student completes a master's thesis that is an original study and the product of the research process. Both the project and the thesis are under the guidance and approval of three faculty members.

Objective
At the end of the course the student will be able to:
      Complete a master's thesis or special research project with the guidance and approval of faculty.

Content Outline
Individual Special Research Project or Master's Thesis That Demonstrates Application of the Research Process

Total Units: 13 units

(case study continues on page 204)

TOTAL UNITS:

Level I:
Theory: 24;——
Clinical: 17
Total Units: 41;
Total Clinical Hours: 720

Level II
Theory: 28–30;——
Clinical: 12
Total Units: 40–42;
Total Clinical Hours: 405 in advanced nursing practice; 540 with the addition of Community
   Health Nursing
Total Units for the Track: 81 to 83

Summary

An analysis of the implementation plan reveals that the course objectives flow from the level objectives and lead to the end-of-program objectives and the overall goal. The courses were reviewed and found to correspond with the KSVM organizing framework and are in logical and sequential order. According to the guidelines for "Assessing the Key Components of a Curriculum," the plan is congruent with its components.

      Noting that the needs assessment indicated a need for staff nurses and clinical specialists in the outreach region, faculty members consult with the teachers in the entry-level MSN track for their opinion on the preparation of the students for entry-level staff positions and as clinical specialists. Indeed, the last three semesters of course work and clinical practice contain content at the advanced level such as the state board requirements for clinical specialists including knowledge and skills in clinical practice, clinical leadership, consultation, research, staff development, and client education. Additionally, the last two semesters focus on a selected clinical specialty in acute and chronic care with 405 total clinical hours of practice. If the community health nursing experience takes place within the selected clinical specialty, students are eligible for state and national certification as clinical specialists. However, the faculty strongly recommends a postgraduate year of clinical practice in that specialty. It is concluded that the program will meet nursing practice demands and the need for nurses in the region currently and in the future.

      From a practical point of view, the track meets all of the criteria for the distance education program except that each course needs an analysis as to the method of delivery to make the program financially feasible. Because this is primarily an administrative task, the faculty offers the following recommendations to the administration:

1. Review each theory course for the possibility of offering it through web-based courses for both the on-campus and distance site. This would help to ease the need for double the number of teachers. However, it is cautioned that the class enrollments must not exceed 30 for the Level One courses and 15 for the Level Two courses.

(continued)

2. If theory courses are not appropriate for web-based platforms, consider the use of interactive televised classes for both campuses. The enrollment cap is less stringent for this type of class.

3. Consider offering theory from the clinical skills courses through web-based platforms with practice labs taking place on site or in the clinical settings to which students are assigned.

4. Recruit master's- and doctorate-prepared nurses in the off-campus region to supervise student clinical experiences under the supervision of an experienced full-time clinical faculty member.

Conclusion

Faculty concludes that the entry-level MSN track is compatible with the proposed distance education program. They present their recommendations to administration and stand ready to assist in its implementation.

DISCUSSION QUESTIONS

1. Which components of the curriculum do you believe have the most impact on the implementation of the curriculum?

2. Why do you or why do you not believe a theoretical framework from nursing should serve as the organizing framework of the curriculum?

3. Why do you agree or disagree with the principle of faculty control of the curriculum?

LEARNING ACTIVITIES

Student Activities

1. Using the "Guidelines for Assessing the Key Components of a Curriculum or Educational Program," assess the educational program in which you are enrolled for the components of the curriculum. Are they easily identified? What resources do you need to locate them?

2. Attend one or more curriculum committee meetings and identify which of the components of the curriculum are addressed. Observe faculty members' interactions, their commitment to curriculum development and evaluation, and the role they play in developing or revising the curriculum. Note evidence of the routes of approval for any changes to the curriculum.

Faculty Activities

1. Using the "Guidelines for Assessing the Key Components of a Curriculum or Educational Program," assess the educational program in which you teach for the components of the curriculum. Are they easily identified? What resources do you need to locate them?

2. When you attend the next curriculum committee meetings, identify which of the components of the curriculum are addressed. Observe faculty members' interactions, their commitment to curriculum development and evaluation, and the role they play in developing or revising the curriculum. Note evidence of the routes of approval for any changes to the curriculum.

REFERENCES

Abriam-Yago, K., Yoder, M., & Kataoka-Yahiro, M. (1999). The Cummins model: A framework for teaching nursing students for whom English is a second language. *Journal of Transcultural Nursing, 10*(2), 143–149.

American Association of Colleges of Nursing. *Accreditation standards, accreditation procedures, and program review guidelines.* Retrieved June 2, 2004, from http://www.aacn.nche.edu/Accreditation/index.htm

American Association of Colleges of Nursing. (1998a). *Essentials of baccalaureate education for professional nursing practice.* Washington, DC: Author.

American Association of Colleges of Nursing. (1998b). *Essentials of master's education for advanced nursing practice.* Washington, DC: Author.

Armstrong, M. L., & Gessner, B.A. (1999). Does baccalaureate nursing education for registered nurses foster professional reading? *Journal of Professional Nursing, 15*(4), 238–244.

Bauerhaus, P. I., & Auerbach, D. (1999). Slow growth in the United States of the number of minorities in the RN workforce. *The Journal of Nursing Scholarship, 31*(2), 179–183.

Berlin, L. E., Stennett, J., & Bednash, G. D. (2002). *2001-2202 salaries of instructional and administrative nursing faculty in baccalaureate and graduate programs in nursing.* Washington, DC: American Association of Colleges of Nursing.

Bowles, K. (2000). The relationship of critical-thinking skills and the clinical judgment skills of baccalaureate nursing students. *Journal of Nursing Education, 39*(8), 373–376.

Bureau of Health Professions, Health Resources and Services Administration, Division of Nursing. (2002). *The national sample survey of registered nurses.* Washington, DC: Author.

Bureau of Health Professions, Health Resources and Services Administration, Division of Nursing. (2004). Retrieved June 3, 2004, from http://bhpr.hrsa.gov/nursing

Chinn, P. L., & Kramer, M. K. (1999). *Theory and nursing. Integrated knowledge development* (5th ed.). St. Louis, MO: Mosby.

Cloutterbuck, J. C., & Cherry, B. S. (1998). The Cloutterbuck minimum data matrix: A teaching mechanism for the new millennium. *Journal of Nursing Education, 37*(9), 385–393.

Comley, A. L. (1994). A comparative analysis of Orem's self-care model and Peplau's interpersonal theory. *Journal of Advanced Nursing, 20*(4), 755–760.

Csokasy, J. (2002). A congruent curriculum: Philosophical integrity from philosophy to outcomes. *Journal of Nursing Education, 41*(1), 32–33.

Daggett, L. M., Butts, J. B., & Smith, K. K. (2002). The development of an organizing framework to implement AACN guidelines for nursing education. *Journal of Nursing Education, 41*(1), 34–37.

DeAngelo, L. (2001). *Students learning, and race-based public policy. A look at diversity curriculum and co-curriculum.* Paper presented at the Annual Meeting of the American Educational Research Association, Seattle, WA.

Diaconis, L. K. (2001). *Changing directions: The lived experience of registered nurses who return to school for a baccalaureate degree in nursing.* Unpublished doctoral dissertation, University of Maryland.

Encyclopedia Britannica. *Philosophy.* Retrieved February 7, 2003, from Encyclopedia Britannica Online. http://www.eb.com

Espeland, K., & Shanta, L. (2001). Empowering versus enabling in academia. *Journal of Nursing Education, 40*(8), 342–346.

Failla, S., Maher, M. S., & Duffy, C. A. (1999). Evaluation of graduates of an associate degree nursing program. *Journal of Nursing Education, 38*(2), 62–68.

Fawcett, J. (1984). The metaparadigm of nursing: Present status and future refinements. *Image, 16,* 84–87.

Fitzpatrick, J. J. (1998). Building community: Developing skills for interprofessional health professions education and relationship-centered care. *Journal of Nurse Midwifery, 43*(1), 61–65.

Gagan, M. J., Berg, J., & Root, S. (2002). Nurse practitioner curriculum for the 21st century: A model for evaluation and revision. *Journal of Nursing Education, 41*(5), 202–206.

Griffiths, M. J., & Tagliareni, M. E. (1999). Challenging traditional assumptions about minority students in nursing education: Outcomes from project IMPART. *Nursing and Health Care Perspectives, 20*(6), 90–95.

Grossman, D., Massey, P., Blais, E., Geiger, E., et. al. (1998). Cultural diversity in Florida nursing programs: A survey of deans and directors. *Journal of Nursing Education, 37*(1), 22–26.

Gulitz, E. A., & King, I. M. (1988). King's general systems model: application to curriculum development. *Nursing Science Quarterly, 1*(3), 128–132.

Halter, M. J., & Polet, J. (2002). The place of baccalaureate nursing programs in the liberal arts setting. *Nursing Forum, 37*(1), 21–29.

Health Resources and Services Administration (HRSA), Bureau of Health Professions (2004a). Division of Nursing. *Moving toward elimination health disparities in the United States.* Retrieved June 3, 2004, from http://www.hrsa.gov/OMH/OMH/disparities/

Health Resources and Services Administration Bureau of Health Professions (2004b). Division of Nursing. *Other definitions of cultural diversity.* Retrieved Nov. 3, 2004, from http://bhpr.hrsa.gov/diversity/cultcomp.htm

Hellwig, S. D., & Ferrante, S. (1993). Martha Rogers' model in associate degree education. *Nurse Educator, 18*(5), 25–27.

Hicks, F. D. (2001). Critical thinking: toward a nursing science perspective. *Nursing Science Quarterly, 14*(1), 14–21.

Johnson, B., & Webber, P. B. (2001). *An introduction to theory and reasoning in nursing.* Philadelphia: Lippincott Williams & Wilkins.

Kellogg, K. (1999). Collaboration: Student affairs and academic affairs working together to promote student learning. *ERIC Digest.* Washington, DC: Office of Educational Research and Improvement.

Kim, H. S. (1998). Structuring the nursing knowledge system: A typology of four domains… including commentary by Hinshaw, A. S. & Kim, H. S. *Scholarly Inquiry for Nursing Practice, 12*(4), 367–388.

Koening, J. M., & Zorn, C. R. (2002). Using storytelling as an approach to teaching and learning with diverse students. *Journal of Nursing Education, 41*(9), 393–399.

Kozier, B., Erb, G., & Blais, K. (1997). *Professional nursing practice* (3rd ed.). Menlo Park, CA: Addison-Wesley.

Kuh, G.D. (1995). Out-of-class experiences associated with student learning and personal development. *Journal of Higher Education, 66*(2), 123–155.

Laanan, F. S. (2000). *Beyond transfer shock: Dimensions of transfer students' adjustment.* Paper presented at the Annual Meeting of the American Educational Research Association, New Orleans, LA.

Leininger, M. (2001). Transcultural nursing research to transform nursing education and practice: 40 years. Image: *Journal of Nursing Scholarship, 29*(4), 341–347.

Lenberg, C. B. (1999). The framework, concepts, and methods of the competency outcomes and performance assessment (COPA) model. *Online Journal of Issues in Nursing, 17.*

Lusk, M., & Decker, I. (2001). Moving toward a model for nursing education and practice. *Nursing and Health Care Perspectives, 22*(2), 81–84.

Mallow, G. E., & Gilje, F. (1999). Technology-based nursing education: Overview and call for future dialogue. *Journal of Nursing Education, 38*(6), 248–251.

McEwen, M., & Brown, S. C. (2002). Conceptual frameworks in undergraduate nursing curricula: Report of a national survey. *Journal of Nursing Education, 41*(1), 5–14.

Metcalfe, S. E. (1998). Behaviorism to humanism: The case for philosophical transformations in nursing education. *Nursing Connection, 11*(4), 41–46.

National League for Nursing Accrediting Commission. Standards and criteria. Retrieved June 3, 2004, from http://www.nlnac.org/home.htm

Newman, M. S., Sime, A. M., & Corcoran-Perry, S. A. (1991). The focus of the discipline of nursing. *Advances in Nursing Science, 14*(1), 1–6.

Orem, D. E. (1985). *Nursing: Concepts of Practice* (3rd ed.). New York: McGraw-Hill.

Paillé, M., & Pilkington, F. B. (2002). International perspectives. The global context of nursing: a human becoming perspective. *Nursing Science Quarterly, 15*(2), 165–170.

Peplau, H. (1952). *Interpersonal relations in nursing.* New York: Putman.

Reale, C. N. (2001). Validating nursing credit: An alternative to challenges. *Journal of Nursing Education, 40*(1), 33–36.

Rogers, M. E. (1970). *An introduction to the theoretical basis of nursing.* Philadelphia: F.A. Davis

Sechrist, K. R., Lewis, E. M., Rutledge, D. N., Keating, S. B., & Association of California Nurse Leaders. (2002). *The California nursing work force initiative. Planning for California's nursing work force. Phase III. Final report.* Sacramento, CA: Association of California Nurse Leaders.

Sloand, E., Groves, S., & Brager, R. (2004). Cultural competency education in American nursing programs and the approach of one nursing school. *International Journal of Education Scholarship, 1*(1), Article 6.

Smith, L. S. (2000). Said another way: Is nursing an academic science? *Nursing Forum, 35*(1), 25–29.

Starck, P. L., Warner, A., & Kotarba, J. (1999). 21st century leadership in nursing education. *Journal of Professional Nursing, 15*(5), 265–269.

Taybei, K., Moore-Jazayeri, M., & Maynard, T. (1998). From the border: Reforming the curriculum for the at-risk student. *Journal of Cultural Diversity, 5*(3), 101–109.

Terenzini, P. T., Cabrera, A. F., Colbeck, C. L., Bjorklund, S. A., & Parente, J. M. (2001). Racial and ethnic diversity in the classroom. Does it promote student learning? *Journal of Higher Education, 72*(5), 509–531.

Terenzini, P. T. and others (1995). Influences affecting the development of students' critical thinking skills. *Research in Higher Education, 35,* 23–39.

Terenzini, P. T., Pascarella, E. T., & Blimling, G. S. (1999). Students' out-of-class experiences and their influence on learning and cognitive development: A literature review. *Journal of College Student Development, 40*(5), 10–23.

Thompson, C., & Scheckley, B. G. (1997). Differences in classroom teaching preference between traditional and adult BSN students. *Journal of Nursing Education, 36*(4), 163–170.

Vezeau, T. M., Peterson, J. W., Nakao, C., & Ersek, M. (1998). Education of advanced practice nurses serving vulnerable populations. Nursing & Health Care Perspectives. *19* (3), 124-131.

Vivarais-Dresler, G., & Kutschke, M. (2001). RN students' ratings and opinions related to the importance of certain clinical teacher behaviors. *The Journal of Continuing Education in Nursing, 32*(6), 274–282.

Waddell, D. L., & Stephens, S. (2000). Use of learning contracts in a RN-to-BSN leadership course. *The Journal of Continuing Education in Nursing, 31*(4) 179–184.

Watson, J. (1979). *Nursing: The philosophy and science of caring.* Boston: Little, Brown.

Watson, J. M. (2001). Postmodern nursing and beyond. In N. L. Chaska (Ed.), *The nursing profession: Tomorrow and beyond.* Thousand Oaks, Sage Publications.

Webber, P. B. (2000). *Clinical decision-making: Components, processes, and outcomes.* National Organization of Nurse Practitioner Faculties, Monograph. Washington, DC: National Organization of Nurse Practitioner Faculties.

Webber, P. B. (2002). A curriculum framework for nursing. *Journal of Nursing Education, 41*(1), 15–24.

Undergraduate Curricula in Nursing

Robyn Marchal Nelson, DNSc, RN, and Diane D. Welch, MSN, RN

OBJECTIVES

Upon completion of Chapter 8, the reader will be able to:

1. Contrast the curricular differences between the three different undergraduate educational approaches to nursing.
2. Analyze the advantages and disadvantages of multiple educational approaches and the impact on career mobility.
3. Articulate the difference between prelicensure preparation and degree requirements in nursing education programs.
4. Evaluate the appropriateness of sample nursing curricula in achieving the role differences proposed in the differentiated practice model.
5. Analyze how the innovative curriculum between two educational approaches to nursing education at the undergraduate level addresses the issues of career mobility.

▲ OVERVIEW

A discussion of curriculum development at the undergraduate level in nursing is more complex than in other disciplines. While the elements of effective curriculum development are the same, the mission and goal of a nursing curriculum will not be the same for all undergraduate programs. This chapter addresses prelicensure content that is established through government regulation and monitored by state boards of nursing. All nursing programs must include this content for a graduate to be eligible to sit for the National Council Licensure Examination (NCLEX) to become a registered nurse (RN). The curricular differences and graduation requirements for a diploma, associate degree, and baccalaureate in nursing are reviewed. The issues surrounding career mobility arising from the multiple educational paths to entry into nursing, including articulation, transfer, advanced placement through challenge, and role socialization are presented. The chapter includes a curriculum model that offers seamless articulation between an associate degree and baccalaureate program and addresses many of the barriers to career mobility. The chapter concludes with a discussion of the challenges that exist in the development of a nursing curriculum, specifically at the undergraduate level.

There are three educational approaches to the nursing major at the undergraduate level: the hospital-based diploma program, the community college associate degree program, or the undergraduate baccalaureate program. The common thread for all three programs is the knowledge, skills, and abilities required for licensure and regulated by the board of nursing within each state. This component of the undergraduate nursing curriculum is referred to as the "prelicensure" content. Concurrent with meeting the prelicensure requirements, an educational program includes degree or diploma requirements set by the institution—at the undergraduate level they are the requirements for an associate of science or arts degree at a community college or a baccalaureate at an upper division level college or university.

Prelicensure Preparation for Nursing

Each state has a nurse practice act that legislates practice and education. The Board of Nursing for the state approves an academic program to offer the curriculum leading to licensure as a registered nurse. In contrast to national accreditation, which is voluntary, a program cannot operate without state approval for its graduates to be eligible for the licensure examination. The board visits each program within the state on a set schedule (e.g., every 5 or more years) to determine compliance with the state regulations. All programs, regardless of the degree or diploma conferred, must comply with the state's educational regulations. As an example, the curricular content from California's Nursing Practice Act, Title 16, California Code of Regulations is presented in Box 8.1 (Board of Registered Nursing, 2000).

Education for Nursing in a Diploma Program

The foundation for the hospital-based diploma nursing programs in the United States was the Nightingale School of Nursing established by Florence Nightingale in London in 1860. In the 1870s, several nursing programs similar to the Nightingale School of Nursing opened in New York, Boston, Philadelphia, New Haven, and Chicago (Ellis & Hartley, 1998). In the first nursing schools, the curriculum was not standardized. There was little classroom experience or theory presented, and the nursing students provided free labor in the hospitals. The students often worked 12 hours a day, 7 days a week, during which they learned skills through hands-on

▲ **B O X 8 . 1**   **California Board of Registered Nursing Required Curriculum**

1426. Required Curriculum; Prior Approval

a. The curriculum of a nursing program shall be that set forth in this section. A program's curriculum shall not be implemented or revised until it has been approved by the board.

b. The curriculum shall reflect a verifying theme, which includes the nursing process as defined by the faculty, and shall be designed so that a nurse who completes the program will have the knowledge and skills necessary to function in accordance with the minimum standards for competency set forth in Section 1443.5.

c. The curriculum shall consist of not less than fifty-eight (58) semester units, or eighty-seven (87) quarter units, which shall include at least the following number of units in the specified course areas:

1. Art and science of nursing, thirty-six (36) semester or fifty-four (54) quarter units, of which eighteen (18) semester or twenty-seven (27) quarter units will be in theory and eighteen (18) semester or twenty-seven (27) quarter units will be in clinical practice.

2. Communication skills, six (6) semester or nine (9) quarter units. Communication skills shall include principles of verbal, written, and group communication.

3. Related natural, behavioral, and social sciences, sixteen (16) semester or twenty-four (24) quarter units.

d. Theory and clinical practice shall be concurrent in the following nursing areas: medical–surgical, maternal/child, mental health, psychiatric nursing, and geriatrics. Instruction will be given in, but not limited to, the following: personal hygiene, human sexuality, client abuse, cultural diversity, nutrition (including therapeutic aspects), pharmacology, legal, social, and ethical aspects of nursing, nursing leadership and management.

e. The following shall be integrated throughout the entire nursing curriculum:

1. Nursing process;

2. Basic intervention skills in preventive, remedial, supportive, and rehabilitative nursing;

3. Physical, behavioral, and social aspects of human development from birth through all age levels;

4. The knowledge and skills required to develop collegial relationships with health care providers from other disciplines;

5. Communication skills including principles of verbal, written, and group communications;

6. Natural sciences including human anatomy, physiology, and microbiology; and

7. Related behavioral and social sciences with emphasis on societal and cultural patterns, human development, and behavior relevant to health-illness.

f. The course of instruction shall be presented in semester or quarter units under the following formula:

1. One (1) hour of instruction in theory each week throughout a semester or quarter equals one (1) unit.

2. Three (3) hours of clinical practice each week throughout a semester or quarter equals one (1) unit.

Title 16. California Code of Regulations, Division 14, Article 3, 2000.

experience. Upon graduation from their programs, the students were granted diplomas in nursing (Catalano, 2003).

In the early 1950s, the National League for Nursing (NLN) assumed the responsibility for accrediting schools of nursing. Many diploma schools chose not to obtain NLN accreditation because they had to comply with standards requiring specific courses of study and preparation of faculty at the baccalaureate or higher degree in nursing levels. As a result, many schools closed (Catalano, 2003). In the early 1960s, numerous diploma schools gained NLN accreditation and began to affiliate with colleges and universities. Their emphasis was still on extensive experience in hands-on care in the acute hospital setting, but the students gained the opportunity to take academic courses. Graduates of a number of these programs were awarded Associate Degrees in Nursing.

According to 2002 NLN statistics, there are 70 accredited diploma programs, the total 86 programs still open in the United States (NLNAC, 2003). The accredited programs meet the standards of NLN accreditation and provide a high quality of nursing education with special emphasis on clinical skills in acute care settings. Most diploma schools in the United States are located in the Midwest and the Eastern sections of the United States. The majority of these programs are affiliated with colleges and universities that enhance the opportunities for students to concurrently earn associate degrees in nursing. In some cases, students have the choice of going through the generic diploma curriculum and graduating with a diploma in Nursing or taking the general education courses in a college concurrently with their nursing courses and graduating with an Associate of Science (AS) or Associate of Arts (AA) in Nursing. The curricula often appear quite similar to that of associate degree nursing programs, especially in those programs that affiliate with colleges. The primary difference noted is the additional clinical hours found in 3-year diploma programs.

Associate Degree Nursing Curriculum

A pilot program conducted by Mildred Montag at Teacher's College in Columbia University prepared "technical" level nurses (Montag, 1951). These technical nurses graduated from associate degree nursing programs in community colleges and demonstrated the ability to provide safe care in acute settings and functioned well within health care teams. Although the curriculum was technically oriented, it had a theoretical base with science and general education courses. As a result of the additional college courses and after much discussion by educators and state boards of nursing, it was decided that the associate degree in nursing (ADN) students were eligible for the registered nurse (RN) licensing examination instead of the licensed practical nurse/licensed vocational nurse (LPN/LVN) examination (Catalano, 2003).

The curricula in ADN programs include social and biologic sciences as well as general education courses such as mathematics, oral and written communications, and certain political science requirements. By integrating these courses and the four semesters of nursing courses into the curriculum, an ADN program often takes 3 years to complete. The total number of units may range from 60 to 90 for the associate degree. Box 8.2 illustrates an example of an ADN curriculum in California. In this program there are six units (18 hours each week) of clinical experience each semester within the nursing courses. Most of the clinical hours are in the acute care setting; however, there are several experiences in ambulatory care throughout the curriculum. It is a curriculum that is commonly accepted for articulation to baccalaureate programs

▲ **BOX 8.2**   **Sample ADN Curriculum**

Prerequisites:	Anatomy and Physiology	8–10 units
	Microbiology	4 units
	English Composition	3 units
	Psychology (Introduction)	3 units
	Nutrition	3 units
	Human Growth and Development	3 units
1st semester:	Fundamentals of Nursing/Medical–Surgical Nursing	10 units
	Oral Communication	3 units
2nd semester:	Medical–Surgical Nursing	8 units
	Maternity Nursing	3 units
	Sociology or Cultural Anthropology	3 units
3rd semester:	Medical–Surgical Nursing	3 units
	Pediatric Nursing	4 units
	Psychiatric Nursing	4 units
	American Institutions	3 units
	Physical Education	1 unit
4th semester	Medical–Surgical Nursing (incorporates critical care, leadership and management, and home health)	10 units
	Humanities Elective	3 units
	TOTAL	**82 UNITS**

throughout California. In essence, it provides an almost seamless track for the associate degree graduate pursuing higher education.

Baccalaureate Preparation—Generic and RN Completion

Historically, generic (*an entry-level program to prepare students for professional practice and eligibility for licensure*) undergraduate nursing programs were developed using a traditional biomedical model identical to hospital settings (e.g., medical–surgical, pediatrics, labor, and delivery). Although course titles changed in an attempt to conceptualize the educational experience around the population served and its needs and to reflect an integrated approach or a nursing model, the prelicensure curriculum often remained focused on the biomedical model. Non- or postlicensure content, defined as baccalaureate core competencies, reflects additional professional concerns, such as an introduction to research, health care and professional issues, and community health. These competencies are usually not required for eligibility to take the licensure examination.

The lack of a consistent nomenclature for undergraduate nursing curricula complicates smooth articulation and transfer among programs, including baccalaureate to baccalaureate and associate degree to baccalaureate. For example, one baccalaureate curriculum may be a nursing process model and integrate the clinical specialties throughout the program. Another program may separate clinical specialties such as Family and Child Health Nursing, Geriatric Nursing, Adult Health Nursing, Community Health, and Mental Health Nursing. With these varying course titles and curricula plans, it becomes difficult to determine which content in the courses and the level in which it is presented is equivalent to content and level from another program.

An example of a generic baccalaureate curriculum is presented in Box 8.3. The Bachelor of Science in Nursing is designed as a four-year, minimum-132-unit program with

---

▲ BOX 8.3   Degree Requirements for the Bachelor of Science in Nursing (BSN)

Units required for Major: 93–96
Minimum total units required for the BSN: 132

A. Required Preclinical Courses (31 units)
When possible, students are encouraged to apply their preclinical courses to General Education requirements.

(3)	ENG001A	College Composition
(3)	PSYC001	Introductory Psychology
(5)	CHEM006B	Organic Chemistry
(4)	BIO022	Introductory Human Anatomy
(4)	BIO131	Systemic Physiology
(4)	BIO139	Microbiology
(3)	FACS113	Nutrition and Metabolism
(3)	CHDV030	Human Development Across the Lifespan
(2)	NURS014	Pharmacology

B. Required Clinical Nursing Courses (59–62 units)

1. Required Lower-Division Courses (13 units)

(3)	NURS011	Introduction to Professional Nursing
(5)	NURS012	Nursing Care of Adults
(2)	NURS015	Introduction to Clinical Nursing Practice
(1)	NURS016	Physical Assessment of the Adult
(2)	NURS017	Concepts and Practices of Gerontological Nursing

2. Required Upper-Division Courses (46 units)

(6)	NURS123	Nursing Families in Complex Illness
(1)	NURS128	Therapeutic Interpersonal and Group Communication
(5)	NURS129	Mental Health Nursing
(1)	NURS136	Nursing the Childbearing Family: Skills and Assessment
(5)	NURS137	Nursing the Childbearing Family
(5)	NURS138	Nursing the Childrearing Family
(1)	NURS139	Nursing the Childrearing Family
(6)	NURS143	Leadership and Management in Nursing Practice
(5)	NURS144	Community Health Nursing
(2)	NURS150	Research in Nursing
(1)	NURS155	Senior Forum
(3)	NURS156	Selected Senior Practicum in Nursing
(3)	NURS169	Reasoning Development in Health Care Sciences
(2)	NURS191	Service-Learning in Nursing

C. Additional Graduation Requirements (3 units)

(3) A course in societal-cultural patterns before certification of eligibility for state licensure.

a foundation of general education and prerequisite courses. The art and science of nursing is organized and sequenced over five semesters with a focus on individuals to groups and communities, moving from dependent to independent to interdependent role functions, emphasizing the needs of self then others, and requiring clinical decision making in situations with fewer variables (simpler) to more complex clinical scenarios. Each course is a full semester and clinical practica range from 90 hours minimum up to 180 hours per course. The curriculum culminates in a collaborative community health and leadership service-learning requirement, which is a type of capstone experience designed to demonstrate achievement of the summative program outcomes. The student moves with a cohort group in a linear manner through the curriculum with little opportunity for electives because the 132 units for the degree are met through the required general education (GE) (51 semester units), prerequisite requirements that include 14 units not counted for GE, and the major courses (minimum 59 units). Another source of units not shown in the curriculum are courses referred to as "prerequisites to the prerequisites." These are courses required by the discipline (for example, Biological Sciences, Social Sciences, or Chemistry) that offer the required nursing prerequisite. For example, Nursing requires Anatomy; however, Biology requires General Biology before Anatomy.

By way of comparison, Box 8.4 shows the baccalaureate curriculum from Brigham Young University (BYU) College of Nursing (2003), which retains some of the traditional aspects of nursing curricula but integrates community health throughout the curriculum and introduces electives that respond to the changing health care delivery system. Examples of electives include international/transcultural courses, alternative and complementary therapies, school health, home health, and rural health.

While community college and university nursing programs are charged to include community-based experiences (Ayers, Bruno, & Langford, 1999; National League for Nursing, 1993), BYU eliminated community health as a separate course. Health promotion/disease prevention, population focus, societal issues, health care policy and finance, and spirituality are threaded throughout the curriculum. The BYU faculty believes that community concepts "must be practiced in all settings for care, not just those outside of the hospital in 'community-based' settings" (Conger, Baldwin, Abegglen, & Callister, 1999, p. 311). For this curriculum, the hospital no longer becomes the central focus of the curriculum (Baldwin, Conger, Abegglen, and Hill, 1998).

▲ A COLLABORATIVE MODEL FOR PROFESSIONAL NURSING PREPARATION

The curriculum of a community college program generally takes a minimum of 3 years to complete (Zerwekh & Claborn, 1997). There is a misconception by the public that a "2-year nursing program" takes just 2 years to complete. Health care is so complex that even an Associate Degree in Nursing must include a foundation in general education as well as a strong preparation in clinical nursing if the graduate is to become a competent practitioner. A university program that has very similar prerequisites and additional upper-division general education requirements takes a minimum of 4 years, in many cases just one more semester than the time a student will spend in a community college program. An RN from a diploma or community college program who returns to complete the baccalaureate generally spends a minimum of another 2 years to complete the baccalaureate. (It is no wonder diploma and community college graduates are reluctant to return to school!)

▲ **BOX 8.4**   **Brigham Young College of Nursing—An Integrated Community Health Curriculum**

Nursing Course Descriptions (Required courses)

NURS 180 – Preview of Nursing (1 credit)
Defines and explores nursing as a potential career opportunity.

NURS 294 – Health Assessment and Health Promotion (4 credits)
Prerequisite: acceptance to nursing major and concurrent enrollment in NURS 296 and 298.
Emphasis on health promotion, health maintenance, and therapeutic communication. Acquisition and application of health assessment knowledge and skills.

NURS 296 – Introduction to Community Health Nursing (3 credits)
Prerequisite: acceptance to nursing major and concurrent enrollment in NURS 294 and 298.
Acquisition and application of basic community health nursing concepts. Emphasis on health of groups and/or populations.

NURS 298 – Nursing Care of Older Adults (5 credits)
Prerequisite: acceptance to nursing major and concurrent enrollment in NURS 294 and 296.
Acquisition and application of basic nursing skills with older adults in residential and inpatient settings.

NURS 300 – Pharmacology in Nursing (2 credits)
Prerequisite: NURS 294, 296, 298, and concurrent enrollment in NURS 330.
Introduction to common categories of drugs, their action, use, desired and undesired effects, and implications for nursing care.

NURS 320 – Nursing Research (2 credits)
Prerequisite: Advanced Writing, STAT 221 or other statistics course, NURS 294, 296, 298, 300, and 330.
Analysis and critique of research in nursing practice. Must be taken before NURS 490.

NURS 330 – Nursing Care of Adults With Acute and Chronic Illnesses (9 credits)
Prerequisite: NURS 294, 296, 298, and concurrent enrollment in NURS 300.
Acquisition and application of knowledge and skills necessary to provide nursing care to the adult patient and acute and chronic illness.

NURS 340 – Nursing Care of the Childbearing Family (4 credits)
Prerequisite: NURS 294, 296, 298, 300, 330, and concurrent enrollment in NURS 350 and 400.
Care of childbearing families from diverse backgrounds. Emphasis on health promotion, assessment, and interventions related to complicated and uncomplicated pregnancy and birth.

> ### ▲ BOX 8.4 Brigham Young College of Nursing—An Integrated Community Health Curriculum (continued)
>
> **NURS 350 –** Nursing Care of the Childrearing Family (4 credits)
> Prerequisite: NURS 294, 296, 298, 300, 330, and concurrent enrollment in NURS 350 and 400.
> Care of children and their families from diverse backgrounds. Emphasis on health promotion/illness prevention, care of acute and chronic illness, and growth and development.
>
> **NURS 400 –** Global Health and Human Diversity (4 credits)
> Prerequisite: NURS 294, 296, 298, 300, 330, and concurrent enrollment in NURS 340 and 350.
> Theory and practice of nursing in diverse populations within a global context.
>
> **NURS 460 –** Psychiatric Nursing (3 credits)
> Prerequisite: NURS 294, 296, 298, 300, 330, 340, 350, 400, and concurrent enrollment in NURS 470.
> Nursing care for clients with complex psychiatric disorder.
>
> **NURS 470 –** Nursing Care of Adults in Crisis (7 credits)
> Prerequisite: NURS 294, 296, 298, 300, 330, 340, 350, 400, and concurrent enrollment in NURS 460.
> Nursing intervention for individuals and families in crisis.
>
> **NURS 480** Nursing Senior Seminar (1 credit)
> Prerequisite: NURS 294, 296, 298, 300, 320, 330, 340, 350, 400, 460, 470, and concurrent enrollment in NURS 490.
> Focuses on the characteristics of the nursing profession and professional behaviors and values. Includes a review of nursing history.
>
> **NURS 490** Capstone (8 credits)
> Prerequisite: NURS 294, 296, 298, 300, 320, 330, 340, 350, 400, 460, 470, and concurrent enrollment in NURS 480.
> Clinical synthesis experience with focus on planning, delivering, and managing patient care in complex environments. Leadership components will be incorporated into clinical.

In an attempt to reduce the time to degree, reduce redundancy, facilitate completion of the baccalaureate, capitalize on the strengths within individual programs, and maximize the resources available between the two programs, a curriculum was designed that is seamless between Sacramento City College (SCC), a community college, and California State University Sacramento (CSUS), a state-supported university. The curriculum can be completed in 4 years with 132 units. The student receives both the associate of science (AS) and the bachelor of science (BS) degrees simultaneously. The community college student is required to take one additional prerequisite (organic chemistry), attend one additional semester in nursing (five semesters rather than four), and complete nine additional upper-division general education units. Box 8.5 shows the curriculum indicating the AS and BS requirements. The similarities in the general education and prelicensure content are obvious.

▲ BOX 8.5   Collaborative Model for the Preparation of the Registered
             Nurse at the Baccalaureate Level

The model curriculum meets the general education requirements for both the associate of science (AS) or bachelor of science (BS) degrees. Beside each course is an indication of which program requires the course. It is clear that there is little difference for the first 3 years.

Freshman Year

1st Semester	Degree	2nd Semester	Degree
Inorg.Chem.	BS	Org. Chem.	BS
Math or Stat.	AS/BS	Anat. Physio.	AS/BS
Speech	AS/BS	Psychology	AS/BS
English 1A	AS/BS	Crit. Think.	AS/BS
Sociology or Anth.	AS/BS	Am. Inst.	AS/BS

Sophomore Year

1st Semester	Degree	2nd Semester	Degree
Microbiology	AS/BS	N10 (SCC)	AS/BS
Anat. Physio.	AS/BS		
Nutrition	AS/BS	Life Span/Hum. Dev.	AS/BS
N 11 (CSUS) (Replaces N90 at SCC)	AS/BS	Phys. Ed.	AS
Pharmacology	BS	World Civ.	AS/BS

Summer semester for GE if desired by student.

Junior Year

1st Semester	Degree	2nd Semester	Degree
N20 (SCC)	AS/BS	N30 (SCC)	AS/BS
GE	AS/BS	Humanities	BS

Summer semester for GE if desired by student.

Senior Year

1st Semester	Degree	2nd Semester	Degree
*N143 (CSUS)	AS/BS	N191 (CSUS)	BS
N144 (CSUS)	BS	N155 (CSUS)	BS
Humanities	BS	N156 (CSUS)	BS
*N143 will meet N40 for SCC	BS	N169 (CSUS)	BS
NURS111B (bridge course)		N150 (CSUS)	BS
Upper-Division GE	BS	Foreign Lang.	BS

Summer semester 2004 CSUS student may choose to take NURS150 and/or upper-division GE.

Total Units: 132 required for BS from CSUS; students would also receive ADN at completion of the program.

▲ **BOX 8.5** **Collaborative Model for the Preparation of the Registered Nurse at the Baccalaureate Level** (continued)

Titles for Nursing Courses Included Above

N10 (SCC)	Fundamentals of Idealth and Nursing Care
N11 (CSUS)	Introduction to Professional Nursing
N14 (CSUS)	Pharmacology
N20 (SCC)	Nursing and Health Maintenance Through Adult Years
N425 (SCC)	Nursing Complex Health Problems Throughout the Life Cycle
N111B (CSUS)	Bridging Concepts for Returning Nurses
N143 (CSUS)	Leadership and Management (to be merged with N40 at SCC)
N144 (CSUS)	Community Health
N150 (CSUS)	Nursing Research
N155 (CSUS)	Senior Forum
N156 (CSUS)	Senior Practicum
N169 (CSUS)	Reasoning Skill Development in Health Care
N191 (CSUS)	Service Learning in Nursing

General Education Requirements Met Through Proposed Collaborative

(All but 9 units upper-division GE may be met at community college)

Area A–Basic Subjects (9 units)

A1	Speech (3 units)
A2	English (3 units)
A3	Critical Thinking (3 units)

Area B–Physical Universe (12 units)

B1	Inorganic Chem. (5 units)
B2	Anthro. (3 units)
B3	Inorganic Chem. lab
B4	Math or Statistics (3 units)
B5	Organic Chem. (5 units)

Area C–Arts and Humanities (12 units)

C1	World Civ. (3 units)
C2	Intro to Art (3 units)
C3	Humanities (3 units)
C4	Foreign Language (3 units)

Area D–Individual and Society (15 units)

D1	Sociology (3 units) and Psychology (3 units)
D2	N167 (3 units)
D3	American Institutions (3 units)
D4	Race/Ethnicity/Multicultural Course (3 units)

(*box continues on page 220*)

▲ **BOX 8.5** **Collaborative Model for the Preparation of the Registered Nurse at the Baccalaureate Level** (continued)

Area E–Understanding Personal Development (3 units)

Life Span/Human Development (3 units)
Phys. Ed. (1 units)

Nine (9) Units Upper-Division GE (one course must be advanced study)

N169 (3 units)
FACS113 (3 units)
Additional 3-unit course

This was started as a pilot program initially; students were selected from the applicant pool to CSUS and were enrolled in Nursing 11, Introduction to Professional Nursing, and Nursing 17, Concepts and Practices of Gerontological Nursing. The students selected for the collaborative pilot were admitted to SCC for three semesters and then transferred to CSUS in the fourth clinical semester. To complete the requirements for the ADN during this semester, students were required to pay fees to both institutions, because Nursing 40 Complex and Multiple Patient Care at SCC was taken concurrently with Nursing 143, Leadership and Management in Nursing Practice, and Nursing 144, Community Health Nursing, at CSUS. Although it was hoped that the students would take courses concurrently at CSUS while enrolled at SCC to promote socialization, class schedules for Nursing 405, 415, and 425 during the first three clinical semesters made it too difficult (if not impossible). An alternative was enrollment in the "bridge course" Nursing 111B, Bridging Constructs for Returning Nurses, once the students enrolled at CSUS to validate competence and facilitate socialization. Students could take the NCLEX upon completion of the fifth semester of clinical nursing.

Ideally, a student in a collaborative curriculum pays only one fee as an enrolled student in the California higher education system, takes courses concurrently on both campuses throughout the program, and is socialized optimally to professional practice. Admission and progression through a collaborative program does not convey that the student is "finished" upon completion of a community college program, but rather that the student will move to the university for the last year. With distance technology, it is possible that every community college program could "connect" to a university for completion of the baccalaureate requirements. The Total Curriculum Plan (see Figure 8.1) shows how the curriculum meets the prelicensure requirements of the California Board of Registered Nursing for theory and clinical courses.

Another model for collaboration between two types of nursing programs exists between California State University Los Angeles (CSULA) and four community colleges. Students complete 1 year of prerequisites and general education before admission to the community college nursing program, where they complete 16 to 20 semester units of nursing content, typically fundamentals and medical–surgical nursing. The students transfer to CSULA for 2 years of upper-division baccalaureate nursing and general education. The students do not complete the ADN program in this model (J. Papenhausen, personal communication, June 2003).

State of California

Department of Consumer Affairs
Board of Registered Nursing

REQUIRED CURRICULUM:
CONTENT REQUIRED FOR LICENSURE

EDP-P-06 (Rev. 03/01)

Submit in DUPLICATE.

Program Name: CSU Sacramento and Sacramento City College Collaborative Program Type of Program: ☐ Entry-Level Master ☐ Baccalaureate ☐ Associate Requesting new curriculum approval: ☐ Major ☐ Minor Date of Implementation: 1/1/02; 2/3/03 forms resubmitted to accurately reflect revision of EDP-P-06/TCP Academic System: ☐ Semester __15–18_____ weeks/semester ☐ Quarter _____ weeks/quarter	**For Board Use Only** Approved by:_____ _____ _____, NEC Date:_____ _____ _____ ☐ BRN Copy ☐ Program Copy

REQUIRED FOR LICENSURE AS STATED IN SECTION 1426

	Semester Units	Quarter Units	Current BRN- Approved Curriculum CSUS	SCC	Proposed Curriculum Revision Collaborative
Nursing	**36**	**54**	45	43	49
Theory	(18)	(27)	(25)	(18)	(23)
Clinical	(18)	(27)	(20)	(25)	(26)
Communication Units	6	9	6	6	7
Science Units	16	24	29	26	34
TOTAL UNITS FOR LICENSURE	**58**	**87**	80	75	90
Other Degree Requirements			52	7	44
TOTAL UNITS FOR GRADUATION			132	82	134**

(*figure continues on page 222*)

F I G U R E 8 . 1 Total curriculum plan for the collaborative curriculum between a community college and a state university.

List the course number(s) and title(s) in which content may be found for the following required content areas:

REQUIRED CONTENT	Course Number	Course Titles
Alcohol & Chemical Dependency	N30	Nursing in Complex Problems Across Life Cycle
Personal Hygiene	N10	Fundamentals of Health and Nursing Care
Human Sexuality	N10, N20	N20-Nursing and Health Maintenance During Adult Year
Client Abuse	N30	Nursing in Complex Problems Across the Life Cycle
Cultural Diversity	N10, N20, N30, N40	N40-Complex and Multiple Care Nursing
Nutrition	FCS10 or FACS113	Nutrition; Nutrition and Metabolism
Pharmacology	N14	Pharmacology
Legal Aspects	N11	Introduction to Professional Nursing
Social/Ethical Aspects	N10, N11, N20, N30, N40	Fund of Health and Nursing Care; Intro to Professional Nursing; Nursing & Health Maintenance During Adult Life; Complex and Multiple Care Nursing
Management/Leadership	N40, N143	Leadership and Management (Planned integration of N40)

Information needed to evaluate transcripts of applicants for licensure (Section 1426, Chapter 14, Title 16 of the California Code of Regulations) is listed in the left column below. Indicate the name(s) and the number(s) of the course(s) which include this content.

REQUIRED CONTENT	Course Number	Course Titles	Units
NURSING			
Medical–Surgical	N10, N20, N40	Fundamentals of Health and Nursing Care; Complex & Multiple Care Nursing	10, 11, 10
Obstetrical	N30 & N136	Nursing in Complex Problems Across the Life Cycle; Nursing the Childbearing Family	11, 1
Pediatric	N30 & N139	Nursing in Complex Problems Across the Life Cycle; Nursing the Childrearing Family	11, 1
Psych/Mental Health	N30 & N128	Nursing in Complex Problems Across the Life Cycle; Therapeutic Interpersonal & Group Communication	11, 1
Geriatrics	N10, N20, N40	Fundamentals of Health and Nursing Care; Nursing and Health Maintenance During Adult Year; Complex and Multiple Care Nursing	10 11 10
Pharmacology	N14	Pharmacology	2
Nursing Foundation	N11	Intro to Professional Issues	3

FIGURE 8.1 Continued

BASIC SCIENCES			
Anatomy	Bio 25 2A/6A, 2B/6B	Introductory Human Anatomy Inorganic and Organic Chemistry	4 or 5 10
Physiology	Bio 26	Systemic Physiology	4 or 5
Microbiology	Bio 6 or Bio 139	General Microbiology	4
Societal/Cultural Pattern	Soc 1 or Anth 2	Intro to Cultural Anthropology Principles of Sociology	3 3
Psychology	Psych 1	Introductory Psychology	3
Human Development	FCS38	Human Development	3
Nutrition	FCS10	Nutrition and Metabolism	3
COMMUNICATION			
Group	Speech 1, N128	Speech Comm.; Therapeutic Interpersonal & Group Communication	3, 1
Verbal	Speech 15	Speech Communication	3
Written	English 1A	College Composition	3
		TOTAL UNITS	90

FIGURE 8.1 Continued

In 1970 the *National Commission for the Study of Nursing and Nursing Education* (Lysaught, 1970) recommended that:

> Junior and senior collegiate institutions collaboratively develop programs and curricula that will preserve the integrity of these institutions and their aims while facilitating the social and professional mobility of the nursing student (p. 110).

The previously described models meet the intent of the 1970 recommendation. There will continue to be even more collaborative models in an attempt to transition all nursing graduates to a minimum of a baccalaureate. Another interesting proposal is the awarding of baccalaureates by community colleges (Evelyn, 2003). In these instances, education codes must be changed, upper-division level courses added, faculty qualifications be comparable, and fees made consistent with a university education .This sort of arrangement could result in baccalaureate preparation for all registered nurses.

▲ ARTICULATION BETWEEN ACADEMIC PROGRAMS

The concept of articulation between academic institutions refers to the equivalency of a course taken at one institution that is required for admission to another institution and would be accepted for credit if the student transferred. A common scenario is articulation between a community college and a 4-year university; given the fact that a large percentage of nurses are prepared in community colleges, articulation is a very important issue in nursing education. Community college courses are classified at the lower-division level, meaning that courses generally taken in the first and second years of college are foundational to a major and total up to 60 units. Four-year universities offer both lower-division and upper-division courses. By definition, upper division implies that courses are taken in the third and fourth years of college or university, that is, the junior and senior years. They usually number 60 units and are largely the major requirements and some upper-division general education courses. The type and number of units transferable to a 4-year university limit graduates from diploma and community college programs. Many state educational systems have a formalized articulation process between the community college and the state university system, ensuring transferability of the required lower-division courses. Box 8.6 shows an example of the transfer agreement between a California community college and a state university for the prerequisites and the 13 units of lower-division courses into the baccalaureate program.

If there were more nursing units at the lower-division level in the baccalaureate program, the transfer of credits in nursing from the community college could be facilitated. Nursing faculty needs to anticipate the potential transfer/articulation issues when developing a nondegree or lower-division nursing program or an upper-division curriculum, which incorporates RNs returning to school for the baccalaureate.

▲ ADVANCED PLACEMENT OR CREDIT BY EXAMINATION

The workplace of a registered nurse often dictates the need for additional education to prepare for a new role or to be eligible for a desired position. Diploma graduates do not possess an academic degree and the nursing units completed in a hospital-based program are not transferable to an institution of higher education. The general education courses required by all prelicensure programs, including diploma programs, are often offered through neighboring academic institutions to create units that are transferable. In the past, a graduate of a diploma program not affiliated with an academic institution applied to an associate degree or baccalaureate program with as many as 90 credit hours, of which none was considered transferable. An example of how a community college can assist a diploma student is the student who enrolls for two semesters of course work at a community college as a re-entry student. The student takes general education and any missing prerequisite requirements for a BS program and after he or she satisfactorily completes 24 to 30 units, the community college posts 30 additional units in recognition of non-traditional prior learning. The diploma graduate RN is then eligible to apply to a BS program having 60 transferable lower-division units.

A graduate from a community college faces different challenges. While all units are potentially transferable, the 4-year university or regional accrediting agencies may limit the number of lower-division units that are accepted toward the baccalaureate. For example, in California, a community college transfer is limited to 70 transferable units. There is no stipulation as to which 70 units, so if a student completed the required lower-division general education and lower-division nursing major requirements with 72 to 80 units, the student does not have to retake a particular content course at the upper division. Rather, the student takes 50 units at the upper-division level in both general education and the major, going beyond the

---

▲ BOX 8.6   **Articulation Agreement Between a Community College and a State University**

Articulation Agreement by Major: Nursing
Effective with the fall 2002 catalog, the following lower-division courses are required for the major. Students eligible for earlier catalog rights should consult with their advisors and may follow the requirements effective for their catalog year.
See the CSUS catalog for a complete explanation of all lower/upper-division major requirements (www.csus.edu/catalog/).

From: Napa Community College   To: CSU Sacramento

A. REQUIRED PRECLINICAL COURSES:
   A grade of "C" or better is required for all preclinical Nursing courses.

ENGL120	Reading and Composition 1	(3)	ENGL1A	COLLEGE COMPOSITION	(3)

PSYC120	General Psychology OR	(3)	PSYC1	INTRO PSY-BASIC PROCESSES OR	(3)
PSYC123	Social Psychology (For Nursing Major Only)	(3)	PSYC5	INTRO PSY-INDIV+SOC PROCS	(3)

CHEM111	Introduction to Organic and Biological Chemistry	(4)	CHEM6B	INTRO ORGANIC+BIOL CHEM	(5)

BIOL218	Human Anatomy AND	(5)	BIO22	INTRO HUMAN ANATOMY AND	(4)
BIOL219	Human Physiology (For Nursing Majors Only) OR	(5)	BIO131	SYSTEMIC PHYSIOLOGY (See Comment #1 & #4)	(4)
BIOL218	Human Anatomy AND	(5)	BIO25	Human Anatomy and Physiology I AND	(4)
BIOL219	Human Physiology	(5)	BIO26	Human Anatomy and Physiology II	(4)

BIOL220	General Microbiology OR	(5)	BIO139	GENERAL MICROBIOLOGY	(4)
BIOL151	Intro Med Micro (For Nursing Majors Only)	(5)		(See Comment #1 & #4)	

BIOL103	Nutrition Today (For Nursing Majors Only)	(3)	FACS113	NUTRITION AND METABOLISM (See Comment #1 & #4)	(3)

PSYC125	Human Development (For Nursing Majors Only)	(3)	CHDV30	HUMAN DEVELOPMENT	(3)

HEOC101	Pharmacology (See Comment #2)	(3)	NURS14	PHARMACOLOGY	(2)

(box continues on page 226)

▲ **BOX 8.6**　　**Articulation Agreement Between a Community College and a State University** (continued)

B. REQUIRED LOWER-DIVISION CLINICAL NURSING COURSES:
　A grade of "C" or better is required for all clinical Nursing courses.

NURS141	Introduction to Nursing	(7)	NURS11	Intro to Prof. Nursing	(3)
NURS142	Nursing in Health Alterations I	(4)			
NURS141	Introduction to Nursing	(7)	NURS12	NURSING CARE OF ADULTS	(5)
NURS142	Nursing in Health Alterations I	(4)			
NURS141	Introduction to Nursing	(7)	NURS15	INTRO CLIN NURS PRACTICE	(2)
NURS142	Nursing in Health Alterations I	(4)			
NURS141	Introduction to Nursing	(7)	NURS16	PHYSICAL ASSESS OF ADULT	(1)
NURS142	Nursing in Health Alterations I	(4)			
NURS141	Introduction to Nursing	(7)	NURS17	CONCPT+PRACT OF GERO	(2)
NURS142	Nursing in Health Alterations I	(4)			

C. ADDITIONAL GRADUATION REQUIREMENTS:
　A course in societal-cultural patterns is required prior to certification of eligibility for state licensure.
　(See Comment #5)

SOCI120	Introduction to Sociology	(3)	SOC1	PRINCIPLES OF SOCIOLOGY	(3)
	OR			OR	
ANTH121	Introduction to Cultural Anthropology	(3)	ANTH2	INTRO CULTURAL ANTHRO	(3)

Comments:

1. The courses listed as acceptable in lieu of CSUS courses are acceptable preparation for the CSUS Nursing major only. If a course in Anatomy, Physiology, Microbiology, or Organic Chemistry is not listed, then any transferable course (each with Lab) is also acceptable.
2. Due to new licensure recommendations, applicants to the Fall 1997 and later clinical Nursing programs must have completed (as a prerequisite for entry into the upper-division clinical program) a course in Pharmacology, regardless of catalog rights.
3. NURS10, Health Care, PHYS2, Topics in Elementary Physics, plus a Statistics course are strongly recommended preparation.
4. BIO131, BIO139, and FACS113 are upper-division courses at CSUS; courses completed at a community college are lower division and meet subject matter requirements only. Upper-division credit cannot be granted.
5. The courses listed are two examples of acceptable societal-cultural patterns or diversity courses. Please see the CSUS catalog for additional options or contact the Division of Nursing for additional information.
6. The above major preparation agreement is subject to periodic change and revision. Please check with a counselor every semester to obtain current information about possible changes in the curriculum and/or articulated courses.

Approved: _____　_____
　　　　　　　　Department Chair　　　　Date　　　　　　Articulation Officer　　　Date

lower-division preparation. Herein is the issue in nursing education—that is, how a baccalaureate program addresses the issue of prelicensure content that is lower division at a community college and may be taught partly or wholly at the upper division level in the university program. This issue and the lack of recognition of comparability and acceptance of prelicensure course work between the different educational approaches in undergraduate nursing results in an alarming statistic: Only 20% of community college nursing graduates return for the BS degree (Sechrist, Lewis, & Rutledge, 1999).

RN completion programs, also called "two plus two" (2+2), were developed to facilitate advanced placement. Box 8.7 shows a sample curriculum of this type of program from California State University—Fullerton (2003). A total of 124 semester units are required for the BS degree. The program builds on the prelicensure preparation of the RN. Prerequisites required for admission may be completed in the prelicensure program, but if not, are taken prior to admission to the BS program. RN completion programs have been very popular and successful because the returning RN feels his or her initial educational preparation is valued and none of the prelicensure content is repeated.

Traditional generic (freshman-to-senior nursing major) baccalaureate programs also admit RN-to-baccalaureate students. National accrediting bodies require that baccalaureate programs validate courses taken in another prelicensure program. The Credit by Examination or the challenge process accomplishes this. An example is an RN-to-baccalaureate completion

---

▲ BOX 8.7   **Baccalaureate Plan of Study for the Returning RN in a Two-plus-Two Program**

Junior Year: First Semester

Nursing 300, Nursing Theories: Bases for Professional Practice (3)
Nursing 302, Assessment and Planning for Nursing Scholarship (2)
Nursing 305/305L, Professional Nursing I (Laboratory/Clinical) (3, 2)
Nursing 307, Health Promotion: Parent–Child Nursing (3)
General Education (3 units)

Junior Year: Second Semester

Nursing 320, Process of Teaching in Nursing (2)
Nursing 353, Alterations in Health Status: Applications in Nursing (4)
Nursing 355/355L, Professional Nursing II (Laboratory/Clinical) (3, 2)
Nursing 357, Health Promotion: Adult-Aged Nursing (3)
General Education (3)

Senior Year: First Semester

Nursing 400/400L, Professional Dimensions of Nursing (2,1)
Nursing 402/402L, Community Health Nursing (Clinical) (3, 3)
General Education Statistics (upper-division) (3)

Senior Year: Second Semester

Nursing 450/450L, Nursing Research (2,1)
Nursing 453/452L, Leadership/Management in Professional Nursing (Clinical) (3, 3)

student who takes a standardized or teacher-made examination requiring a passing score before credit is posted for the equivalent prelicensure course in the baccalaureate program. In many cases, it had been 15 to 20 years since the RN studied for the National Council Licensure Examination (NCLEX). There was anxiety and anger on the part of students about the need to study specific psychiatric disorders or perinatal nursing, particularly if the RN worked in critical care and needed the baccalaureate for admission to a graduate program.

To encourage RNs to return to school, university nursing programs, which were not designed specifically for RN-to-baccalaureate completion students, offer courses to "bridge" from the diploma or associate degree preparation (see Box 8.8, NURS 111A, Transitional Concepts for Professional Nursing [3 units], and NURS 111B, Bridging Concepts for Returning Nurses at CSUS [3 units]). Within these bridge courses, role socialization issues are addressed and validation that the RN possesses the requisite knowledge, skills, and abilities to succeed in the baccalaureate core is completed through a portfolio process. Upon completion of the bridge units, the RN receives credit for the prelicensure courses offered at the upper-division level. For example, in the CSU Sacramento (CSUS) advanced-placement curriculum, the RN receives 24 upper-division units for advanced medical–surgical nursing, mental health, pediatrics, and obstetrics. The RN-to-baccalaureate completion student now has 30 upper-division units completed toward the degree through the two completion courses and portfolio. Box 8.8 shows the Advanced Placement Curriculum for an RN-to-baccalaureate student attending CSUS.

The role of prior work experience applied toward a degree is another curricular issue. The amount and type of clinical experience a nurse possesses upon returning to school for a baccalaureate is a curricular challenge. Diploma and community college graduates are traditionally prepared for specific positions in the acute care setting, often referred to as more structured roles. While the baccalaureate program typically adds community health, research, health policy, case management, and community collaboration, the senior practicum hours for students are often in acute care settings for the purpose of skill acquisition. A technically competent RN generally doesn't need 300 hours of clinical experience in an acute care setting. An alternative to the senior practicum is to substitute the development of a project in response to an agency need from an evidenced-based practice perspective or to substitute the required undergraduate course with a graduate course exploring issues and ethics in health care. The latter can challenge the RN and encourage him or her to return for the master of science degree.

▲ COMPETENCY-BASED ROLE DIFFERENTIATION IN NURSING

National projections from a number of entities indicate a nursing shortage that is expected to increase in severity in the future. Nursing leadership throughout the United States has examined approaches to try to meet the critical need for more nurses and, at the same time, nurses who are prepared to function in the increasingly complex health care system. There is a need to differentiate among the levels of nursing education and clinical competencies of nurses, including competencies gained through experience. In 1991, the California Strategic Planning Committee for Nursing (CSPCN) was formed as a "virtual" consortium representing nearly

---

▲ **B O X 8 . 8**   **Advanced Placement Curriculum for an RN BS Student in a Generic Program**

Transferable Units from Community College Nursing Program (10 units total)

- ▲ N12 Nursing Care of Adults (5 units)
- ▲ N15 Introduction to Clinical Nursing Practice (2 units)
- ▲ N16 Physical Assessments of the Adult (1 unit)
- ▲ N17 Concepts and Practices in Gerontological Nursing (2 units)

Challenge Credit Given (24 units total) by Completion of N111A, Transitional Concepts for Professional Nursing, and N111B, Bridging Constructs for Returning Nurses

- ▲ N123 Nursing Families in Complex Illness (6 units)
- ▲ N128 Therapeutic Interpersonal and Group Communication in Nursing (1 unit)
- ▲ N129 Mental Health Nursing (5 units)
- ▲ N136 Nursing the Childbearing Family: Skills & Assessment (1 unit)
- ▲ N137 Nursing the Childbearing Family (5 units)
- ▲ N138 Nursing the Childrearing Family (5 units)
- ▲ N139 Nursing the Childrearing Family: Skills & Assessment (1 unit)

Required Core Courses: Transition Bridge Courses

- ▲ N111A Transitional Concepts for Professional Nursing (3 units)
- ▲ N111B Bridging Constructs for Returning Nurses (3 units)

Senior-Level Courses (28 units total)

- ▲ *N143 Leadership and Management in Nursing Practice (6 units)
- ▲ N144 Community Health Nursing (5 units)
- ▲ N150 Research in Nursing (2 units)
- ▲ N155 Senior Forum (1 unit)
- ▲ **N156 Selected Senior Practicum in Nursing (3 units)
- ▲ N169 Reasoning Development in Health Care (can be used as upper-division general education) (3 units)
- ▲ N191 Service Learning in Nursing (senior project) (2 units)

* Work experience may be used for clinical hours at instructor's discretion; project development requirement.
** RN BS students with 3 years of experience may attend a graduate course as a substitute for this course.

40 nursing groups throughout the state. The mission of CSPCN was to "establish master plans for the nursing workforce and education to ensure an adequate supply of nurses prepared to meet healthcare needs of the population and for the demands of the industry" (Fox, Walker, Bream, & the Education/Industry Interface Work Group of the California Strategic Planning Committee for Nursing/Colleagues in Caring, 1999, p. 1)

One of the outcomes of the work accomplished by CSPCN was a framework for competency-based role differentiation in nursing. The framework, developed in collaboration with representatives from nursing service, nursing education, and numerous organizations that represented nurses throughout California, includes competencies expected of graduates of RN and licensed vocational nursing (LVN) programs. The competencies specifically address the LVN role (licensed practical nurse [LPN] in many states), the RN care provider, the RN care coordinator, and the advanced-practice nurse.

The RN care provider is defined as the nurse "who provides direct care to clients and their families" (i.e., the staff nurse) (Fox et al., 1999, p. 29). Within this role, the RN functions as provider of care, advocate, teacher, and supervisor of assigned staff. The RN care coordinator "functions outside the direct care arena and functions across the health care continuum in a variety of settings" (Fox et al., 1999, p. 5). This role encompasses, for example, case manager, unit manager, quality improvement coordinator, clinical educator, and risk manager. The advanced-practice nurse role includes the clinical nurse specialist, nurse anesthetist, nurse midwife, and nurse practitioner whose roles are expansions of baccalaureate and master's practice. Within each of these roles and functions, the competencies illustrate degrees of expertise from novice to expert as described in 1996 by Benner, Tanner, and Chesla (as cited in Fox et al., 1999) and are based on the current scopes of practice in California.

The perception is that determining the expected competencies for the LVN/LPN and RN provides guidance for nursing service administrators to utilize nursing personnel at their optimum level of education and within their scopes of practice. The model also serves as a framework for nursing curricula. Highly motivated and self-directed nurses can accomplish successful movement along the continuum from novice to expert without necessarily obtaining a higher degree. An important element of this framework is the belief that nurses, through education and/or experience, can gain competencies in the various roles and progress from one level to another.

▲ ROLE SOCIALIZATION, ACCELERATED PROGRAMS, AND CAREER MOBILITY

A discussion of the educational approach to preparing a professional nurse, the requisite curriculum, and the time to complete the degree must include some thoughts on role socialization and role attainment. Nurse educators use the term "generic" program when referring to students enrolled in a traditional nursing program leading to their first degree or diploma in nursing and their first exposure to the nursing role.

A generic program provides a standard foundation from which all graduates can build. The term generic has been extended to include generic master of science and doctoral programs in nursing for people who enter nursing for the first time at those levels. Generic education begins the process of professional socialization, which includes serious involvement and a rigorous course of study "over a *sustained* time with guidance from mentors who are inquirers, continuous learners and exquisite practitioners" (Schlotfeldt, 1977). Professional education in all fields involves a preprofessional period of exposure to the arts and sciences. There is a relationship between the amount and type of liberal arts and professional courses. The graduate of a professional program goes beyond the mastery of skills to identifying gaps in knowledge, providing structure to nonstructured and unpredictable situations, and testing hypotheses in support of evidenced-based practice. The trend toward accelerated programs for rapid completion of entry-level programs initially in response to the shortage, as well as career mobility options for RNs to earn the baccalaureate or higher degrees, should raise questions as to the sufficiency of time to be socialized into the role of a professional nurse. Thus, curriculum planners need to take into account and apply socialization theories and concepts to ensure that students are prepared for professional roles and responsibilities.

Career mobility must be addressed when developing a nursing education curriculum. Prelicensure community college programs typically include 80 lower-division semester units of general education and nursing, and completion of the baccalaureate requires a minimum of 40 additional units at the upper-division level largely in nursing. A seamless transition between educational programs requires that nursing courses and their sequence distinguish between the lower and upper divisions of undergraduate education. The innovative collaborative models previously discussed represent an approach to seamless transitioning with recognition of what each program does best.

▲ UNDERGRADUATE NURSING CURRICULA IN THE FUTURE

If undergraduate nursing faculty members continue to hold on to traditional, time-honored approaches to curriculum development and clinical education, they will miss the opportunity to recast, revitalize, and restructure for the future of nursing (Tagliareni & Mengel, 2001). The educational approach to a basic nursing education is not simple, uncomplicated, or even clear. Prior to the critical nursing shortage, which is projected to continue well into 2010, Lindeman (2000) posited that the direction of nursing education would be influenced greatly by market-driven economic policy, technology, demographics, and the knowledge explosion. Adding a nursing shortage to the influence of market forces on curriculum changes some of the implications.

While Lindeman forecasted a market-driven, competitive system of higher education, the competition appears to be for the graduates of any basic nursing program. Entrepreneurial organizations and traditional educational programs that traditionally offer RN completion or advanced-practice education are quickly entering the marketplace to offer LVN/LPN-to-RN programs or generic associate degree and baccalaureate programs. Collaboration between education and service to support preparation of more graduate RNs has in some cases focused on preparing a licensed RN as quickly as possible for the lowest cost to provide care at the bedside. This approach to nursing education does not address the need for a sustained educational experience to achieve a professional role or the fact that the emphasis in health care shifted to community-based care delivery.

The Pew Health Professions Commission (O'Neill & Pew Health Professions Commission, 1998 p. iii) expressed concern that educational programs were preparing graduates for yesterday's health care system and not for the demands of the new health care system. The Commission supported differentiated practice as an outcome of different educational programs and suggested the number and types of nurses prepared should reflect regional health care needs, not institutional or political needs. This is consistent with the work of the California Strategic Planning Committee for Nursing (Sechrist, Lewis, & Rutledge, 1999), which identified the need for more baccalaureate- and master's-prepared graduates.

A second driving force identified by Lindeman (2000) is technology, both in the delivery of health care and in the delivery of an educational program. Education is available through virtual universities and critical care practice is provided in a virtual intensive care unit (ICU). While educators argue that the traditional classroom setting increases interaction, decreases procrastination, provides immediate feedback, and is more meaningful, proponents of distance learning cite cost effectiveness, convenience, and flexibility in support of a new pedagogy (Leasure, Davis, & Thievon, 2000). There appears to be some concern emerging with regard to the credibility and rigor of a nontraditional approach to nursing education versus a residential program that enhances traditional delivery supported by technology. Prelicensure RN programs that require no clinical experience in the program exist (ACNL, 2004). Basic RN programs are offered totally online using resident preceptors (California State University Dominguez Hills Division of Nursing, 2004). The use of preceptors for clinical nursing education raises the issues of mentoring and role modeling in professional role preparation.

Delivering a nursing curriculum via distance or distributive education requires faculty to accept a new set of assumptions. Learning outcomes must be the same as in the traditional classroom. Faculty members will assume a new role—"guide on the side versus sage on the stage"—and to learn how to teach all over again. Effective distance education does not mean merely putting lecture notes on a website and monitoring a chat room. Not all students adapt easily to new technology such as replacing face-to-face communication with synchronous or asynchronous chat or using e-mail attachments for submission of papers. See Chapter 14 of this text for a detailed discussion of distance education in nursing.

Shifting demographics was the third force on Lindeman's (2000) list. Implications for curriculum development focus on the need to prepare students to deliver care to a diverse and older population who may subscribe to alternative and complementary therapies. The curriculum must be designed to meet the needs of a growing number of students with diverse learning styles, variable English language skills, and learning disabilities. The fourth driving force is the knowledge explosion. Lindeman cites a quote from Eleanor Sullivan that is relevant to the discussion of nursing curricula for the future:

> The 19th century university model, still common today, is obsolete. This model championed scholarship over application and lecture without discussion, was professor-centered rather than student-centered, and used a cumbersome system of self-governance. The forces of change are many and complex. They include the demand for public accountability of how society's money is spent, demographic changes, student demand for relevant experiences, the impact of economics, and technological advances. All are changing the face of higher education such that it will never be the same (Sullivan, 1997, p.144).

The implications for curriculum development in undergraduate nursing are cited throughout the literature. In addition to the recommendation that nursing curricula move away from the traditional, illness-centered approach to a community-based focus, Bowen, Lyons, and Young (2000) set forth six skill areas that they believe enable the professional nurse to succeed in the real world of health care, that is, a world of patients with increasing acuity, limited resources both fiscal and human, and an environment that does not support the professional practice essential for quality care. Those six skill areas that must be threaded throughout any nursing curriculum are:

1. The development of effective, accurate oral and written communication
2. A sense of internal control over a dynamic practice arena
3. Political savvy to influence health policy

4. Leadership
5. Crisis management
6. Organization, priority setting, and time management strategies

Lindeman (2000) summed up the challenges facing curriculum development in undergraduate nursing by saying that it is imperative for nurse educators "to give up notions of control and predictability and learn to enjoy change and ambiguity. Like it or not, it is indeed a new world" (p. 6).

▲ THE UNIVERSITY OF VICTORIA EXPERIENCE— THE EMANCIPATORY CURRICULUM

A significant departure from the traditional nursing curriculum, which focuses on the content necessary for licensure, is the curricular approach called emancipatory education that appeared in the literature beginning in 1989 (Bevis & Watson, 1989). As the term implies, the curriculum focuses on "emancipation, empowerment, and liberation from the oppressive structures of traditional education" (Schreiber & Banister, 2002, p. 41).

The philosophy of the University of Victoria School of Nursing's, British Columbia, Canada, curriculum is based on feminism, phenomenology, and critical social theory. Hiring a number of new faculty members supportive of this approach to nursing education facilitated implementation of this nontraditional curriculum. There is a significant power shift in this curriculum. Students are free, actually encouraged, to challenge course assignments, due dates, and the value of the course. Complaints are viewed as indications that the students feel heard and may actually be the basis for a student project that leads to curriculum revision. Students are free to learn at their own pace and determine how learning will be measured. Poor performance or failure is viewed as an opportunity for growth. The faculty role is one of coach and mentor; however, a faculty member insecure in the role may feel vulnerable. The emphasis is on teaching, which may take precedence over administrative functions, and competes with the time required for scholarship. Faculty members in this curriculum believe they are better able to respond to the rapidly changing health care environment when learning is grounded in context, not content, and they believe this approach is the future of nursing education (Schreiber & Banister, 2002).

▲ SUMMARY

Chapter 7 reviewed the three traditional types of nursing programs for entry into practice in the United States: diploma, associate degree, and baccalaureate. Sample curricula for associate degree and baccalaureate programs were described. Some of the problems, issues, and challenges for accommodating nurses who wish to continue their education in baccalaureate and higher degree programs were reviewed and an exemplar curriculum for blending an associate degree and a baccalaureate program was presented. A competency-based role differentiation model to define levels of practice from the LPN/LVN to advanced practice was offered as a way in which to recognize both the education and clinical experience of nurses. The model can also serve as a guide for curriculum development. Finally, the issues and challenges for nurse educators in the future were described.

DISCUSSION QUESTIONS

1. To what extent is it realistic to think or expect that an RN returning to school will experience a change in his or her professional role concept within a few short semesters after the initial education experience?
2. To what extent should the transition from prelicensure preparation in a diploma program or community college be seamlessly articulated with a baccalaureate nursing program?
3. To what extent should the multiple approaches in nursing education, particularly at the undergraduate level, be viewed as career changes with no presumption of comparability or articulation?
4. How does a differentiated practice model support the continuation of multiple approaches to entering the field of nursing?
5. What changes must occur in an undergraduate nursing curriculum to meet the demands of the health care system?

LEARNING ACTIVITIES

Student Activities

1. Review the basic nursing education program you attended for examples of facilitation or barriers to transfer or articulation between the different approaches to undergraduate nursing education.
2. Discuss with colleagues prepared at the diploma, associate degree, or baccalaureate levels the similarities and differences in the prelicensure and the baccalaureate curricula. Compare your educational experience with your colleagues.
3. Compare your undergraduate preparation with the competencies expected in the role differentiation between the different educational approaches.

Faculty Activities

1. Analyze the curriculum of your nursing program for the facilitators of or barriers to articulation or transfer of credits for students into your program or for graduates of your program into higher levels of education. Develop strategies for removing the barriers you find and improving transfer of credit or articulation agreements.
2. In what ways does your nursing program recognize differentiated practice at various levels of education?

REFERENCES

Association of California Nurse Leaders. (2004). Position statement on non-clinical pre-licensure nursing education. ACNL: Sacramento, CA. Author.

Ayers, M., Bruno, A., & Langford, R. (1999). *Community-based nursing care: Making the transition.* St. Louis: Mosby.

Baldwin, J. H., Conger, C. O., Abegglen, J. C., & Hill, E. H. (1998). Population focused and community-based nursing: Moving toward clarification of concepts. *Public Health Nursing, 15*(1), 12–18.

Bevis, E. O., & Watson, J. (1989). *Toward a caring curriculum: A new pedagogy for nursing.* New York: National League for Nursing Press.

Board of Registered Nursing. (2000). *Required curriculum: Prior approval.* Title 16. California Code of Regulations, Division 14, Article 3.

Bowen, M., Lyons, K. J., & Young, B. E. (2000). Nursing and health care reform: Implications for curriculum development. *Journal of Nursing Education, 39*(1), 27–33.

Brigham Young College of Nursing. (2003). Advisement Center Program Guide. Retrieved June 20, 2003, from http://nursing.byu.edu/advisement/ academicprogram/undergraduate.htm

California State University Dominguez Hills Division of Nursing. Dominguez Online Bachelor of Science Nursing. (2003). Retrieved October 25, 2004, from www.csudh.edu/dominguez online/bsn/bsnwork.htm

California State University–Fullerton. (2003). Baccalaureate plan of study. Retrieved July 12, 2003, from http://www.fullerton.edu/catalog/academic_departments/nurs.asp#bs_in_nursing

Catalano, J. (2003). *Nursing now! Today's issues, tomorrow's trends* (3rd ed.). Philadelphia: F.A. Davis.

Conger, C. O., Baldwin, J. H., Abegglen, J., & Callister, L. C. (1999). The shifting sands of health care delivery: Curriculum revision and integration of community health nursing. *Journal of Nursing Education, 38*(7), 304–311.

Ellis, J., & Hartley, C. (1998). *Nursing in today's world: Challenges, issues, and trends* (6th ed.). Philadelphia: Lippincott.

Evelyn, J. (2003, April 11). Making waves in Miami. *The Chronicle of Higher Education,* , A34-35.

Fox, S., Walker, P., Bream, T., and the Education/Industry Interface Work Group of the California Strategic Planning Committee for Nursing/Colleagues in Caring. (1999). *California's framework for competency-based role differentiation in nursing.* Sacramento, CA: ACNL.

Leasure, A. R., Davis, L., & Thievon, S. L. (2000). Comparison of student outcomes and preferences in a traditional vs. World Wide Web-based baccalaureate nursing research course. *Journal of Nursing Education, 39*(4), 149–154.

Lindeman, C. A. (2000). The future of nursing education. *Journal of Nursing Education, 39*(1), 5–12.

Lysaught, J. P. (1970). *An abstract for action.* New York: McGraw-Hill.

Montag, M. I. (1951). *The education of nursing technician.* New York: G.P. Putnam's Sons.

National League for Nursing Accrediting Commission. (2003). Home Page. Retrieved July 9, 2003, from http://www.nlnac.org/ AboutNLNAC/whatsnew.htm

National League for Nursing. (1993). *A vision for nursing education.* New York: The League.

O'Neill, E. N., & the Pew Health Professions Commission. (1998). *Recreating health professional practice for a new century.* San Francisco, CA: Pew Health Professions Commission.

Schlotfeldt, R. M. (1977). Educational requirements for registered nursing. *Entry into registered nursing—Issues and problems.* New York: National League for Nursing.

Schreiber, R., & Banister, E. (2002). Challenges of teaching in an emancipatory curriculum. *Journal of Nursing Education, 41*(1), 41–45.

Sechrist, K. R, Lewis, E. M., & Rutledge, D. N. (1999). *Planning for California's nursing work force: Phase II final report.* Sacramento, CA: Association of California Nurse Leaders.

Sullivan, E. J. (1997). A changing higher education environment. *Journal of Professional Nursing, 13*(3), 143–149.

Tagliareni, M. E., & Mengel, A. (2001). Broadening clinical education in basic nursing programs. In J. M. Dochterman & H. K. Kennedy (Eds.), *Current issues in nursing.* St. Louis: Mosby.

Zerwekh, J., & Claborn, J. C. (1997). *Nursing today: Transition and trends* (2nd ed.). Philadelphia: W.B. Saunders Co.

Graduate Curricula in Nursing

Kathleen Huttlinger, PhD, RN, and
Diana L. Biordi, PhD, RN, FAAN

OBJECTIVES

Upon completion of Chapter 9, the reader will be able to:

1. Evaluate the historical development and role of graduate nursing education in the United States.
2. Differentiate between undergraduate and graduate curricula and master's and doctorate curricula.
3. Analyze the types of master's and doctoral programs.
4. Identify the key external and internal frame factors that affect the development of graduate nursing programs.
5. Evaluate some of the outcome measures that apply to graduate education.
6. Analyze some of the key issues facing graduate education, currently and in the future, including nursing's fit within academe, the faculty shortage, faculty workload, and economic and resource influences.

9

▲ OVERVIEW

Developing master's and doctoral level nursing programs presents a variety of challenges, many of them unique and quite different from those of undergraduate programs. This chapter describes the major features of graduate education in nursing and begins with a brief historical overview. It is followed by descriptions of those external and internal frames that influence program development, decisions regarding the curriculum development, and the program's evaluation. Issues facing graduate education are discussed, including their impact on addressing the faculty shortage in nursing and the demand for expanding nursing science to provide a knowledge base for evidence-based practice. Samples of graduate education curricula are included in the figures throughout the chapter.

▲ HISTORICAL DEVELOPMENT OF MASTER'S AND DOCTORAL NURSING EDUCATION

Master's Degree Education

As discussed in Chapter 1, the evolution of nursing education in the United States reflects the needs of society and the nursing profession and the demands of the health care system (Meleis, 1988). In terms of education, nursing in academe is relatively young, with the majority of baccalaureate and graduate nursing programs only being about 25 years old, although a few have existed for 50 and even 75 years.

Societal and subsequent health care demands led to the early development of master's level nursing education programs at Western Reserve (Case Western Reserve) in the early 1920s. Yale University's program was founded after the Rockefeller Foundation and the Goldmark Reports recommended that nursing education be placed in institutions of higher education (Committee for the Study of Nursing Education, 1923) and that the society and health care of that time needed nursing professionals who were "educated" rather than "trained." At the same time, nurse educators across the country stressed that nursing faculty needed postbaccalaureate education to ensure a quality education. Whereas the early Master's of Nursing degree (MN) at Yale built upon bachelor's degrees in science, arts, or philosophy and offered a 30-month course of study toward the master's degree, the MN at Western Reserve built upon a strong baccalaureate nursing curriculum. Others such as Vanderbilt University and the University of Chicago soon followed these two early graduate programs. However, even with the pioneering efforts of these few colleges, the number of graduate nursing programs remained small for the next 25 years or so.

From the end of World War II and into the late 1970s, graduate nursing education emphasized three primary areas: the preparation of nursing educators and administrators, clinical nurse specialists, and nurse practitioners. During the years from 1945 to 1960, nursing education at the graduate level focused on preparing educators and administrators. The 1960s and 1970s saw a very rapid rise of technology in health care followed by the opening of critical care units and treatment centers. The rapid infusion of technology along with the emergence of Medicare brought about a need for nurses who were able to manage patient care that went beyond preparation at the baccalaureate level. Therefore, nurse educators were faced with answering questions that addressed whether master's level nurses should function as educators, administrators, clinical specialists, or a combination of all three (Hawkins & Thibodeau, 1993; Bell, 2003).

Most graduate programs responded to these questions by developing core curricula and clinical education tracks that emphasized specific clinical areas, such as maternal child, pediatrics, medical–surgical, case management, midwifery, nurse anesthetist, education, psychiatric–mental health, community health, or nursing administration, a pattern which is still reflected in many nursing education programs today (Bell, 2003; Walker et al., 2003). A typical master's curriculum featured several required core courses such as Nursing Theory, Research, and Professional/Health Care Issues along with clinical specialty courses.

Other programs developed ways to combine a master's degree in nursing with other disciplines. Most notable of these are the master's in nursing degree with a business administration master's (MSN/MBA) in schools of business and community health or nurse practitioner specialties with public health (MSN/MPH) in schools of public health (Bell, 2003)

During the 1960s and 1970s, market forces in health care placed pressure on nursing to respond to a need for clinical specialists, consultants, patient educators, and staff developers. At the same time, there was a critical shortage of pediatricians and primary care providers in rural Colorado (Gortner, 1991; Walker et al. 2003). This need was met by the development of an advanced-practice nurse, the nurse practitioner, whose "education and training extended beyond the basic requirements for licensure" (Ford & Silver, 1967). Functions of the nurse practitioner included the diagnosis and management of common acute illnesses as well as disease prevention and management of stable, chronic illnesses (Safreit, 1992). Although these early "postlicensure" education programs varied in terms of educational requirements, present nurse practitioner programs fall under accreditation, certification, and curricular guidelines, and are generally offered at the master's or postbaccalaureate level.

Hanson and Hamric (2003) examine advanced-practice nursing by tracing its history, its definition, and trends in graduate education and certification. In visioning the future, the authors advocate a standardized core curriculum for advanced-practice roles, standardization of curricula and certification examinations, and the need to develop a cohesive view of advanced practice to ensure its legitimacy in the health care system.

Doctoral Degree Education

Early doctoral programs in nursing were few and varied in degree emphasis. Columbia University began offering the education doctorate (EdD) for nurses in 1924, which was followed by the PhD in nursing at New York University in 1934. However, the need for master's-prepared nurses and for doctoral-prepared nurses became evident after World War II and was prompted by legislative and political policy decisions at national, state, and local levels (Marriner-Tomey, 1990; Jones & Lusk, 2002). During the 1950s and 1960s, the federal government offered a program to help stimulate the research preparation of nurses and to provide financial support for their research efforts. It sponsored the nurse-scientist graduate training programs in 1962, which promoted PhDs for nurses in cognate disciplines such as biology, physiology, psychology, and philosophy. These programs flourished during the late 1960s and until 1976, when the last federal grant to support this effort ended (Marriner-Tomey, 1990).

The end of the 1970s and early 1980s saw an increase in doctoral programs across the United States, from five in 1965, to 88 at the time of this writing (AACN, 2004).

There are presently four different kinds of doctoral degrees awarded in nursing (Meleis, 1988; AACN, 2003). These are the Doctor of Philosophy (PhD), the Education Doctorate (EdD), the Doctorate in Nursing Science (DNSc), and the Nursing Doctorate (ND). The focus of the doctorate and the advantages of each kind are often debated, but in general, it is believed that the PhD represents a research degree with emphasis on advancing the clinical research that underlies nursing practice (Jones & Lusk, 2002). The DNSc and ND are considered professional degrees with an emphasis on research in terms of clinical applications. The EdD has a focus on education with the intent that research is aimed at problems that deal with nursing education. The idea of separation of research and practice is, to some degree, a false dichotomy but is nevertheless the line of demarcation between the types of degrees (AACN, 2002a). The focus of the doctoral program is an important consideration in developing the curriculum for a program, and the implications for its development are discussed later in this chapter (see Figure 9.1 for a sample PhD in nursing curriculum plan).

On another note, the present and future nursing shortage is also reflected in schools of nursing where large numbers of nursing faculty have retired or will soon retire. To document the crisis, the National League for Nursing conducted a 2002 survey of U.S. RN and graduate programs for information on their faculty. Of the 1,419 programs surveyed, with a return rate of 77%, there were 1,106 vacant positions representing a vacancy rate of 6% for baccalaureate and higher degree programs and 5.5% for Associate Degree in Nursing (ADN) programs. Two-thirds of the faculty were 45 to 60 years old and only 25% were 31 to 45 years of age. The majority of faculty in ADN programs held master's degrees, and of their part-time faculty, 44.1% held a baccalaureate. About half of the faculty in the baccalaureate and higher degree programs held doctorates, and 22.4% of the diploma program faculty held baccalaureates. To compensate for the shortage, 70.2% of the programs hired part-time faculty (NLN, 2003). There is a pressing, if not urgent, need for doctoral programs to offer teaching opportunities for those who wish to pursue faculty positions.

▲ GRADUATE NURSING EDUCATION IN THE 21ST CENTURY

Nursing faculties and administrations across the United States, in conjunction with the National Institute of Nursing Research, have begun a serious examination of the research trajectories and funding of nursing faculty. Compared to other disciplines, nursing faculty are 20 years older than their counterparts when beginning their research, and typically have only one to two major funded grants before retirement. This trend, while cognizant of the relative newness of nursing research, does not bode well for a strong research firmament for nursing as a profession, nor does it provide a cadre of researchers within a particular field of study. In addition, it limits the availability of qualified research faculty mentors for graduate students. To demonstrate the dearth of graduate-prepared nurses, the Division of Nursing's report on the registered nurse population in 2000 reported that 22.3% of the workforce held the diploma in nursing, 34.3% the ADN, 32.7% the baccalaureate, 9.6%

```
FULL-TIME
3–4 YEARS

Yr 1 Sem 1        History & Philosophy of Nursing Science
                  Quantitative Research
                  Methods in Nursing
                  Statistics I

Yr 1 Sem 2        Theory Construction & Development in Nursing
                  Qualitative Research Methods in Nursing
                  Statistics II or Cognate
                  Introduction to Nursing Knowledge Domains

Yr 2 Sem 1        Nursing Science Seminar
                  Statistics II or Cognate
                  Cognate
                  Advanced Methods for Nursing Research

Yr 2 Sem 2        Nursing Science Seminar II
                  Nursing and Health Care Policy
                  Cognate

Yrs 3 & 4         Examination for Candidacy for Doctoral Dissertation
                  Dissertation Prospectus
                  Dissertation I & II

PART-TIME
5–6 YEARS

Yr 1 Sem 1        History & Philosophy of Nursing Science
                  Statistics I

Yr 1 Sem 2        Theory Construction & Development in Nursing
                  Statistics II

Yr 2 Sem 1        Quantitative Research Methods in Nursing
                  Cognate

Yr 2 Sem 2        Qualitative Research Methods in Nursing
                  Introduction to Nursing Knowledge Domains

Yr 3 Sem 1        Advanced Methods for Nursing Research
                  Choose from below
                  ▲ Measurement in Nursing Research
                  ▲ Application of Qualitative Methods in Nursing Research
                  ▲ Grant Development and Funding
                  ▲ Program Evaluation in Nursing
                  ▲ Other (to be announced)

                  Nursing Science Seminar I
                  Course developed to fit student needs, e.g.:
                  ▲ Family Theories & Nursing Research
                  ▲ Nursing & Women's Health
                  ▲ Stress, Coping, & Social Support and Nursing Research
                  ▲ Other

Yr 3 Sem 2        Nursing Science Seminar II
                  Nursing & Health Care Policy

Yr 4 Sem 1        Cognate
                  Cognate

Yrs 4, 5          Examination for Candidacy for the Doctoral Dissertation
(and beyond if    Dissertation Prospectus
necessary)        Dissertation I & II
```

FIGURE 9 . 1   Kent State University and the University of Akron joint PhD in nursing (JPDN) curriculum plans: Full- and part-time plans. (Note: All courses are 3 semester credit hours.)

the master's, and 0.6% the doctorate. Of the master's group, 21% held a master's in other related fields and 51% of the doctorates were in related fields (USDHHS, HRSA, Bureau of Health Professions Division of Nursing, 2002).

In an attempt to offset these problems, nursing programs are promoting accelerated or "Fast-Track" degrees for outstanding students, so that the time spent moving from the baccalaureate to master's or doctorate may be shorter. In addition, the AACN (2002a) cites 34 accelerated master's programs in late 2002, with at least 18 others in the planning stages. Most of these accelerated programs are geared to meeting the learning needs of individuals with undergraduate degrees in disciplines other than nursing and are considered entry-level programs. Examples of programs meeting this need are Yale University, the University of Iowa, Samuel Merritt College (see Figure 9.2 for its curriculum plan), Marquette University, and DePaul University to name a few. See Figure 9.3 for a curriculum plan for a traditional master's degree nursing program to compare it to an entry-level program.

Under pressure for accountability for more effective resource distribution and handling of personnel shortages, nursing took the lead in developing and planning new ways for earning the master's and doctorate in nursing and new ways to deliver graduate programs (AACN 2003; Armstrong, Johnson, Bridges, & Gessner, 2003). Although it has not yet happened, it is projected that future doctoral curricula may themselves be shortened, so that what is now an accelerated master's or even the baccalaureate-to-doctorate becomes a norm, much as is the case in other academic disciplines (McCarty & Higgins, 2003). Several of these types of nursing programs are offered currently. In addition to accelerated (Fast-Track) programs, new clinical specialties at the master's level are gaining in popularity. Examples include nursing informatics, case management, transcultural, and parish nursing. There are other specialties such as forensic nursing and ambulatory care that may one day be included as master's program offerings.

▲ EXTERNAL FRAME FACTORS AND GRADUATE NURSING EDUCATION

The external frame factors that influence the planning and development of a graduate nursing program include the surrounding environment, geographic location, community and professional support, proximity of other graduate nursing programs, regulatory agencies, and political constituents. The environment surrounding the nursing unit is an important consideration when developing a graduate nursing program. The surrounding environment includes all of those "external" factors that lie outside of the nursing unit that could influence and impact the development of any new program. These environmental factors include the geographic area in which the unit is located and the local and surrounding communities that may impact or be impacted by the proposed program.

The geographic location of the proposed program, especially in terms of urban versus rural location, may have a direct influence on how the program is implemented. For example, a more rural or remote location where there are issues of transportation and access for students might lend itself to distance or Web-based learning modalities, while a more urban location might be able to offer its program during weekdays or evenings. As discussed

Semester I

N518	Pharmacology	2 units
N519	Pathophysiology	3 units
N524/524L	Health Assessment	3 units
N534/534L	Mental Health Nursing	6 units
N542L	Nursing Skills I	1 unit
Total		15 units

Semester II

N546/546L	Nursing Care of Adults and Older Adults	10 units
N543L	Nursing Skills II	1 unit
N501	Access and Presentation of Health Care Information	1 unit
Total		12 units

Semester III

N566/N566L	Nursing Care of Critically Ill Adults	4.5 units
N556/556L	Nursing Care of Pediatric and Youth Populations	5.5 units
N540/N540L	Reproductive Health Care	6 units
Total		16 units

Semester IV

N594L	Clinical Internship	6 units
N560	Leadership, Management, and Organizational Behavior in Health Care Delivery Systems	3 units
N562	Professional, Legal, and Ethical Issues	3 units
Total		12 units

Semester V

N601	Research Methods	3 units
N564	History and Theories of Nursing	3 units
N570/N570L	Community Health Nursing	6 units
Total		12 units

Semester VI

N302	Nurse Practitioner Issues Seminar I	1 unit
Employment as a Registered Nurse for 400 hours		

Semester VII

N300	Family Nursing	3 units
N301	Advanced Health Assessment	3 units
N320	Advanced Pathophysiology	3 units
Total		9 units

Semester VIII

N304	Primary Health Care I	3 units
N307	Ambulatory Pharmacy for Nurse Practitioners	3 units
N308A	Clinical Practicum (90 hours)	2 units
N602	Analysis of Health Policy Issues	3 units
Total		11 units

Semester IX

N303	Nurse Practitioner Seminar II	1 unit
N305	Primary Health Care II	4 units
N308B	Clinical Practicum (270 hrs)	6 units
Total		11 units

Semester X

N306	Primary Health Care III	2 units
N309	Internship (270 hrs)	6 units
N605/606	Thesis/Special Project	3 units
Total		11 units

F I G U R E   9 . 2　Sample curriculum of an entry-level MSN program.

ADULT HEALTH PRIMARY CARE NURSE PRACTITIONER		
YEAR 1 FALL SEMESTER		
Course #	**Name**	**CHRS**
N60041	Advanced Assessment for Adults	3
N60206	Ambulatory Diagnostics	2
N60204	Health Care Issues in Aging (optional for students interested in gerontology)	(3)
BSCI60495	Advanced Physiology	3
	TOTAL	**8 (11)**
YEAR 1 SPRING SEMESTER		
Course #	**Name**	**CHRS**
N60042	Primary Health Care I	5
N60101	Theoretical Basis in Nursing	3
N60441	Advanced Pharmacology	3
	TOTAL	**11**
YEAR 1 SUMMER SEMESTER		
Course #	**Name**	**CHRS**
N60044	Nurse Practitioner Practicum	2
N60401	Clinical Inquiry I	3
	TOTAL	**5**
YEAR 2 FALL SEMESTER		
Course #	**Name**	**CHRS**
N60043	Primary Care II	5
N60205	Epidemiology	1
N60402 or	Clinical Inquiry II	2
N60199	Thesis (6 hours of thesis may be substituted for Clinical Inquiry II)	(3)
N60451	Health Care Policy	2
	TOTAL	**10 (11)**
YEAR 2 SPRING SEMESTER		
Course #	**Name**	**CHRS**
N60432	APCNP Role Practicum	4
N60450	Ethics	2
N60199	Thesis (optional)	(3)
	TOTAL	**6 (9)**
	TOTAL PROGRAM CREDIT HRS	**40 (44)**

NURSING OF THE ADULT CLINICAL NURSE SPECIALIST		
YEAR 1 FALL SEMESTER		
Course #	**Name**	**CHRS**
N60041	Advanced Assessment for Adults	3
N60101	Theoretical Basis in Nursing	3
BSCI60495	Advanced Physiology	3
	TOTAL	**9**
YEAR 1 SPRING SEMESTER		
Course #	**Name**	**CHRS**
N60053	Adult Health Nursing Clinical Interventions and Physiological Health	5 3
Nxxxxxx	Nursing Elective (e.g., Pharmacology, Informatics, Health Care)	3
	TOTAL	**8**
YEAR 1 SUMMER SEMESTER		
YEAR 2 FALL SEMESTER		
Course #	**Name**	**CHRS**
N60056	Adult Health Nursing: Clinical Interventions and Psychosocial Health Behaviors	5
N60451 or	Health Care Policy	2
N60450	Ethics	
N60401	Clinical Inquiry I	3
	TOTAL	**10**
YEAR 2 SPRING SEMESTER		
Course #	**Name**	**CHRS**
N60342	CNS Practicum	6
N60451 or	Health Care Policy	2
N60450	Ethics	
N60402	Clinical Inquiry II	2
	TOTAL	**10**
	TOTAL PROGRAM CREDIT HRS	**37**

FIGURE 9.3   Kent State University College of Nursing MSN program plans, full-time study.

in Chapter 5, a needs assessment for the program should reflect and identify the most needed modes of delivery.

There are also geographic implications when recruiting faculty for positions in a graduate program. A few of the things that potential faculty will consider are access to transportation systems for them to engage in research consultation and to attend professional conferences, the availability of local and regional support systems for clinical practice and research, and the presence of colleagues for collaboration. Therefore, if the program is in a rural or more remote area, the nursing unit might have to strategize ways to attract qualified faculty. For example, sometimes programs in rural areas can offer quality of life, low-cost housing and living expenses, or the attractiveness of nearby recreational offerings.

The surrounding community in which the nursing unit lies is another very important factor. The community should promote professional nursing standards and support graduate nursing education. Problems can occur if a nursing unit proposes a graduate program and the local nursing community does not recognize or understand the importance of graduate nursing education. This is in contrast to a community that visibly supports graduate education and where there are active professional nursing groups such as chapters of Sigma Theta Tau and the American Nurses Association that sponsor local and regional conferences with research and scientific presentations.

Clinical agency recognition of the need for graduate nursing education is another important factor. Questions that need to be addressed at the time of assessment and throughout the planning process include:

▲ What kinds of support will the nursing unit receive from community agencies?
▲ Will the agencies lend financial support to the graduate nursing program?
▲ Will they offer in-kind support in terms of adjunct faculty, clinical space, and practice opportunities?
▲ Will they support and encourage, financially and otherwise, their nursing staff that enrolls in graduate programs?
▲ Are there employment opportunities for the master's and doctoral graduates of the program in local agencies?

One other important factor is the proximity of the nearest competing graduate nursing program. If there is another graduate nursing program in the same or nearby community, does the proposed program fulfill a need that is not currently being met? For example, program A, which is planning an MSN program in a CNS track along with a PhD program, would not be competing for students with program B, which has a well-established MSN, family nurse practitioner program. In addition, program A might be housed in a public institution while program B is in a private, secular college, which gives potential students another option from which to choose.

Other external factors include the receptiveness of local health professionals including physicians and other kinds of health care providers, health care agencies, funding groups, and the pool of potential students. At the state level, typical constituents including legislators, academic state or regional boards, and the other nursing programs that are scattered throughout the area might have an interest in, or be affected by, a new graduate nursing program.

Lastly, approval from professional and academic regulatory bodies at both national and state levels is necessary before the program can begin (Biordi & Wineman, 1999). As one can see, developing a nursing program responsive to the needs of the health care system and nursing is merely the beginning of a long odyssey into the development and implementation of a graduate nursing program.

▲ INTERNAL FRAME FACTORS AND GRADUATE NURSING EDUCATION

The idea of the isolated scholar working in an ivory tower is mythic—and wrong. No nursing program at the graduate level, whether master's or doctoral, was ever initiated without consideration of the possible constituents and the stakes they hold. Private or public, the program's nursing constituencies and stakeholders may differ, but all programs must consider who holds the power to impact their program's development and acceptance. Internal frame factors, therefore, consist of the educational unit, college, university, etc., of which the nursing program belongs; the role of graduate education and research within the university; outcomes as they relate to the nursing unit; faculty and faculty workload; and material resources including costs. Assuming that the most basic mandate of a society is the need for competent professional nurses, most graduate nursing programs exist within an academic structure, typically a college or university. Internally, a program is considered within the context of the university mission.

Graduate nursing programs differ from graduate programs in most of the other academic disciplines. Most academic disciplines use master's programs as a starting point for students to funnel into their narrower, doctoral-focused specializations. In nursing, the master's programs are specialized, in-depth programs that concentrate on clinical practice and the clinical relevance of research. The nursing doctoral programs expand on these specialized, clinical bases, while expanding the students' worldview within the context of theory and research. Thus, the nursing master's program tends to specialize in one particular focal area while the doctorate tends to expand ideas about a particular specialty or phenomenon.

Interestingly, as doctoral programs proliferated and competed for research sites, the research function of the master's program shifted from the "production" of nursing research toward the "utilization" of nursing research, with a resultant focus on evidence-based practice (Jack, 2002). Nursing is now advocating that those nurses holding or in study for the doctorate are the more appropriate research practitioners. However, the market has not yet caught up to this idea, and many nursing master's graduates in agencies are being called upon to conduct and interpret research, particularly evaluation research. Today, nursing graduate programs at the master's and doctoral levels affirm clinical practice and research across a variety of patients in all kinds of health, home, and community environments, nationally and internationally.

▲ NURSING'S FIT WITHIN THE UNIVERSITY

A graduate program in nursing nestled within the graduate structure of a large university is quite different in its aspects than the nursing graduate program that is embedded in a smaller college, particularly a small liberal arts college. In the larger universities, nursing is frequently one of several health science programs representing the master's and doctoral levels. These programs are often located within a health science center serviced by its hospitals and laboratories. Nursing, in such an environment, often competes for resources and even for students with other health science programs including medicine, pharmacology, public health, social work, occupational or physical therapy, and/or dentistry. Nonetheless, because it is an obvious fit into health professions, nursing is accepted readily into such an environment, particularly if its faculty can produce the necessary academic products (e.g., significant research, extremely competent faculty and students, sustainable and remarkable community relationships, and program cost recovery). In the smaller programs, nursing is typically one of two or three professional programs (e.g. education and business), and, like them, delivers programs at the baccalaureate or master's levels.

Whether at the small or larger programs, academe traditionally favors the arts and sciences that are still dominated by white, male faculty. The faculty's acceptance of professional programs, particularly feminine occupations such as education and nursing, depends much on the professionals' research facility, program cost, organizational fit with the mission goals of service and teaching, and other social and political relationships, such as faculty gender, tenure, and university corporate issues (Biordi & McFarlane, 2001). While colleges of education are a long-standing tradition within academe, and business programs are acceptable because of their fit and prestige within the societal institution of commerce, nursing had to prove its mettle in only a few short years while establishing its identity as a profession in its own right. Nursing in academe found its niche as it quickly caught up with the research norms of academic colleagues and by building bridges to the community's health sector and labor force (Biordi & McFarlane, 2001).

What many outside of academic administration do not realize, however, is the increasing need for financial and other support as more universities compete for research and meaningful gifts. In the politics of alumni relations, prestige, connections, and wealth are important to the ongoing security of the university. If one examines gift giving, nurses' gifts are rarely among the largest donations. Rather, nursing alumni are often the steadiest of givers of smaller gifts. While professional education and business alumni may be well rewarded within the basic educational and financial structures of the community, nursing is not competitive with them or with other health professionals, such as physicians. Consequently, nursing students and alumni must become more aware of the need to contribute to their alma mater and find ways, such as large class gifts, that create an image to be noted by their university.

▲ CURRICULUM DEVELOPMENT AND OUTCOMES

A curriculum must fit within the mission of the university and program, and it is important to keep in mind that the curriculum is more than a collection of courses designed for particular outcomes. The curriculum includes those learning objectives and experiences that facilitate the desired and expected student outcomes. These experiences often dictate the quality of the program, insofar as the faculty can demonstrate their sagacity, develop outstanding clinical sites, encourage student services and projects of originality and substance, and reach out in practice and research to other cultures and communities. Even as these events become a measure of programmatic quality, education is increasingly accountable for outcomes, rather than maintaining a sole focus on process. Thus, outcome specificity has begun to generate certain clarity of thought and product, which is reflected by its measurement.

At the graduate level, outcomes have been defined in a number of ways, but typically they measure the program's quality and the safe competence of the graduate. There are many ways to view outcomes, and they can vary from the specific to the general. Examples of commonly used outcome measures include course grades or students' achievement of certain roles and certifications in those roles; particular student and program products, such as dissertation research, theses, papers, and projects; evidence of leadership in service arenas and learning communities; and faculty competency. Other programmatic outcomes might demonstrate global outreach, community service projects, or cluster living in learning environments to name a few. Therefore, of importance to any curriculum is the periodic and careful examination for its fit with the mission and goals of the parent institution. Included in the assessment is the program's response to societal mandates that are reflected through its professional relevance and competence of the graduates. In general, the nursing faculty determines these goals and the curriculum and reviews both on a periodic basis.

▲ CURRICULUM AND FACULTY

A dialectic exists between societal and market needs, faculty availability, specialties, and the graduate curriculum. The choice of curriculum dictates the kind of faculty, and the targeted number of students dictates the size of the faculty needed. However, choice of faculty members should include an assessment of the individual's knowledge, personal goals, fit within the mission and culture of the organization, and an ability to manage students effectively and humanely. Based on the assessment, the administration and existing faculty make informed decisions for adding to the faculty cadre. Organizational culture is difficult to change, but leadership by senior faculty and administration has much to do with prevailing ethos. However consciously they may do so, leadership sets an ongoing tone that becomes critical to the choice of faculty and the subsequent reputation of a program.

Many programs' faculties believe that diversity of faculty preparation and ethnicity help students grasp and understand larger views of their world. In fact, the idea is still propounded that faculty members should hold graduate degrees from more than one institution, and not narrowly confine their education to a single program regardless of its quality. In general, this norm holds true in that most programs prefer to have faculty with a variety of backgrounds, holding degrees that represent a variety of philosophies and theoretical approaches to teaching, learning, and scholarship. However, as faculty shortages began, and as learning opportunities expanded within the professional careers of students and faculty, this norm of variety in graduate degrees was successfully challenged.

▲ FACULTY AND WORKLOAD DISTRIBUTION

Master's and doctoral programs differ in the number of faculty needed to implement the curriculum in an effective manner. As such, the faculty-to-student ratio for master's programs varies by clinical specialty with nurse practitioner, nurse midwives, and nurse anesthetist programs typically requiring lower faculty-to-student ratios than some of the other specialties such as education, administration, or management. In addition, the aforementioned advanced-practice and clinical specialty ratios may be mandated by state as well as national accreditation standards to maintain a certain faculty-to-student ratio. The ratio becomes even more complex when factoring in a thesis requirement, which can dramatically increase the workload of faculty who supervise or mentor thesis students. Data on thesis faculty-to-student ratios are not easily available, but from these authors' experiences, the number of thesis students successfully managed by a faculty member per year averages about five maximum.

Although a faculty-to-student ratio has not been advocated for doctoral nursing programs, informal surveys indicate that in most programs, faculty tend to assume between one and four or five doctoral students as academic or dissertation advisees (C. Wynd & D. Biordi, personal communication, February 2003). Therefore, the number of students accepted into a graduate program requires a careful administrative analysis and match between the availability of faculty who are not only clinically prepared but are active participants in programs of research as well.

Administrators must distribute faculty workload so that faculty's clinical practice and other teaching responsibilities across the educational levels of their programs are adequately met. In this age of the graying professoriate and with fewer doctoral-prepared faculty available for teaching and research, faculties are increasingly torn between taking in higher numbers of students to meet future professional needs and the immediate needs of enrolled students, scholarship activities, and service obligations. Graduate faculty-to-student ratios are critical to graduate programs and are typically established by nursing regulatory agencies at one faculty member to six to eight students.

In both doctoral and master's programs, part-time faculty, adjunct faculty, and graduate student assistants assist the faculty. Master's programs, in particular, use adjunct faculty and preceptors that provide the majority of practice sites for the advanced-practice nurses. Moreover, they frequently donate their time and practice to the service of the program, often without recompense of any sort. However, as competition for clinical sites increases, programs are seeking to symbolically or tangibly reward their preceptors and adjunct faculty, using such rewards as certificates, continuing education, or honoraria. In an effort to contain costs, nursing programs, like other programs, have increasingly resorted to the use of part-time faculty, particularly for undergraduate programs and clinical coverage. The numbers of part-time faculty vary, but in some instances, up to half of nursing faculty is part time (Gosnell & Biordi, 1999; NLN, 2003).

While part-time faculty may solve the immediate problem of clinical coverage, issues of communication, commitment, and articulation increase exponentially. Graduate students are more often distributed through graduate and undergraduate programs, either as teaching assistants (TAs), research assistants (RAs), or general-use graduate assistants (GAs). Originally modeled on the bench scientist apprenticeship, graduate assistants function in different ways in nursing programs. They are usually distributed throughout the educational program at both graduate and undergraduate levels. RAs and TAs can assume some or all of the percentage of work normally assigned to a full-time faculty member, thus freeing the faculty for research, grantsmanship, administration, or other duties.

Graduate faculty teaching load (assignments) must be adjusted owing to the increased contact time with students who are participating in seminars, testing nursing theories and research findings, and generating new research. In addition, advanced-practice education requires faculty expertise and time for arranging clinical preceptorships, supervising students and their mentors, and maintaining their own clinical practice as credible clinicians. While many of these latter activities apply to undergraduate education as well, graduate level experiences are compounded by the need for individual clinical placements versus group assignments.

For the viability of a graduate program, ample research opportunities and resources must be available to students and faculty. Technology support and assistance from expert staff are necessary to aid students and faculty and to find resources for financial support, writing grant proposals, managing grants, and the conduct of research such as human subjects review, collection and analysis of data, and preparing reports.

▲ MATERIAL RESOURCES

Other important analyses for the support of graduate programs include break-even or greater revenue-to-cost ratios (which include student enrollments); classroom, office, storage, and laboratory space; health care agencies and their facilities; adequate library support; research, grant, and technology transfer support; and technology. Revenues come from multiple streams. In some public universities, revenues are generated by tuition and tuition subsidization by tax dollars, which relate to the numbers and levels (baccalaureate, master's, or doctoral) of students actually enrolled (rather than admitted). Other typical revenues flow from general funds, special donations, foundations, or endowments. Space, as one of the most sacred resources in any university, is a premium for nursing programs, which like the sciences and unlike the humanities require expensive laboratories, research space, and classrooms. The level of library support is established in each region and state and is reviewed for adequacy for nursing's unique curriculum by state review boards, or if in a private school, within the parameters set by that school. Faculty research and teaching needs are facilitated by certain material supports supplied by the university, such as in-house research grants, travel funds, research showcases, and research space. Although they are not strictly material support in that they support a human resource, funds for graduate assistants are critical to the research mission. These funds flow from direct and indirect funding from grants, as well as from tax dollars, endowments, and scholarships. As indicated previously, graduate assistants can function in an apprentice to a full teaching mode and are critical to the success of the mission of the programs of which they are a part.

Beyond even these typical costs is the growing need for technology. With the advent of advanced sciences and associated laboratory equipment, the computer, and now, distance learning, most programs are increasingly allocating very large portions of their budget to ever-changing technology. Universities are still learning the costs of implementation, maintenance, and disposal of high technology, and some are getting out of the business of providing these high-technology items. Rather, they are interning or outsourcing their students to commercial laboratories.

Lastly, the American Association for Colleges of Nursing (AACN) annually sponsors a doctoral forum where issues of program direction, quality, funding, and educational pedagogy and trends are discussed by deans and doctoral program directors from across the nation.

One need that the AACN responded to was the development of parameters that can be used by existing doctoral programs to evaluate their own effectiveness and as guidelines for those institutions planning a doctoral program (C. Anderson, personal communication, January 2003). One of the proposed parameters was the suggestion of $2 million as a minimum funding base. Members of the AACN believe that this is a minimum amount that is needed to provide an adequate research base in a doctoral program. This sum reflects the faculty's level of research funding, future research trajectories, and the confidence that they muster from established funding agencies. The research itself becomes the foundation for student–faculty interaction so necessary in a graduate doctoral program.

▲ GRADUATE CURRICULUM AND EVALUATION

Societal need for accountability in education and especially in professional programs is increasing. Therefore, any planning phase for graduate education programming should include evaluation from the very beginning. Although there is a variety of evaluation schemes that have been used in the past, there is a movement in higher education and in nursing education from rather static models to more dynamic models of evaluation, which now include examination of the organization's own goals and their realization. Whatever model is being employed, in nursing, at least the following areas are examined for quality: mission, resources, curricula, faculty qualifications and performance, and student performance (outcomes). Both the AACN and the National League for Nursing (NLN) have developed criteria that reflect "essential" or core standards for all master's degree programs as well as for advanced practice. In addition, most advanced practice specialties (e.g., midwifery, anesthesia) have specific accreditation demands. Also, various state professional and educational boards require certain standards to be met and verified before implementation of a program or its continuance.

While most program evaluation applies to the master's programs, doctoral programs are typically examined at institutional or state levels. As yet in nursing, there are no "formalized" professional accreditation requirements for doctoral programs, but there is a growing interest in establishing a review process that ensures quality. To that end, nursing programs have begun to identify "Quality Indicators" of doctoral programs, drawing on extant faculty and programs (AACN, 2002b). Similar to master's program outcomes, doctoral indicators of quality curriculum include resources, institutional support, governance, faculty performance, and student performance. These indicators are increasingly being used in lieu of more widespread or institutionalized evaluation models

Evaluation and Cost

Today's colleges and universities, both public and private, are faced with tremendous across-the-board financial cutbacks so that faculties are challenged to "do more with less." One of the "costs" that needs to be included in the planning phase for any new graduate nursing program is the projected cost of accreditation. These costs range far beyond annual fees for being a member of an accreditation agency and include such things as an evaluation fee, a new applicant fee, and a new program fee (AACN, 2002c). Importantly, these fees do not include the outlay of resources

▲ TABLE 9.1	Costs of Accreditation	

College of Nursing at New University 25 FTE Faculty College Resources Needed for New MS Program Accreditation		
Item	**Time needed**	**Amount**
1. Faculty release for report preparation; .5 release; PhD-prepared	12 months	$43,000
2. 2, Part-time adjunct faculty to replace "released" faculty; MS–prepared (to teach clinical sections)	9 months	$25,000
3. Temporary secretarial support to meet accreditation needs; .5 FTE	12 months	$17,500
4. Supplies, duplication, binding, etc.		$5,000
5. Hotel, transportation for visitors (N = 3) (Hotel & board: 3 rooms @ $170/day/3 × 3 = $1,530) (Airfare: $625 average R T × 3 = $1,875)		$3,405
Total		$82,905

incurred by the applicant institution to prepare for a national accreditation. See Table 9-1 for an example of the cost of accreditation. Also, Chapter 12 discusses in detail the process of accreditation and its impact on the institution as well as quality of the program.

▲ SUMMARY

In summary, graduate-level nursing education programs present a variety of interesting and unique challenges. The historical development of graduate nursing education incorporated societal, technological, and professional needs resulting in present day programs that vary from the very traditional to those that are innovative. The chapter described types of master's and doctoral programs and differentiated research activities for both levels. It also presented the argument for master's level research activities focused on the utilization of evidence-based practice research findings with the doctorate level focused on production of new theories and findings in clinical practice and nursing science.

External and internal factors are key elements that must be addressed when planning for any graduate-level program, as are the material resources and costs involved from planning to the implementation of the program and including accreditation costs at national and state levels and faculty workload. Implementing a doctoral program must also include a research base funding level within the college that supports both faculty and doctoral students. Needless to say, careful planning is a key to successful implementation and ongoing maintenance and quality.

DISCUSSION QUESTIONS

1. Identify strategies that can be used to attract qualified faculty to your institution. What are the strengths that your program offers that potential faculty would find desirable?
2. In light of increasing competition for scarce resources for research, what are potential sources of nongovernmental research support that you can identify?
3. Compare and contrast the development of a graduate nursing education program in a private and public university. What similar factors must each consider? What factors are different?

LEARNING ACTIVITIES

Student Activities

Divide your group into two debate teams and debate the pros and cons of the following two issues related to graduate education:

1. Entry-level programs at the graduate level (master's and doctorate) versus the undergraduate level (baccalaureate). Support your arguments from the literature as well as personal experience.
2. The differences and value of the PhD versus the DNSc or ND. Support your arguments from the literature as well as personal experience.

Faculty Activities

Collect data on the make-up of your faculty on the following characteristics:

1. Part-time and full-time percentages
2. Vacancies
3. Average age and predicted retirements with the next 5 and 10 years
4. Clinical and functional specialties representation
5. Percentages of master's and doctoral degrees and their majors

Analyze your findings for their match to your current and future program needs. Based on your analysis, what problems can you foresee for their effect on the quality of the program? What strategies do you plan to solve these problems immediately, in the near future, and in the long term?

REFERENCES

American Association of Colleges of Nursing (AACN). (2002a, August). Accelerated programs: The fast-track to careers in nursing. *AACN Issue Bulletin.* Washington, DC: Author.

American Association of Colleges of Nursing (AACN). (2002b). Indicators of quality in research-focused doctoral programs in nursing. *Journal of Professional Nursing, 18*(5), 289–294.

American Association of Colleges of Nursing (AACN). (2002c). *Commission on Collegiate Nursing Education fee structure.* Washington, DC: Commission on Collegiate Nursing Education.

American Association of Colleges of Nursing (AACN). (2003). Seeking clarities in the complexities of doctoral education, January 29–February 1. Sanibel Island, FL: Author.

American Association of Colleges of Nursing (AACN). (2004). Institutions offering doctoral programs and nursing degrees conferred. Retrieved June 6, 2004, from http://www.aacn.nche.edu/Education/index.htm

Armstrong, M. L., Johnson, B. A., Bridges, R. A., & Gessner, B. A. (2003). The impact of graduate education in reading for lifelong learning. *Journal of Continuing Education in Nursing, 34*(1), 19–25.

Bell, L. (2003). Specialty roles and specialty education. *Journal of Pediatric Healthcare, 17*(2), 105–111.

Biordi, D. L., & McFarlane, E. A. (2001). Academic role and faculty development. In N. L. Chaska (Ed.), *The nursing profession* (pp. 809–823). Thousand Oaks, CA.: Sage Publications.

Biordi, D. L., & Wineman, N. M. (1999). *The joint PhD in Nursing between Kent State University and the University of Akron: Executive summary, proposal and consultant report.* Kent, OH: Kent State University.

Committee for the Study of Nursing Education (Josephine Goldmark, Secretary). (1923). *Nursing and nursing education in the United States.* New York: Macmillan Co.

Ford, L. C., & Silver, H. K. (1967). The expanded role of the nurse in child care. *Nursing Outlook, 15*, 43–45.

Gortner, S. R. (1991). Historical development of doctoral programs: Shaping our expectations. *Journal of Professional Nursing, 7*(1), 45–53.

Gosnell, D. J., & Biordi, D. L. (1999). Personnel resource distribution for nursing programs in Carnegie classified research I and II doctoral institutions. *Journal of Professional Nursing, 15*(1), 44–51.

Hanson, C. M., & Hamric, A. B. (2003). Reflections on the continuing evolution of advanced practice nursing. *Nursing Outlook, 51*(5), 203–211.

Hawkins, J. W., & Thibodeau, J. A. (1993). Advanced practice roles: Nurse practitioner/clinical nurse specialist. In J. W. Hawkins & J. A. Thibodeau (Eds.), *The advanced practitioner. Current practice issues* (3rd ed., pp. 1–41). New York: Tiresias Press.

Jack, B. (2002). The final hurdle: Preparation for the PhD via examination. *Nursing Research, 10*(2), 66–76.

Jones, C. B., & Lusk, S. L. (2002). Incorporating health services research into nursing doctoral programs. *Nursing Outlook, 50*(6), 225–231.

Marriner-Tomey, A. (1990). Historical development of doctoral programs from the middle ages to nursing education today. *Nursing & Health Care, 11*(3), 133–137.

McCarty, M., & Higgins, A. (2003). Moving to an all graduate profession: Preparing preceptors for their roles. *Nursing Education Today, 23*(2), 89–95.

Meleis, A. (1988). Doctoral education in nursing: Its present and its future. *Journal of Professional Nursing, 4*(6), 436–446.

National League for Nursing. (2003). *Nurse Educators 2002. Report of the faculty census survey of RN and graduate programs.* By Rosenfeld, P., Kovner, C., & Valiga, T. M. New York: NLN.

Safreit, B. J. (1992). Health care dollars and regulatory sense: The role of advanced practice nursing. *Yale Journal of Regulation, 9*(2), 417–487.

USDHHS, HRSA, Bureau of Health Professions, Division of Nursing. (2002). *The registered nurse population: March 2000: Findings from the national sample survey of registered nurses.* Washington, DC: HRSA.

Walker, J., Gerard, P. S., Bayley, E. W., Coeling, H., Clark, A. P., & Dayhoff, N. A. (2003). A description of clinical nurse specialist programs in the United States. *Clinical Nurse Specialist, 17*(3), 50–57.

Curriculum and Program Evaluation

▼

Sarah B. Keating, EdD, RN, FAAN

5

▲ OVERVIEW

Section 5 analyzes theories, concepts, and models that apply to the evaluation of nursing education programs and curricula. Although evaluation appears to be the last step in curriculum development, it occurs throughout the process of curriculum development and implementation. Information from evaluation activities provides the impetus for major and minor changes that must take place to maintain an up-to-date and high-quality curriculum. Most evaluation models in nursing education are linked to assessing the achievement of program or curriculum goals and objectives. These are very useful and provide feedback for improving quality; however, there are many other indicators for measuring the success or failure of an education program or curriculum. Current economic and educational systems in the United States place an emphasis on outcomes and total quality management—that is, continually assessing the program, correcting errors as they occur, and continually improving the quality of the program.

Earlier evaluation models in nursing focused on the process phases for delivering education. They spoke of student-centered teaching and learning processes. Faculty's role was to enable the learner to become actively involved in the educational process and in self-directing to acquire new knowledge, behaviors, attitudes, and skills. Outcomes were linked to and measured by meeting the goals and objectives of the program and the curriculum. These processes continue to be vital parts of curriculum development and evaluation; however, there is a need for other types of information to measure outcomes and a demand by consumers for information on the quality of the program.

▲ THE ROLE OF FACULTY, STUDENTS, CONSUMERS, AND ADMINISTRATORS IN EVALUATION

As is true for curriculum development, the faculty is key to the choice of the evaluation methodologies that guide the processes of curriculum and instruction and the assessment of the outcomes. Students are an important part of the evaluation process and should be part of the planning process. Their performance and satisfaction are critical to the evaluation of the program and curriculum. Consumers of the program include employers of the graduates, alumni, students and their families, nursing staff, clients and, yes, even faculty, staff, and administrators. Consumer opinions on the program and curriculum are valuable and serve as a barometer of the program's match to the needs of the health care system, health care professions, and the educational system.

The role of administrators is to provide the financial resources necessary for evaluation and consultation (internal or external expertise) to assist faculty in developing and implementing plans for evaluation. Administrators must see to it that there is adequate support staff for the ongoing collection of data and analyses, and they have responsibility for ensuring that the findings are disseminated in a timely fashion to stakeholders and for follow-up on the recommendations. These activities contribute to the total quality management of the educational program.

▲ PROCESS (FORMATIVE) AND OUTCOME (SUMMATIVE) EVALUATION

For the purposes of this text, the terms *process* and *formative* evaluation are considered the same. *Formative evaluation is the assessment that takes place during the implementation of the educational program and curriculum. Formative evaluation activities measure the processes and progress along a continuum toward the goal of the educational program.* Formative evaluation measures include assessing the students, the curriculum, and the program according to their progress toward the end product. Often, the objectives of the program that represent the steps toward the final goal serve as guidelines for the evaluation. Examples of student assessment measurements include tests, clinical performance, presentations, classroom and online participation, and papers or other writing assignments. Examples of formative evaluation measures for the curriculum and program include course and faculty performance evaluations; review of course syllabi and their delivery; and faculty and committee review of courses, cost analyses, and data regarding enrollments and completion of courses. While these measures satisfy the meeting of goals and objectives, they are categorized as formative measures of evaluation.

Current and future demands for high-quality education programs indicate the need to measure "outcome," "summative," or "end-point" results. For the purposes of this text, these terms are used interchangeably. Outcome evaluation is similar to "goal-based" evaluation, which compares the results of the educational process to the prestated overall goal(s) of the program. For example, the overall goal of a nursing program might be "to prepare caring and competent professional nurses to meet the health care needs of the populace." Measures for studying the achievement of this goal include the graduates' care of clients and their levels of competency. Ways in which to collect data for these measures could include surveys of the graduates' employers as to the graduates' competency, the clients' satisfaction with the care provided, and the graduates' perceptions of how well the program prepared them for practice in meeting the needs of their clients.

Frequently, these outcome measures are identified as "summative" evaluation. *Summative evaluation takes place at the end of the program and measures the final outcome. However, in systems nomenclature, summative evaluation takes place after a system terminates or "dies," so that one could say that for all living systems, evaluation is formative. However, in education, summative evaluation is often linked to the fulfillment of the goal(s) or purpose of the program.*

Traditional outcome evaluation processes for measuring educational outcomes linked the quality of the program to the mission, goals, and objectives of the program. Currently, however, outcome evaluation goes beyond the stated goals and may include other items to measure program products, for example, graduation rates, NCLEX results, career success for its graduates, and cost effectiveness. Examples to measure these outcomes include reports on pass rates for the licensure examination, graduates' accomplishments in leadership roles and as change agents, demonstrated professional commitment such as membership in professional organizations, graduates' rates for continuing education and their pursuit of postgraduate education, and a financially secure program.

Many of the evaluation models reviewed in this section are described in systems theory language that is very similar to the nursing process (i.e., assessment, problem identification, planning, implementation, and evaluation). These frameworks and models contribute to the critical steps of developing, evaluating, and revising programs and curricula. They also serve as master plans for evaluation to assist faculty, administrators, and consumers to measure the quality of the program and its graduates and compare it to others.

▲ THE MASTER PLAN OF EVALUATION

With today's emphasis on outcomes, the evaluation process is essential to measuring success, establishing benchmarks, and continually improving the quality of the program. Because institutions need to meet accreditation standards, professional discipline expectations, and consumer demand, most institutions have a master plan of evaluation or assessment. The master plan may use an evaluation model or criteria set by accrediting bodies, or it may use both. The plan provides the guidelines necessary for collecting information to prepare required reports such as program review, accreditation, marketing, and demonstrating the worth of the program to the parent institution and the community. Institutions use the results of evaluation to improve the program, demonstrate excellence, and market their programs.

▲ ACCREDITATION AND PROGRAM APPROVAL

Consumers (students, families, alumni, and employers of graduates) of educational programs should verify that the institution is accredited. A degree awarded by an accredited college or university testifies to its quality, and many other accredited institutions do not recognize degrees or college credits from nonaccredited institutions. Graduation from an accredited institution can also determine eligibility for federally sponsored programs and rank in the military. These facts are especially important to persons who are assuming leadership and education roles in nursing. The "buyer beware" adage applies here.

Accreditation is the process that education programs and curricula undergo to receive recognition for meeting basic standards or criteria set by national, regional, or state organizations. Although it is voluntary, most programs undergo accreditation to demonstrate their quality to the consumers of their products. The U.S. Department of Education is the driving force behind accreditation and approves both regional education accrediting bodies as well as specialty accrediting agencies.

Quality nursing programs participate in regional accreditation and must abide by state regulations as well. Each state's board of nursing, education department, or other regulating body reviews the program and makes site visits to approve it. *Program approval is a process whereby regulating bodies review programs to ensure consumer safety. Nursing education programs are subject to the state regulations that are usually administered by the State Board of Nursing.* Approval is necessary to allow the graduates of the program to take state boards or the licensure examination (NCLEX). Nurse educators must keep in mind that the primary role of the state agency is to ensure consumer safety.

Chapter 10 reviews theories, concepts, and models of evaluation and discusses some common evaluation models and professional standards that can be adapted as master plans for educational programs. Chapter 11 presents a few examples of the utility of these models in total quality management in education, and Chapter 12 discusses accreditation and program approval processes in detail.

Master Planning for Program and Curriculum Evaluation: Systematic Assessment and Evaluation

Sarah B. Keating, EdD, RN, FAAN

OBJECTIVES

Upon completion of Chapter 10, the reader will be able to:

1. Compare common definitions, concepts, and models of quality assurance and program evaluation.
2. Evaluate common theories, concepts, and models for their application to program and curriculum evaluation.
3. Justify the rationale for a master plan of evaluation for educational programs.
4. Analyze several models of evaluation for their utility as master plans of evaluation.
5. Analyze some of the tools available for curriculum and program evaluation.
6. Apply the guidelines and major components of evaluation for developing a master plan of evaluation to a nursing education program.

▲ OVERVIEW

Educational evaluation occurs while assessing the program for its quality, currency, relevance, projections into the future, and the need for possible revisions in light of these factors. As is true of all living systems, the curriculum responds to internal and external pressures in the faculty's search for excellence and thus, there is a need for continuous evaluation. According to the classic definition by Worthen and Sanders (1974), *evaluation is the determination of the worth of a thing. It includes obtaining information for use in judging the worth of a program, product, procedure, or objective or the potential for utility of alternative approaches to attain specific objectives* (p. 19).

Nursing education program and curriculum evaluation is evolving from an emphasis in the past on the use of models of evaluation in education to the adaptation of business models to measure productivity, outcomes, cost effectiveness, and quality. Issues from these changes that are raised relate to the increasing emphasis on outcomes and benchmarks to measure quality and the possible loss of equal attention to the processes that lead to the outcomes. One flaw in many of the master plans is the lack of specific plans to follow up on the analyses and their recommendations. Implementing strategies to follow up on the recommendations closes the loop between data collection and actions for changes in the curriculum, thus maintaining a quality program. Chapter 10 introduces common definitions, theories, concepts, and models for program and curriculum evaluation and continues with the justification for master plans of evaluation, suggestions for developing them, and a few samples of evaluation tools.

▲ EVALUATION AND RESEARCH

Frequently, people confuse program evaluation with research. Research is "the activity aimed at obtaining generalizable knowledge by contriving and testing claims about relationships among variables or describing generalizable phenomena. This knowledge, which may result in theoretical models, functional relationships, or descriptions, may be obtained by empirical or other systematic methods, and may or may not have immediate application" (Worthen & Sanders, 1974, p. 19). Research studies are usually categorized into two main types, quantitative and qualitative, and the same applies to evaluation.

Research and evaluation require an overview and statement of the problem followed by the purpose of the study or goal. For research, this takes the form of a problem statement or line of inquiry. Quantitative research may contain a hypothesis and/or a null hypothesis. The purpose of evaluation in education is to judge a program or curriculum; thus, it does not form a hypothesis, but rather states its purpose for evaluation. However, it is possible to conduct an evaluation study that becomes evaluation research. In this case, the study should explore either new methodologies or applications that test evaluation theories, and to qualify as research, the study should contribute new knowledge to the field of evaluation.

▲ THE PROCESS FOR EDUCATIONAL EVALUATION

All faculty members participate in the evaluation of the curriculum and the program through the collection of data, analyses, and the formulation of recommendations for decision making regarding the program. In many schools of nursing there are evaluation committees who lead the process, or in other cases, curriculum committees may be charged with the evaluation of the curriculum and program. Evaluation information and decisions based on the information lead to adjustments to the curriculum plan that result in either minor or major revisions. Revisions to the curriculum can result in the need for reapproval or reaccreditation depending upon the nature of the changes. If the overall mission, purpose, goals, and objectives remain basically intact, it is not usually necessary to undergo reapproval if the program faculty approves the changes. However, major revisions must undergo the usual processes of approval by committees, faculty, the academic senate or other governing body, the administration, and finally, accrediting and regulating bodies. These latter processes were described in Chapter 2 of the text.

▲ COMMON DEFINITIONS OF EVALUATION

"Quality"

To initiate a discussion on evaluation in education, the first term to consider is quality. This term takes on many meanings depending on the context in which it is used. For the purposes of this chapter and in the interest of simplicity, the text will use the second definition of *quality* from Merriam-Webster's Online Dictionary (2004): *a degree of excellence*. Examples of the context of quality include the standards, by which an entity is measured, comparison to other like entities, and consumer expectations.

Quality control refers to the *detection and elimination of components or final products that are not up to standard* (Sallis, 2002, p.17). Examples of quality control from nursing are the decision to eliminate a skill that is no longer relevant to current or future practice and the elimination of a specialty track in a graduate program for which there is no longer a job market.

Quality assurance "*is about consistently meeting product specification or **getting things right the first time, every time**"* (Sallis, 2002, p.17). Total quality management (TQM) for education programs *is used to describe two slightly different but related notions. The first is a philosophy of continuous improvement. The second related meaning uses TQM to describe the tools and techniques... which are used to put quality improvement into action* (Sallis, 2002).

Formative and Summative Evaluation

Scriven (1996) reiterates his definitions of formative and summative evaluation by a discussion of the context in which evaluators use the terms to assess educational programs. He describes formative evaluation as *intended—by the evaluator—as a basis for improvement*. For example, in nursing, the faculty compares students' grades in prerequisites to their grades in nursing courses to determine if certain levels of achievement in prerequisites influence grades in nursing. Scriven describes summative evaluation *as a holistic approach to the assessment of a program, which can use results from the formative evaluation*. Continuing with the examples from nursing, a faculty can evaluate the development of critical thinking skills in its graduates as a product of the educational program. In this instance, these skills need to be measured both before and after the program to determine an increase in the skills.

Both formative and summative types of evaluation "involve efforts to determine merit or worth, etc." (Scriven, 1996, p. 6). Scriven also points out that summative evaluation can serve as formative evaluation. For example, if a nursing program finds that graduates' clinical decision-making skills are weak (summative evaluation), it can use that information to analyze the program (formative evaluation) for its strategies to promote these skills throughout the program and make improvements as necessary.

Goal-Based and Goal-Free Evaluation

Additional definitions commonly used in evaluation are goal-based evaluation and goal-free evaluation. Scriven (1974) moved away from program evaluation, which focused only on the examination of program goals and intended outcomes (goal-based), to an alternative method that examined the actual effects of the program. These effects (goal-free evaluation) include the intended effects, unintended effects, side effects, and secondary effects. An unintended effect in nursing education might be an increase in the applicant pool owing to the community's interactions with students in a program-sponsored, nurse-managed clinic. While this was not a stated goal of the program, it was a positive, unintended outcome.

Goal-free evaluation has the benefit of an evaluation that should be bias free. The evaluator, who is an expert in education and evaluation and has no previous knowledge about the program, observes the program or curriculum and assesses it for its quality in delivery and the assumed outcomes from it. These observations are then compared to the stated goals, objectives, and implementation plan for differences between the intended and unintended program processes and outcomes. This method can be a powerful tool for evaluating the program and identifying factors that were not thought of by the program planners.

▲ ANALYSIS OF THE STRUCTURE OF THE CURRICULUM

Analyzing the structure of the curriculum provides information to help the program evaluate its effectiveness and judge its worth. The classic three-part structure of an undergraduate curriculum consists of 1) general education requirements, 2) the major, and 3) electives (Carnegie Foundation, 1977; WASC, 1997). Each institution determines the general education requirements that every graduate must complete. The nature of the institution determines the spirit of general education; for example a small liberal arts college will emphasize the liberal arts while a research institution might emphasize the sciences and research.

No matter the emphasis, general education requirements in most institutions include the sciences, social sciences, liberal arts, government and politics, economics, mathematics, and communications. Although a majority of the general education requirements take place in the lower division (i.e., freshman and sophomore or community college levels), most undergraduate baccalaureate programs require upper-division general education courses as well. Associate degree and baccalaureate programs usually require a hefty assortment of general education requirements, some of which can be double-counted in the nursing major and all of which provide a baseline for developing scholarship and responsible citizenship.

Electives are the courses that students choose to supplement their major and general education requirements. In many institutions, a prescribed number of electives may be required to ensure a broad education for the students. In other institutions, the numbers of electives may not be specified. Either way, electives fill in the additional number of credits over and above general education and the major to complete the degree. Professional programs such as nursing seldom have space for many electives, which can be unfortunate because it reduces the exposure of students to other disciplines' perspectives.

The major is discipline specific and can be both lower and upper division or upper division only. Nursing often has a problem in transferring lower-division nursing courses into upper-division level programs. The Council of Higher Education Accreditation's Fact Sheet #4 provides a framework for the responsibilities of institutions to meet transfer of credit (CHEA, 2003). Graduate programs have similar common components such as core nursing courses, cognates (supporting courses usually from other disciplines), and clinical specialty or advanced roles courses (e.g., advanced practice, administration, education, case management, etc.). Assessing the effects general education or, in the case of graduate education core courses, electives have on the major is part of the total evaluation of the program and curriculum.

▲ THE UTILITY OF STANDARDS

Owing to many accreditation and program approval standards or criteria, educational programs usually have master plans of evaluation in place to facilitate the process of collecting and analyzing data. These data relate to the standards expected for accreditation and the goals and objectives of the program. There are other groups that set educational standards for programs. The AACN has two statements, *The Essentials of Baccalaureate Education and the Essentials of Master's Education for Advanced Practice Nursing* (AACN, 1998, 1996). The Council for Associate Degree Nursing of NLN issued a document called *Educational Competencies for Graduates of Associate Degree Programs* (CADN/NLN, 2000). The National Organization of Nurse Practitioner Faculty has an extensive list of recommendations for nurse practitioner programs (NONPF, 2004). The American Nurses Association has a list of scope of practice standards for many of the specialties in nursing. Education programs can use these in developing and evaluating their curricula and specialty tracks (ANA, 2004).

▲ THE DEVELOPMENT OF A MASTER PLAN OF EVALUATION

With today's emphasis on outcomes, the evaluation process is essential to measuring success, establishing benchmarks, and continually improving the quality of the program. A master plan of evaluation is used to provide data for faculty decision making as part of an internal review and for meeting external review standards. Owing to the need to meet accreditation standards, professional discipline expectations, and consumer demand, most institutions have a master plan of evaluation. For total quality management in a nursing education program, it is important to have a master plan that continually monitors the program so that adjustments can be made as the program is implemented. It is equally important to measure outcomes in terms of meeting the intentions, goals, and objectives of the program and certain benchmarks that help to pinpoint the quality of the program.

When developing a master plan of evaluation, one of the major tasks to integrate into the plan is to meet accreditation or program approval standards. These standards or criteria are the baseline requirements of the profession to ensure that programs are of sufficient quality to meet the expectations of the discipline. They also demonstrate to the public that a program is recognized by expert external reviewing bodies and thus, the quality of its graduates meets professional standards. Graduation from an accredited program is usually one of the admission standards for continued degree or education work. Many funding agencies for programs require accreditation because it indicates that the program is of high enough quality to assume the responsibility for the administration of grants and completion of projects.

Most accrediting agencies require that a program have a master plan of evaluation. Even if it is not required, a master plan helps to identify the components that need to be evaluated, who will do the data collection and when, what methods of data analysis will be employed, and the plans for responding to and following up on the findings and recommendations from the assessment. Having a master plan of evaluation in place greatly facilitates these processes when submitting accreditation self-study reports, program approval reports, or proposals for funding (CCNE, 2004; NLNAC, 2004).

The master plan must specify what is being evaluated, and an organizing framework is useful so that as nearly as possible, no crucial variable is omitted for review. Additionally, it is important to identify the persons who will:

1. Collect the data.
2. Analyze the findings.
3. Prepare reports.
4. Disseminate the reports to key people.
5. Set the timelines for collection, analysis, and reporting of the data.

Finally, there must be a feedback loop in place for recommendations and decision making. Reports from the evaluation should include:

1. Identification of existing and potential problems.
2. Previously unidentified or new needs.
3. Successes and why.
4. Recommendations for improvement or discontinuance of a program, or proposals for new programs.
5. Action plans for changes that include the people responsible and timelines.

Table 10.1 provides guidelines for developing a master plan of evaluation and the major components to be assessed for evaluation. In addition to including the curriculum and its components, it incorporates external and internal frame factors (Johnson, 1977), the infrastructure, the core curriculum, students, alumni, and human resources. As indicated in the table, these are only the major components. It is possible that as educational evaluation evolves, other components will emerge. The elements within each component are not listed. Each institution must determine which elements fall under the major components.

Adaptation of Models of Evaluation to Master Plans of Evaluation

The following discussion presents some of the classic models of evaluation that have been adapted as organizing frameworks for master plans of evaluation in education. Chapter 11 presents several models as examples of master plans.

▲ TABLE 10.1 Major Components and Guidelines for Developing a Master Plan of Evaluation

Component	Action Plans						Follow-up Plans	
	Responsible Party	When and How Often	Instruments/Tools for Data Collection	Data Findings & Analysis	Criteria, Outcomes, or Benchmarks	Reports & Recommendations	Maintain & Monitor or Improve	By Whom, How, & When
External Frame Factors (Johnson, 1977)								
Internal Frame Factors (Johnson, 1977)								
Infrastructure Systems Buildings								
Facilities								
Support systems								
Student services								
Financial								
Administration								
Core Baccalaureate Curriculum Prerequisites								
General education								
Electives								
Nursing major								
Core Graduate Curriculum Prerequisites								
Cognates								
Core nursing courses								
Specialty/functional courses								
Curriculum Components Mission/vision								
Organizational framework								

(table continues on page 266)

▲ **TABLE 10.1** Major Components and Guidelines for Developing a Master Plan of Evaluation (continued)

Component	Action Plans					Follow-up Plans	
	Responsible Party	When and How Often	Instruments/Tools for Data Collection	Data Findings & Analysis	Criteria, Outcomes, or Benchmarks	Reports & Recommendations	Maintain & Monitor or Improve	By Whom, How, & When
Philosophy							
Overall purpose/goal							
End-of-program and level objectives							
Implementation plan							
Students							
Applications							
Enrollments							
Achievement							
Graduation							
Alumni							
Human Resources							
Milieu							
Administrators							
Faculty							
Staff							
Colleagues							

STAKE'S MODEL: THE COUNTENANCE OF EDUCATIONAL EVALUATION

Although Stake's (2004) paper "The Countenance of Educational Evaluation" was originally written in 1967, it remains applicable to today's evaluation scene. It discusses two major functions that evaluators perform in the process of program or educational evaluation. One function is that of describing the program undergoing evaluation. Stake states that some evaluators stop at this point. However, the other function is to render judgment on the quality of the program. Some educators leave that judgment to the evaluators, while others prefer to make their own judgments based on the description provided by the evaluator. Accreditation is an example in nursing of passing judgment on a program by outside evaluators. As stated in Chapter 2 of this text, it is the faculty's responsibility to monitor the curriculum as it is implemented and to collect and analyze data that relate to its outcomes. Thus, faculty has the primary role for developing and following the master plan of evaluation, and when recommendations from the evaluation indicate revisions, faculty determines if an outside evaluator or consultant is appropriate for assisting in identifying problems and formulating plans for curriculum change.

Stake's (2004) model for evaluation could be adapted as a master plan of evaluation for a nursing education program. He suggests a matrix of three components for organizing the data that are collected during an evaluation. The components are described as antecedents, transactions, and outcomes. Antecedents are defined as the factors that exist prior to the program's implementation. Examples from nursing are the prerequisite social sciences, sciences, and communication courses required for entering the nursing major. Transactions are the processes that occur during the course of the educational program. Examples from nursing include the interactions that occur during theory classes and the clinical experiences for students and their teachers, preceptors, nursing staff, etc. Outcomes are the final product of the educational experience and the extent to which the graduates meet the program goals.

Two other concepts discussed by Stake are congruence and contingencies. Congruence looks at the processes and outcomes that occur in the curriculum and if what was intended by the curriculum plan is actually happening. Contingencies are the relationships among the variables in the curriculum and their effects on the processes and outcomes. An example of congruence from a nursing curriculum is the intention to produce caring, compassionate nurses. In this case, an evaluator looks at students' learning experiences for evidence of opportunities to express caring and compassion for the clients for whom they care (process). Additionally, there should be an objective that measures graduates' behaviors in caring and compassion (outcome).

As an aside, Beck (1999) reviewed the literature to identify tools that measure caring and found 11 quantitative instruments. An analysis of the instruments revealed that there are multiple dimensions of caring; thus, evaluators who wish to measure caring should review the various tools to determine which one(s) apply to their situation.

Examples of contingencies in nursing are the prerequisites of Anatomy and Physiology. It is possible that students' achievement in these prerequisites could influence their performance in the nursing major. Evaluators of the program might ask the question: To what extent do grades in these prerequisites influence the students' achievement in pathophysiology and health assessment?

If a master plan of evaluation is based on Stake's model, it should include a matrix that addresses each of the three major components, that is, antecedents, transactions, and outcomes, and then compares the congruence for each of these components to what was planned, what happened in actuality, and why. The components are also examined for planned and unplanned contingencies. The information collected according to the matrix provides the data for measuring success and making decisions relative to the quality of the program and the need for change.

Donabedian: Structure, Process, and Outcome

Donabedian (1986, 1996) developed a classic model for evaluation in nursing and health care composed of three major parts: structure, process, and outcome. This model easily adapts to a master plan of evaluation for a nursing education program. Structure includes the internal and external frame factors (Johnson, 1977) that encompass and support the program as well as the program plan or curriculum. Process is the implementation of the curriculum, and outcomes measure the quality and extent to which the graduates meet the intentions of the program.

Sallis: Total Quality Management

Sallis (2002) discusses the Total Quality Management (TQM) model applied to education. The model focuses on the student and involves a commitment on the part of all of the people involved in the educational process. The consumers are intimately involved in the educational process, and for nursing this implies students, faculty, staff, administrators, employers of the program's graduates, and the clients whom the graduates serve. Sallis describes the upside down hierarchy of management indicating that quality starts at the grassroots level and the role of administration is to support the institution's people in the delivery of a quality educational program. The model is appropriate to a master plan of evaluation in nursing education; however, as Sallis warns, it requires "a change of culture. This is notoriously difficult to bring about and takes time to implement. It requires a change of attitudes and working methods" (p. 25).

Sperhac and Goodwin: Example of an Eclectic Model

Sperhac and Goodwin (2003) describe various evaluation tools that were used to assess a pediatric nurse practitioner curriculum. Among them were the Context Input Process and Product (CIPP) model described by Stufflebeam* (2000) and used by their school of nursing as a master plan of evaluation; surveys of alumni, graduates, and their employers; the American Association of Colleges of Nursing (AACN, 1996) *Essentials of Master's Education*; and the standards of the Association of Faculties of Pediatric Nurse Practitioner and Associates Program (1996). All of these data points provided information for the faculty that led to revision of courses (including core courses) and clinical experiences. The revisions were based on analyses of the data and geared toward improving the learning outcomes for students and to meet the expectations of the practice setting. This model is an example of an eclectic model through the use of several models of evaluation, standards, and outcome measures to assess a specific curriculum in nursing.

---

* Stufflebeam's model as applied in nursing is described in detail in Chapter 11.

Benchmarking

More recently, programs are setting benchmarks by which they can measure their own success and standards of excellence or compare themselves to similar institutions. Benchmarking can be used in competition with other programs for recruiting students or seeking financial support, or it can be used to motivate the members of the institution to strive toward excellence. Yet another function of benchmarking is the ability to collaborate with another institution in sharing strengths with each other to continually improve both programs. Benchmarks can include the financial health of the institution; applicant pool; admission; retention and graduation rates; commitment to diversity; student, faculty, staff, and administrators' satisfaction rates; and so forth.

The American Association of Colleges of Nursing (AACN, 2004) offers this service to its member colleges. It collects information from participant institutions and compiles it into an anonymous report. For a fee, other institutions can access the information to compare themselves to other similar programs. Benchmarking responds to the emphasis on outcomes, and as Sallis (2002) succinctly states, "Benchmarking is about bridging the gap between where we are and where we want to be" (p. 101).

Additional references for possible models of evaluation to serve as frameworks for master plans can be found in the Cumulative Index of Nursing and Allied Health Literature (CINAHL) http://www.cinahl.com (2004) and teacher-education literature in the Educator's Reference Desk: http://www.eduref.org (2004). As in research, evaluation has many models from which to choose. The selected model provides the framework or guidelines for the evaluation process. It includes a design for collecting the information that will yield data to be analyzed. The analysis includes the use of many statistical tools and can be the same as those used in research. They include quantitative and qualitative procedures such as content analysis; case studies; factor analysis; multiple regressions; descriptive statistics; and calculations of the means, modes, and medians. The findings are summarized, and as in research, recommendations are put forth. This is crucial information for the program or curriculum undergoing evaluation and is used to provide the feedback loop for continually improving the quality of the program or curriculum.

▲ TOOLS FOR EVALUATION

The following discussion describes some of the tools that evaluators may use when implementing the master plan of evaluation. It includes tools that are useful for collecting and analyzing information that relates to process, formative, or structural evaluation and others that apply to summative or product and outcome evaluation.

Formative or Process Evaluation Tools

Evaluation methods include many of the same measures and instruments utilized in research. Formative and/or process evaluation strategies include course evaluations; student achievement measures; staff, student, administration, and faculty satisfaction measures; impressions of student and faculty performance by clinical agencies' personnel; assessment of student services and other support systems; critical-thinking development and other standardized tests such as gains in knowledge and skills; NCLEX readiness; satisfaction surveys of families of students; and cost effectiveness of the program. Antecedent or input evaluation items include entering grade point averages (GPAs) or Scholastic Achievement Test (The College Board, 2004), ACT (2004), and Graduate Record Examination (GRE) (2004) scores for applicants and accepted students; retention and/or attrition rates; scholarship, fellowship, and loan availability; and endowments and grants for program development and support. As Scriven (1996) points out, these measures help to predict and guide summative, outcome, or product evaluations.

Tools to measure input, support systems, processes, and outcomes are plentiful, and it is strongly recommended that faculty and administrators review the literature for tools that demonstrate reliability and validity. Faculty should review the literature rather than developing new tools that have not been subjected to statistical analyses. Examples of instruments that exist are surveys, appraisal forms, interview schedules, videotaping formats, standardized tests, satisfaction measures, course evaluation forms, and student and faculty performance evaluation forms. The following discussion presents some examples from the literature of formative evaluation methods.

Examples of Formative Tools

- ▲ Fawcett and Alligood (2001) conducted an extensive review of various research instruments and tools used in nursing that were derived from the Science of Unitary Human Beings (Rogers, 1970). They analyzed the instruments as to their usefulness in research and clinical practice and categorized them. Many of these tools can be applied to nursing education as well.
- ▲ A review of critical-thinking instruments is found on the National Center for Educational Statistics Tests for Critical Thinking Skills (2004) Web site, http://nces.ed.gov/npec/evaltests/ctskilltest.asp?ItemNo=45. Newer, nursing-specific assessment tests are available that evaluate students' critical-thinking skills upon entrance, gains throughout the program, and NCLEX readiness. One example of such a program is the Assessment Technology Incorporated program (ATI) (2004), which can be found at http://www.atitesting.com/CriticalThinking.asp.
- ▲ The development of communication skills is at the heart of interpersonal relationships between nurses, clients, and other health team members. Ravert, Williams, and Fosbinder (1997) describe an instrument that measures interpersonal relationship skills of nurses that was based on patient impressions of nurses. The instrument was subjected to various statistical analyses and is one that could be useful in measuring students' and graduates' skills in communications and interpersonal relationships.
- ▲ A description of the use of videotaping is described by Spiers, Costantino, and Faucett (2000) and has possibilities for the evaluation of student performance and faculty teaching effectiveness. A videotape often captures environmental factors and interactions among people that can otherwise be lost. It can prove to be a very useful tool for curriculum process evaluation activities.
- ▲ Jeffreys, Massoni, O'Donnell, and Smodlaka (1997) analyzed student course evaluation tools reported in the literature, and their results provide useful information as it relates to the need for empirical data related to course evaluations. They conclude that if the tools are subjected to statistical analyses and found to be reliable and valid, they can be used to

identify the strengths and weaknesses in the curriculum and ways in which the program can be improved.

▲ Faculty teaching effectiveness is an essential element for determining the quality of the implementation of the curriculum. Crawford (1998) surveyed National League for Nursing–accredited baccalaureate schools of nursing for reports on the use of classroom observation instruments to evaluate faculty. She found that most schools use observation as one of the tools for evaluating faculty; however, reliability and validity of the tools were lacking. She concluded that classroom observation could be a powerful tool for evaluating teaching effectiveness, but that the lack of consensus on the purpose of it (i.e., performance evaluation or professional development), and the myriad methods related to it constrain its usefulness in faculty evaluation.

▲ Moody (1996) raised the specter of the faculty shortage in nursing and studied faculty satisfaction by surveying schools of nursing with doctorate programs. With a 60% return rate and the use of two standardized job satisfaction instruments and three researcher-developed tools, Moody found that the factors most influencing faculty satisfaction were salary, degree level of nursing students, and length of annual contract. Faculty satisfaction influences the quality of the program and its implementation. Findings from this study and periodic assessment of faculty satisfaction should play a part in the evaluation of the process elements of the curriculum.

Summative or Outcome Evaluation Tools

Measures to determine outcomes of the program include follow-up surveys of the success rates of the graduates, including their pass rates on licensure and certification exams, employers' and graduates' satisfaction with the program, graduates' performance, and alumni's accomplishments in leadership roles, accomplishments as change agents, professional commitment, and continuing education rates. Additional outcome measures include graduation rates, accreditation and program approval status, ratings of the program by external evaluators or agencies, research productivity, community services, and public opinion surveys. There is a plethora of instruments available for measuring graduates' performance as an indication of the success of the nursing educational program. Several examples of these studies follow.

Examples of Summative Tools

▲ A measure to study the performance of senior nursing students and new graduates is described by Keating and Sargent (2001) and Keating, Rutledge, Sargent, and Walker (2003). The study was based on the California Competency Based Role Differentiation Model (CBRDM) to test the utility of specific components of the CBRDM (Fox, Walker, & Bream, 1999). The alpha pilot study tested levels of competence in teaching and leadership functions and found that while the sample was small, the CBRDM tool can be used to measure levels of competence in senior students and new graduates.

▲ A study of outcomes for graduate students was conducted by O'Connor, Hameister, and Kershaw (2000) who examined the practice patterns of adult nurse practitioner students. They utilized a variety of nursing taxonomies to describe the students' practice patterns in nursing terminology. The North American Nursing Diagnoses Association (NANDA) and the University of Iowa's Nursing Intervention Classification (NIC) taxonomies were useful in describing nursing diagnoses and interventions of care by nurse practitioner students. The authors recommend continued use of these nursing taxonomies to advance their use as a discipline-specific tool to measure advanced nursing practice.

▲ Kapborg and Fischbein (2002) found that education goals and frameworks have an impact on nursing students and nurses' professional practice. Based on their findings, they argue for the use of a conceptual model for evaluating the effectiveness of a nursing education program. Their findings further validate the need for a master plan of evaluation.

The tools described in this chapter are but a few of those available in the literature. Nurse educators are urged to review the latest literature in search for the best tools for collecting and analyzing data to measure the outcomes and the processes used to reach the outcomes of the educational program. These tools should be congruent with that of the master plan of evaluation.

▲ SUMMARY

Chapter 10 reviewed classic definitions, concepts, and models of evaluation with definitions of commonly used terms. The rationale for a master plan of evaluation was presented as well as several examples of classic frameworks for developing a master plan of evaluation. Types of tools and instruments for data collection for evaluation of educational programs are reviewed from the literature.

Based on the practical aspects of accreditation standards and the recommendations that come from the data collected through an evaluation model, the argument for a master plan is strong. The only issue that remains is the selection of the model. This should be a faculty decision based on its philosophy of nursing education and evaluation and the setting in which the education program is located.

DISCUSSION QUESTIONS

1. Describe how a master plan of evaluation contributes to the external review processes of a nursing education program. Read the classic treatise by Stake (1967), *The Countenance of Educational Evaluation* (at http://www.ed.uiuc.edu/circe/Publications/CIRCE_Publications .html), and describe how Stake's matrix could be adapted to the development of a master plan of evaluation for a nursing program.

2. Justify the use of a total assessment tool/package to measure the development of students' critical-thinking skills throughout a nursing program and upon graduation. Which type of evaluation is more important to curriculum development—formative evaluation that measures processes and progress along the way, or summative evaluation that measures outcomes and the final end product? Explain your rationale.

LEARNING ACTIVITIES

Student Learning Activities

1. Utilizing Table 10.1, develop a master plan of evaluation for the case study of a fictional school of nursing outreach program found in Chapters 5, 6, and 7.

Faculty Development Activities

1. Utilizing Table 10.1, find your school of nursing's or agency's evaluation plan and assess it for any missing components or action plans.

R E F E R E N C E S

ACT. (2004). *Homepage.* Retrieved June 8, 2004, from http://www.act.org/aap

American Association of Colleges of Nursing. (2004). *Data center. Benchmarking project. Questions and answers about performance measures and benchmarking reports.* Retrieved June 8, 2004, from http://www.aacn.nche.edu/Data/bench.htm

American Association of Colleges of Nursing. (1998). *Essentials of baccalaureate education for professional nursing practice.* Washington DC: Author. Retrieved June 8, 2004, fromhttp://www.aacn.nche.edu/Publications/catalog2.htm

American Association of Colleges of Nursing. (1996). *Essentials of master's education for advanced practice nursing.* Washington, DC: Author. Retrieved June 4, 2004, from http://www.aacn.nche.edu/Publications/catalog2.htm

American Nurses Association. *ANA standards.* Retrieved June 8, 2004, from http://nursingworld.org/anp/pdescr.cfm?CNum=15

Assessment Technology Incorporated (ATI) Program. Critical Thinking Exam (2004). Retrieved June 8, 2004, from ATI Critical Thinking: http://www.atitesting.com/productinfo/CriticalThinking.asp

Association of Faculties of Nurse Practitioner and Associate Programs. (1996). *Philosophy, conceptual model, terminal competencies for the evaluation of pediatric nurse practitioners.* Rockville: MD Author.

Beck, C. T. (1999). Quantitative measurement of caring. *Journal of Advanced Nursing, 30*(1), 24–32.

Carnegie Foundation. (1977). *Missions of the college curriculum. A contemporary review with suggestions.* San Francisco, CA: Jossey-Boss Publishers.

Commission on Collegiate Nursing Education. (2004). *Standards for accreditation of baccalaureate and graduate nursing education programs.* Retrieved October 29, 2004 from http://www.aacn.nche.edu/accreditation/NEW STANDARDS.htm

Council of Associate Degree Nursing Competencies Task Force. National League for Nursing with support from the National Organization of Associate Degree Nursing. (2000). *Educational competencies for graduates of associate degree programs.* (G. Coxwell & H. Gillerman, Eds., Rev.). Sudbury, MA: Jones and Bartlett Publishers.

Council of Higher Education Accreditation. (2003). *Research and information sheets. Fact sheet #4. A framework for meeting transfer of credit responsibilities.* Retrieved June 8, 2004, from http://www.chea.org/research

Crawford, L. H. (1998). Evaluation of nursing faculty through observation. *Journal of Nursing Education, 37*(7), 289–294.

Cumulative Index of Nursing and Allied Health Literature (CINAHL). Retrieved June 4, 2004, from http://www.cinahl.com

Donabedian, A. (1986). Criteria and standards for quality assessment and monitoring. *Quality Review Bulletin, 12*(3), 99–100.

Donabedian, A. (1996). Quality management in nursing and health care (pp. 88–103). In J. A. Schemele (Ed.), *Models of Quality Assurance.* Albany, NY: Delmar Publishers.

The Educator's Reference Desk. Home page (2004). Retrieved June 8, 2004, from http://www.eduref.org/

Fawcett, J., & Alligood, M. R. (2001). SUHB instruments: An overview of research instruments and clinical tools derived from the Science of Unitary Human Beings. *Journal of Nursing Theory, 10*(3), 5–12.

Fox, S., Walker, P., & Bream, T. (1999). *California's framework for competency-based role differentiation in nursing.* Report of the Education/Industry Work Group. CSPCN/CIC. Sacramento, CA: Association of California Nurse Leaders.

Graduate Record Examination. (2004). *GRE Web site.* Retrieved June 8, 2004, from: http://www.gre.org/splash.html

Jeffreys, M. R., Massoni, M., O'Donnell, M., & Smodlaka, I. (1997). Student evaluation of courses: Determining the reliability and validity of three survey instruments. *Journal of Nursing Education, 36*(8), 397–400.

Johnson, M. (1977). *Intentionality in education.* (Distributed by the Center for Curriculum Research and Services, Albany, NY.) Troy, NY: Walter Snyder, Printer, Inc.

Kapborg, I., & Fischbein, S. (2002). Using a model to evaluate nursing education and professional practice. *Nursing and Health Science, 4*(1/2), 25–31.

Keating, S. B., & Sargent, A. (2001). Testing California's differentiated practice model through industry & education partnerships. *Nursing Administration Quarterly, 26*(1), 1–5.

Keating, S. B., Rutledge, D. N., Sargent, A., & Walker, P. (Spring 2003). Testing the Model for Competency. *Patient Care Management, 19*(5), 7–11.

Merriam-Webster's Online Dictionary. "Quality" (2004). Retrieved June 8, 2004, from http://www.m-w.com/cgi-bin/ dictionary

Moody, N. B. (1996). Nurse faculty satisfaction: A national survey. *Journal of Professional Nursing, 12*(5), 277–288.

National Center for Educational Statistics Tests for Critical Thinking Skills. National Assessment of College Student Learning: Identifying College Graduates' Essential Skills in Writing, Speech & Listening, & Critical Thinking, (2004). Retrieved June 8, 2004, from http://nces.ed.gov/pubsearch/pubsinfo.asp?pubid=95001

National League for Nursing Accrediting Commission. (2004). 2002 *standards and criteria.* Retrieved June 8, 2004, fromhttp://www.nlnac.org/default1.htm

National Organization of Nurse Practitioner Faculties. (2004). *Evaluation Criteria.* Retrieved June 10, 2004, from http://www.nonpf.com/criteria.htm

O'Connor, N. A., Hameister, A. D., & Kershaw, T. (2000). Developing a database to describe the practice patterns of adult nurse practitioner students. *Journal of Nursing Scholarship, 31*(1), 57–63.

Ravert, P., Williams, M., & Fosbinder, D. M. (1997). The interpersonal competence instrument of nurses. *Western Journal of Nursing Research, 19*(6), 781–791.

Rogers, M. E. (1970). *An introduction to the theoretical basis of nursing.* Philadelphia: F.A. Davis

Sallis, E. (2002). *Total quality management in education* (3rd ed.). London: Kogan Page Ltd.

Scriven, M. (1996). Types of evaluation and types of evaluator. *Evaluation Practice, 17*(2), 151–161.

Scriven, M. (1974). Evaluation perspectives and procedures. In W. J. Popham (Ed.), *Evaluation in education. Current applications.* Berkeley, CA: McCutchan Publishing Corporation.

Sperhac, A. M., & Goodwin, L. D. (2003). Using multiple data sources for curriculum revision. *Journal of Pediatric Health Care, 17*(4): 169–175.

Spiers, J. A., Costantino, M., & Faucett, J. (2000). Video technology: Use in nursing research. *AAOH, 48*(3), 119–124.

Stake, R. (2004). *The countenance of educational evaluation.* Retrieved June 8, 2004, from University of Illinois, College of Education: http://www.ed.uiuc.edu/circe/Publications/CIRCE_Publications.html.

Stufflebeam, D. E. (2000). The CIPP model for evaluation. In D. L. Stufflebeam, G. F. Madaus, & T. Kellaghan (Eds.), *Evaluation models: Viewpoints on education and human services evaluation.* (2nd ed.). Boston: Kluwer Academic Publishers.

The College Board. (2004). *SAT Program. Higher Education.* Retrieved June 4, 2004, from http://www.collegeboard.com/highered/ra/sat/sat.html

Western Association of Schools and Colleges (WASC). (1997). *Handbook of accreditation.* Oakland, CA: Western Association of School and Colleges.

Worthen, B. R., & Sanders, J. R. (1974). *Educational evaluation: Theory and practice.* Belmont, CA: Wadsworth Publishing Company.

Application of Educational Evaluation Models to Nursing

Arlene A. Sargent, EdD, MSN, RN, and
Ellen M. Lewis, MSN, RN, FAAN

OBJECTIVES

Upon completion of Chapter 11, the reader will be able to:

1. Justify the value of outcome-based education for a nursing curriculum.
2. Apply several models of evaluation to the assessment of nursing programs and curricula.
3. Analyze the components of an evaluation model necessary for its successful implementation.
4. Examine the implications for faculty, curriculum committees, students, and employers from implementing an evaluation model.
5. Analyze a case study that utilizes formative and summative evaluation models for its application to curriculum evaluation in advanced-practice nursing.

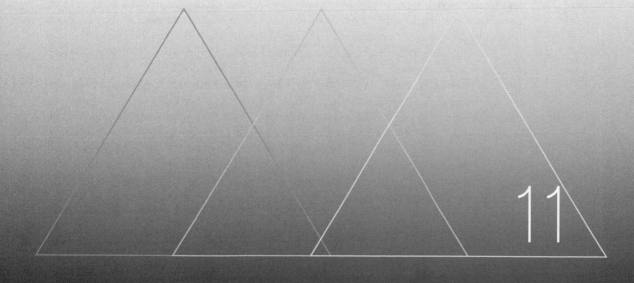

▲ OVERVIEW

Chapter 11 provides an overview of three specific curriculum evaluation models tracing the early behavioral model of Tyler through the commonly used Stufflebeam model, to the more recent Baldrige quality model. These evaluation models provide different ways to measure student outcomes, all with the underlying philosophy of continuous improvement. The evaluation design begins with the premise that nursing competencies are planned as part of a program of study, and that each competency is expressed in terms of goals or outcomes at the completion of the program.

Evaluation models provide a structured approach for the development of a master plan of evaluation and quality improvement. Successful utilization of the models requires commitment and ownership of them by all those involved in the educational process, from top administrators to the lowest staff level. Sections of different existing models can be used if they seem appropriate and can result in the development of an eclectic model of evaluation that fits the educational program or curriculum. Evaluators make choices among models depending on the purpose of evaluation and the desired outcomes from an assessment.

A case study at the end of the chapter provides an example of an actual model of evaluation used to evaluate the curriculum of a nurse practitioner program to measure the students' clinical competence. It integrates the Stufflebeam model of evaluation—Context, Input, Process, and Product (CIPP)—and illustrates formative (process) and summative (output) evaluation techniques.

▲ OUTCOME-BASED EDUCATION

Considering recent changes in health care and education, evaluation models provide guidance to faculty for curriculum assessment by focusing on student outcomes and the learning experiences associated with those outcomes. Answers to questions about outcomes, teaching and learning practices, quality, and academic standards are sought by accrediting bodies, commissions on higher education, academic institutions, schools of nursing, and employers, as well as by students and faculty pioneering new ways of teaching and learning. Outcomes are influenced by multiple educational practices, and the utilization of evaluation models add value to the educational process by providing a structure for determining outcomes and modifying practices.

Outcome-based education is a performance-based approach to curriculum development that offers a powerful and appealing way of reforming and managing nursing education (Harden, Crosby, & Davis, 1999). The emphasis is on the product (i.e., what sort of nurse will be produced), rather than on the educational process. In outcomes-based education, the outcomes are clearly and unambiguously specified. These determine the curriculum content and its organization, the teaching strategies and methods, the courses offered, the assessment process, and the educational environment.

Nursing education must prepare the workforce to ensure that the public receives the nursing care it needs. This is nursing's professional contract with society. The public is concerned with the product that education produces; it is focused on outcomes, not the process. "There is a great chasm between what schools claim they are doing and what is actually achieved in terms of student outcomes" (Lindeman, 2000, p. 7). Utilization of an outcomes-based education model enables educators to have a more accurate analysis of how well the outcomes sought are achieved and to identify what measures need to be implemented to enhance effectiveness.

Schools of nursing need to prepare nurses to practice in an increasingly complex health care milieu with changing public expectations and increasing demands from employers. Outcomes-based education offers many advantages as a guiding principle. It emphasizes relevance in the curriculum and accountability and serves as a guide to student assessment and course evaluation. The clinical effectiveness of nurses depends heavily on their ability to improve quality. In addition, the use of outcomes-based techniques in the curriculum demonstrates evaluation processes to students, and nurses need to know how to collect data on measures of quality and how to use these data to continuously improve the quality of nursing care. It is imperative to ensure that tomorrow's RNs are equipped with the latest knowledge in quality improvement and the skills necessary to improve quality even if, as expected, shortages develop and the composition of the nursing workforce is markedly different than it is today.

▲ EVALUATION MODELS

The use of evaluation models by nursing education programs reflects a commitment to take actions aimed at reducing the waste of resources in education that do not contribute to quality outcomes. The more the nursing curriculum includes the theories and methods of quality improvement, the better prepared nurses are to apply this knowledge to their practice. Assessing and managing student performance is fundamental to the achievement and improvement of curriculum effectiveness. Providing evidence of achievement and certifying the competence of graduates is of fundamental importance in demonstrating program quality (Karlowicz, 2000).

Educational researchers developed a multitude of evaluation models, and nurse educators have much of the information needed to perform comprehensive evaluations of their curricula from their nursing knowledge and practice base. The application of evaluation models assists in developing master plans for evaluation and guiding the process. The following discussion provides an overview of several evaluation models and focuses on two models in greater depth, the CIPP model, which has been a heavily used model in education for several decades, and the Baldrige Evaluation Model, a newer model.

A Classic Model: The Tyler Model

The Tyler Model (Tyler, 1942) is often referred to as the "objectives model" or the "goal-attainment model." It emphasizes consistency among objectives, learning experiences, and outcomes. Tyler identified four principles for teaching:

1. Defining appropriate learning objectives
2. Establishing useful learning experiences
3. Organizing learning experiences to have a maximum cumulative effect
4. Evaluating the curriculum and revising those aspects that did not prove to be effective

Tyler put forward one of the earliest ideas in education leading to the measurement of outcomes by pointing out that a list of program or curriculum objectives indicates both the kind of behavior to be developed in the student and the area of content or life in which the behavior is to be applied.

The CIPP Model

The CIPP approach to evaluation described by Stufflebeam (1971, 2000) is based on the view that the most important purpose of evaluation is not to prove but to improve. It sees evaluation as a tool to help make programs work better for the people they are intended to serve. The model moves away from the view that evaluation is only an instrument of accountability, and instead sees evaluation as a tool to help programs work better for those under instruction. CIPP is an acronym for Context, Input, Process, and Product evaluation, which together comprise the CIPP model (Stufflebeam, 1971, 2000). An overview of these four components and their relationship to objectives, methods, and uses is provided in Table 11.1.

Context evaluation focuses on the identification of strengths and weaknesses of some object (such as a nursing program or a person) to provide direction for improvement. As a result of context evaluation there should be a sound basis for adjusting existing goals and priorities. Context evaluation provides the necessary information for curriculum revision or for a specific component of it.

Input evaluation is primarily to assist educators in bringing about needed changes in the program. While the context provides the agreement that changes need to be made, input evaluation is necessary to determine the best approach. Input evaluation promotes the consideration of alternatives in the context of program or individual needs and evolves into a plan that is appropriate to the program. Input evaluation also allows for the comparison of an existing program to what is being done elsewhere and what is presented in the literature.

Process evaluation allows for ongoing feedback that aids in carrying out a program as it was planned or, if it is found to be seriously flawed, to make revisions accordingly. Process evaluation requires the evaluator to gather data in a regular, unobtrusive way to ensure that the curriculum is on track. This might include visiting and observing student activities, reviewing course syllabi, attending meetings, and meeting with key participants. The evaluator then provides regular feedback on what is learned. This approach allows for changes to be made midcourse to ensure a greater likelihood that end objectives and outcomes will be achieved.

Product evaluation, has as its purpose the measurement, interpretation, and judgment of the attainments of a program. Product evaluation ascertains the extent to which the program meets the needs of the group it is intended to serve. In a school of nursing, various stakeholders are consulted, including students, clinical agencies, community members, faculty, other university departments, and others who are directly affected by the program. Product evaluation speaks to accountability and the degree to which programmatic outcomes are achieved.

Each of the four components of the CIPP evaluation model serves a unique function in providing feedback on various components of curricula. The role each plays depends on the design of the evaluation plan that was decided on initially by the educators. However, the dynamic and interactive qualities of evaluation require flexibility throughout the evaluation process to ensure that the most appropriate evaluative focus continues to be utilized.

The Baldrige Evaluation System

The Malcolm Baldrige Evaluation system (Baldrige National Quality Program, 2000) provides a basis for self-assessment as well as a framework for programmatic and university-wide assessment of performance. The Performance Assessment System is based on a set of core

From Stufflebeam (1983), p. 129.

▲ TABLE 11.1   Four Types of Evaluation

	Context Evaluation	Input Evaluation	Process Evaluation	Product Evaluation
Objective	To define the institutional context, to identify the target population and assess their needs, to identify opportunities for addressing the needs, to diagnose problems underlying the needs, and to judge whether proposed objectives are sufficiently responsive to the assessed needs	To identify and assess system capabilities, alternative program strategies, procedural designs for implementing the strategies, budgets, and schedules	To identify or predict, in process, defects in the procedural design or its implementation, to provide information for the preprogrammed decisions, and to record and judge procedural events and activities	To collect descriptions and judgments of outcomes, to relate them to objectives and context, input, and process information, and to interpret their worth and merit
Method	By using such methods as system analysis, surveys, document reviews, hearings, interviews, diagnostic tests, and the Delphi technique	By inventorying and analyzing available human and material resources, solution strategies, and procedural designs for relevance, feasibility, and economy, and by using such methods as literature searches, visits to exemplary programs, advocate teams, and pilot trials	By monitoring the activity's potential procedural barriers and remaining alert to unanticipated barriers, by obtaining specified information for programmed decisions, by describing the actual process, and by continually interacting with and observing the activities of project staff	By defining operationally and measuring outcome criteria, by collecting judgments of outcomes from stakeholders, and by performing both qualitative and quantitative analyses
Relation to decision-making in the change process	For deciding on the setting to be served, the goals associated with meeting needs or using opportunities, and the objectives associated with solving problems (i.e., for planning needed changes), and for providing a basis for judging outcomes	For selecting sources of support, solution strategies, and procedural designs (i.e., for structural change activities) and for providing a basis for judging implementation	For implementing and refining the program design and procedure (i.e., for effecting process control) and for providing a log of the actual process for later use in interpreting outcomes	For deciding to continue, terminate, modify or refocus a change activity and present a clear record of effects (intended and unintended, positive and negative)

values and concepts that are the foundation for integrating key business requirements within a results-oriented framework. The core values are embedded in seven categories: leadership, strategic planning, customer and market focus, information and analysis, human resource focus, process management, and business results.

1. Leadership

   This category examines how the leadership of organizations addresses values and performance expectations as well as focuses on customers and other stakeholders and empowering, innovating, learning, and influencing organizational directions. The leadership criteria address how an organization carries out its responsibilities to the public and supports its key communities. Figure 11.1 illustrates the stakeholder groups of one college, with students as the primary customers. Faculty and staff function both as customers and as the link between students and the other stakeholder groups, partners and consumers. Consumers consist of employers, health professionals, patients, and the community. Partners are affiliated organizations, feeder schools, donors, alumni, and board members.

2. Strategic Planning

   This category integrates strategic planning and operations management through its work on continuous quality improvement. It includes developing strategic objectives, action plans, and related human resource plans. Measurement includes how plans are deployed as well as how performance is tracked. One college implements this category through the utilization of the Five-Step Process (FSP) and a cross-disciplinary task force synthesized from several clinical planning models (Samuel Merritt College, 1999). The FSP was adopted by the college to create a common terminology and approach to the planning process. The strategic planning process at the college follows the FSP. See Figure 11.2 for a model of the five-step process.

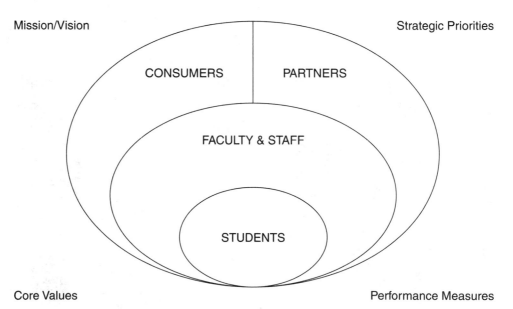

Mission/Vision

Strategic Priorities

Core Values

Performance Measures

FIGURE   11.1   Stakeholder groups. From Samuel Merritt College (1999).

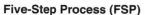

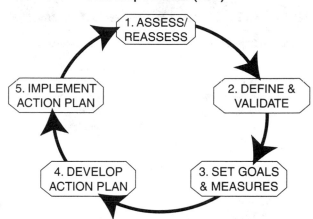

FIGURE 11.2 The five-step process (FSP). From Samuel Merritt College (1999).

3. Student and Stakeholder Focus

This criterion examines how a college determines requirements, expectations, and preferences of students and stakeholders and how it builds relationships with students and determines their satisfaction. In addition to the college defining the criterion, each department within the college identifies its own mission, key processes, major stakeholders, and their requirements. Table 11.2 provides an example of how college objectives can be applied to four key stakeholder groups.

4. Information and Analysis

The fourth category examines a college's performance measurement system and how the college analyzes performance data and information. Data are used as an integral part of the continuous improvement process. Departments and committees track important data and use the resulting analyses to revise processes and improve performance. For example, the undergraduate faculty could track NCLEX licensure pass rates as a key indicator of student learning. These data could be used to develop action plans and track subsequent performance. This same process could be used in analysis and performance review at various levels of the curriculum and department.

5. Faculty and Staff Focus

The fifth category examines how the college/department enables faculty and staff to develop and utilize their full potential and align themselves with the college's objectives. Also examined are the college's efforts to build and maintain a work environment and an employee-support climate conducive to performance excellence, full participation, and personal and college growth.

All faculty and staff contribute to the student focus. The Baldrige process focuses on designing a work environment that best serves students and other stakeholders. Organizational design with a Baldrige framework enhances communication processes and focuses on systems improvement. Performance excellence is emphasized in performance standards, leadership development, new staff orientation, and all components of service to students.

6. Process Management

This category examines the key aspects of a college's process management, including student-focused design, curriculum, and student service delivery. The design and delivery of all of the

▲ **TABLE 11.2**   **Example of College Objectives for Key Stakeholder Relationships**

College Objectives	College Needs	How Needs Communicated
STUDENTS To prepare graduates who represent the college well and serve employers and the community with professionalism	Integrity, talent, and aptitude Personal and financial commitment Active engagement in learning and service Dedication to improving the college	Admission process Orientation and publications College policies Events (convocation, graduation) Faculty/staff contact Advising, counseling, and modeling behaviors
FACULTY/STAFF To create the environment and curriculum that enable students to achieve their educational goals *To attract and retain satisfied faculty and staff to support growth*	Expertise Commitment to college mission and values Active engagement in education and improvement Reliability Commitment to individual role	Position description and orientation Faculty staff handbook and other publications Annual performance evaluation Deployment of climate survey and course evaluation results Faculty/staff development activities Informal feedback Formal recognition and rewards
PARTNERS To link with others whose resources, expertise, and reputation complement and strengthen the college's capacity to fulfill its mission	Effective communication Access to expertise, resources, influence, and markets Continuity of commitment	Contracts Organization structure Events and personal contact Formal and informal communication
CONSUMERS To build and sustain relationships that support and enhance the college and its mission	Goodwill Information Commitments of time, money, and influence to benefit the college	Marketing and advertising Personal contact Events College participation in the community

From Samuel Merritt College (1999), p.12.

curricula changes as well as new programs are reviewed through a process that ensures that they meet defined criteria and have broad support from the faculty and the wider community.

Academic departments determine course sequencing and linkages within and between programs based on the nature of learning experiences, foundation knowledge, and skills required to build new competencies. Departmental curriculum committees examine the whole curriculum and how the content of each course relates to or depends on other courses. Table 11.3 illustrates how evaluation delivery can be monitored in different timeframes.

7. College Performance Results

This category examines the college's performance and improvement in key areas: student and alumni satisfaction, licensure, certification and accreditation results, and graduation and employment rates. Other factors measured under this category include diversity

▲ **TABLE 11.3**   **Approaches to Monitoring Education Delivery**

Minimum Response Time	Measure/Indicator	Users	How Used
Immediate	Learning assessment results Mid-semester course evaluations Student comments Clinical site feedback	Individual faculty Curriculum committees Student services	Assess student learning Counsel individual faculty Maintain or revise curriculum content and teaching methods Adjust curriculum to meet program philosophy and purpose Adjust program and services to meet accreditation standards
Semester	Learning assessment results Faculty evaluations Course evaluations six-semester trend analysis Specialty accreditation findings	Individual faculty Curriculum committees Department chair Academic vice president	Assess student learning Counsel individual faculty Maintain or revise curriculum content and teaching methods Adjust curriculum to meet program philosophy and purpose Adjust program and services to meet accreditation standards
1–3 years	Climate survey results Entry and graduation survey results Alumni survey results Employer survey results Professional clinical competency Financial performance	Academic departments Student services Strategic planning committees	Maintain or revise program design Adjust program philosophy and purpose Maintain or revise admission criteria Determine effective marketing strategies Incorporate healthcare trends in curriculum

From Samuel Merritt College (1999), p. 27.

among students and faculty, faculty scholarship, professional service, and community service. Service learning is measured in terms of its effectiveness in providing all students with a community service experience.

Table 11.4 illustrates how one school of nursing utilized the Baldrige evaluation system in identifying key processes, how these are evaluated, and by whom. The key processes have a direct link to both the college core processes and the institutional mission.

▲ **TABLE 11.4**   **Key Processes For Quality Improvement**

1. **Develop, implement, and evaluate the curriculum to optimize student learning**
2. **Develop more efficient and effective systems for student recruitment, retention, and progression**
3. **Support acquisition, professional development, scholarship, and productivity of faculty and staff**
4. **Provide service to the profession, the college, and the greater community**
5. **Create and maintain a responsive system of governance and collegial work environment**

KEY PROCESS #1: Develop, implement, and evaluate the curriculum to optimize student learning
CUSTOMERS: Students, corporate partners, employers
OUTPUTS: Employable students and marketable curricula
COLLEGE CORE PROCESS: Teaching

Key Quality Indicators	Measurements Required	Measurement Targets	Responsibility/Timeline
a. Current, comprehensive curriculum	Course evaluations	All courses ranked >3.25	Grad/undergrad committees Annual
	Accreditation/external reviews	Full accreditation	Departments Accreditation cycle
	CT data pool	ERI Score >90%	Undergraduate Chair
	BSN senior program evaluation	Score to be determined (TBD)	Annual
b. High-quality instruction	Faculty instructional evaluations	All faculty ranked >3.25	Supervisors and/or peer evaluations Annually and/or end of contract
c. Adequate fiscal and human resources	Student and faculty climate surveys	Satisfaction of both groups >3.25	Dean/admin. Team Annually
d. Marketability of graduates	Licensure rates	NCLEX rate >80%	Institution research, faculty/ dean Annually
	Certification rates	CRNA rate >90%	Director Annually
	New graduate evaluation	Score TBD	UG faculty Annually
e. New program development	College enrollment statistics	Increase of nursing enrollments >10% annually	Dean/nursing administrative council, faculty Annually
f. Program grants	# of submitted grants	TBD	Annually

▲ **TABLE 11.4**   **Key Processes For Quality Improvement** (continued)

KEY PROCESS #2: Student recruitment, retention, and progression
CUSTOMERS: Students
OUTPUTS: Students who move sequentially through the admission process and graduate
COLLEGE CORE PROCESS: Serving students, managing enrollment

Key Quality Indicator	Measurements Required	Measurement Targets/ Standards	Responsibility/Timeline
Recruitment	Conversion rate	Increase qualified applicant pool by 5% annually	Administrative team Annually
Retention	Attrition rates	<4% grad and undergrad	Undergraduate committee/chairperson of undergraduate nursing programs Annually
Progression	Probation rates—measured by GPA	<7% grad and undergrad	Undergraduate committee/ chairperson of undergraduate nursing programs Annually
Advising	Climate survey	90% above 3.5 on climate survey	Undergraduate committee/ chairperson of undergraduate nursing programs Biannually

KEY PROCESS #3: Support acquisition, professional development, scholarship, and productivity of faculty and staff
CUSTOMERS: Faculty, administration, staff
OUTPUTS: Sufficient numbers of faculty and staff, current in their area(s) of expertise, who actively contribute to key departmental processes and outcomes
COLLEGE CORE PROCESS: Managing resources

Key Quality Indicators	Measurements Required	Measurement Targets/ Standards	Responsibility/Timeline
a. Full complement of regular faculty/ staff	Faculty FIAs Staff positions filled	90% FTE filled by regular faculty 100% staff positions filled	Dean/search committee chair Annual review of faculty contracts November
b. Support for scholarly work	Faculty Climate Survey	>3.25 on relevant items. 100% faculty meet contracted goals for scholarly work	Dean Annually during budget cycle

(*table continues on page 286*)

▲ TABLE 11.4	Key Processes For Quality Improvement (continued)		

Key Quality Indicators	Measurements Required	Measurement Targets/ Standards	Responsibility/Timeline
b. Support for scholarly work (continued)	Faculty Evaluation, Section IV	Continuous output	Dean/program directors Annually—Spring
	Body of scholarly work by School of Nursing		Dean Annually
	Evidence of research funding	Additional grants funded	Dean Annually
c. Faculty orientation mentoring program for faculty/staff	Internal orientation evaluation tool	>3.25	Program directors End of first semester for new faculty
	Internal evaluation tool	>3.25	Dean Annually
d. Professional development opportunities	Plan for distribution of CE funds	Completed plan 90% F/T faculty attends activities	Faculty Prior to budget submission Annually
	Regular SMC development programs	9 programs/year	Faculty development committee Annually
	Tuition reimbursement for doctoral studies	3–5 faculty/year.	Dean Annually

KEY PROCESS #4: Provide service to the profession, the college, and the greater community
CUSTOMERS: College, community service organizations, corporate interests
OUTPUTS: Effective services or products available to external stakeholders
COLLEGE CORE PROCESS: PARTNERING

Key Quality Indicators	Measurements Required	Measurement Targets/ Standards	Responsibility/Timeline
a. Nursing membership on college committees	Data from annual Faculty Evaluation Summary Form (FESF)	Nursing fills 35% of all college committees	Faculty Annually
b. Faculty membership in school committees/task forces/meetings	Data from annual Faculty Evaluation Summary Form (FESF)	All faculty successfully complete "service" requirements on FESF	Faculty/Dean Annually
c. Program or service to community entities	Community satisfaction survey results	Contract of Memorandum of Understanding (MOU) renewals	Faculty/Admin team Annually

▲ TABLE 11.4	Key Processes For Quality Improvement (continued)		

Key Quality Indicators	Measurements Required	Measurement Targets/ Standards	Responsibility/Timeline
d. Formal liaisons with external agencies	Corporate satisfaction survey results	Contract or MOU renewals	Faculty/Admin team Annually
e. Membership and/or leadership positions in local/state or national professional organizations	Annual Faculty Evaluation	100% faculty membership in minimum of one professional organization	Dean Annually

KEY PROCESS #5: Create and maintain a responsive governance system and work environment
CUSTOMERS: Faculty
OUTPUTS: A system of communication and decision making that is clearly understandable, relevant to need, has high user satisfaction ratings, and contributes positively to the academic community
COLLEGE CORE PROCESS. NO APPLICABLE CORE PROCESS

Key Quality Indicators	Measurements Required	Measurement Targets/ Standards	Responsibility/Timeline
a. Written bylaws or governance guidelines	Faculty climate survey or other suitable survey instrument	>90%	Faculty Biennially
b. Written communication guidelines	Faculty climate survey or other suitable survey instrument	>90%	Faculty Biennially
c. Collegial community	Climate survey or other suitable survey instrument	>90%	Faculty/staff Biennially

The utilization of an evaluation model has to take into account a variety of constituents and contexts. All evaluation models should address:

▲ The evaluation question
▲ The evaluation criteria
▲ The evidence to be used in the evaluation (the types of questions or test instruments that are going to be used)
▲ The role subjective judgment is to play in the evaluation
▲ A plan for implementing the evaluation design

The analysis of teaching methodologies and learning resources is ongoing. Evaluation must continue from the time of program development until it is determined that the entire curriculum is achieving expected results. Evaluation occurs in the same timeframe as revision activities.

It is the faculty's responsibility to identify which model of evaluation works best for its program. The need for faculty to validate and enhance curriculum efficiency and effectiveness through evidence-based quality strategies to provide cost-effective education and quality health care providers has never been more crucial.

▲ SUMMARY

Evaluation of health care education is fundamental to demonstrating and improving quality. The application of evaluation models as master plans of evaluation can be used in documenting competencies and ensuring their attainment. To prove and improve quality and to meet the requirements of regulatory bodies and agencies, those involved in the design and implementation of evaluation strategies must be open to new ideas, flexible in the selection of potential data sources, and willing to take advantage of different models and available technology. Furthermore, they must be able to design a package of complementary measures appropriate to the range of courses, students, health care practitioners, and clinical and educational settings in which they learn and practice. In this way, not only will the quality of programs be proved and improved, but also employers and other stakeholders can be confident that health care professionals will be fit for purpose, practice, and award.

C A S E   S T U D Y

▼

Standardized Patient Technology in Formative and Summative Evaluation of Nurse Practitioners

Ellen M. Lewis, MSN, RN, FAAN

Overview

Clinical evaluation processes, which utilize the standardized patient (SP), a person who is trained to portray an actual patient by simulating an illness, are becoming the "gold standard" for performance-based assessments (U.S. Medical Licensing Examination, 2004). Unlike real patients, SPs can be available at any time and in any setting. The use of SPs is a known technology for helping the learner obtain interpersonal, communication, interviewing, counseling, assessment, physical exam, and patient management skills. The Objective Structured Clinical Evaluation (OSCE), a formative assessment of student performance, and the Clinical Practice Exam (CPX), a summative assessment of student performance, use SPs and are well documented as valuable tools in the teaching and evaluation of interviewing, physical examinations, and interpersonal skills of medical students and residents (Barrows, 1987; Colliver & Williams, 1993; Klass et al., 1992; Reznick, Blackmore, & Cohen, 1993; Swanson, Norman, & Linn, 1995; Van der Vleuten & Swanson, 1990; Vu & Barrows, 1994). It has also been reported that administration of serial assessments can detect interval learning (Prislin, Giglio, Lewis, Ahearn, & Radecki, 2000) and that SPs allow "teachable moments" to be created rather than waiting for them (Nagoshi, 2001).

Recent literature suggests that nursing is beginning to incorporate similar SP modalities in formative and summative evaluation processes. The Bart's Nursing OSCE (Nicol & Freeth, 1998) was developed in response to the changing nature of clinical placements, changing length of stays, and expanding work assignments and was designed as a formative tool to assess clinical skills through the observation of simulated practice in the realistic setting of a skills center. The Student Clinical Performance Scale was developed to standardize faculty assessment of videotaped SP encounters (Miller, Wilbur, Montgomery, & Talashek, 1998).

The Clinical Competency Evaluation (CCE) provides another performance feedback mechanism to nurse practitioner students and identifies benchmarks to validate student advancement (Stroud, Smith, Edlund, & Erkel, 1999). Interaction with SPs provides customized and immediate clinical learning for graduate nursing students (O'Connor, Albert, & Thomas, 1999). Gibbons et al. (2002) demonstrated that summative and formative uses of the SP pedagogical model have benefits that traditional methods of education and evaluation lacked.

In the mid-1990s, the faculty members of the Department of Family Medicine at the University of California, Irvine, College of Medicine Family Nurse Practitioner (UCICOMFNP) program were asked to be observers in OSCEs for third-year medical students and family medicine residents. After experiencing the richness of the OSCE and the incorporated tenets of the Context,

(case study continues on page 290)

Input, Process, and Product (CIPP) (Stufflebeam, 2000) model of evaluation, the faculty members were interested in improving their program for students and in assessing the application of classroom learning in a simulated clinical environment.

Believing that the most important purpose of evaluation is not to prove but to improve, faculty members determined that they would pilot an OSCE for the students enrolled in the program as a formative evaluation process. They also felt these assessments would augment the student's clinical evaluations by their preceptors and faculty evaluations during clinical site visits when students are observed in various patient encounters. The following describes the program's experience in utilizing both the OSCE and CPX as evaluation tools.

UCICOMFNP Program Description

The UCICOMFNP program is located in Southern California in a suburban setting, rich in ethnic and cultural diversity. It has a dual track curriculum with a rigorous 13-month postmaster's certificate program and a specially defined six-semester track in which graduate students from California State University, Fullerton, obtain core specialty courses. All students receive a certificate of completion from UCICOM after they meet all program requirements. In addition to classroom instruction, all students rotate through a variety of clinical settings, including university-based clinics, community clinics, managed care organizations, and private practice sites.

All FNP faculty members in the program have active clinical practices, and all students are required to successfully complete one clinical rotation with UCICOMFNP faculty. The UCICOMFNP program has access to a premier "state-of-the-art" student-training center. The center was developed to teach and assess the clinical skills of medical students, residents, MDs, and other health care professionals in an environment that simulates an actual clinical setting. Participants are monitored and videotaped as they interact with SPs or actual patients to evaluate their clinical performance and competency related to obtaining a medical history, conducting an appropriate physical examination, counseling, and developing treatment management plans. The center has a well-developed SP program and personnel to train SPs and support faculty in teaching, assessment, and research activities. FNP students also have access to "Harvey," a computerized cardiology-training simulator, a revolutionary teaching tool capable of simulating 98% of the pathology seen in cardiovascular disease. The UCICOMFNP faculty members use the student-training center in the clinical instruction and assessment of FNP students.

Formative Evaluation: OSCE and OSCE Administration

An OSCE consists of a six- to eight-station examination, which utilizes SPs and is designed to assess a specific clinical skill or competency. UCICOMFNP's OSCE is conducted in the student-training center. At the beginning of each academic year, faculty members plan a date to administer the OSCE. This date is partially determined by the completion of approximately 300 hours of clinical rotations by most students. Another determinant is the availability of faculty members to participate in the event, because it is critical that they observe the students to give formative feedback. Three months prior to the scheduled OSCE, faculty members select cases they want presented in the exam. The cases selected are, for the most part, reflective of what the students have learned to date in terms of

(continued)

physical exam, interviewing, information sharing, and beginning differential diagnostic skills. The case presentations can be acute or chronic, or they can require a great deal of information sharing, such as diabetes or smoking cessation. The goal is to have cases that most often present in primary ambulatory care. The cases and supporting exam materials, such as performance checklists, are selected from an established case bank in the College of Medicine.

The checklists, which are developed by the case author(s), are instruments that have a relatively high degree of interrater reliability among faculty and SPs. SPs and/or instructors that record the student's performance during each station complete these checklists. The checklist items are scored as "done" or "not done." Some checklists with physical exam items may indicate a third category, which would be that the student attempted to perform the maneuver but did it "incorrectly." Faculty members review and modify the case checklists, if necessary, prior to each exam to ensure that they are reflective of FNP practice standards and guidelines. Student training center personnel recruit, train, and schedule the SPs for the event and are responsible for setting up and taking the exam down. All the SPs receive between 4 and 6 hours of training and are paid for training and performance time.

On the day of the exam, students come to the student-training center and receive an orientation by a member of the FNP faculty covering what to expect and addressing student's questions or concerns. Student-training center staff members proctor and time the OSCE. During the OSCE, faculty observes student performance from the monitoring room, which has video technology and is located in the student-training center. All student encounters are videotaped. At each station, during the SP encounter, the student has a primary task to accomplish. The student may be asked to perform a focused physical exam, obtain a history, counsel the patient, or complete any combination of these tasks. Specifically, instructors assess history-taking skills from the perspective of organization, quality, and interpersonal communication. When observing physical exam skills they evaluate technique, completeness, and organization. When the case presentation requires a great deal of information sharing, the faculty members observe whether appropriate information is provided, ease and clarity of communication, interpersonal skills, the ability to recognize "red flags," and the need for physician collaboration and/or referral.

All assessments are timed and each encounter lasts 10 minutes. Students then receive 5 minutes of SP and faculty feedback in the patient room. The SP is asked to give the student 1 minute of feedback related to communication skills, and then the faculty member who observed the encounter discusses the student's performance. SPs and faculty members are encouraged to give the student positive reinforcement for the skill or competency demonstrated and to give formative feedback on how the student could improve performance. Students are also asked for comments on any challenges they had in accomplishing the station objective(s). While the instructor is giving formative feedback, the SP completes a paper checklist to record the student's performance during the encounter. After the feedback session is completed, the student rotates to the next station and the process is repeated.

After the students complete four stations, they receive a 15-minute break and then continue in the exam. When the students have completed all the stations, they return to the student waiting room for a debriefing by faculty. At this time, no specific case content, checklist, or student performance is discussed. Faculty members discuss, in general terms, what they observed most students doing well and where some students need to focus further to develop practice competency. They also

(*case study continues on page 292*)

solicit the students' opinions on the value of the OSCE. Students always want to have more of these types of experiences because they value faculty input and they want to be sure they have the skills and knowledge to safely move forward in caring for their patients. Students are encouraged to set up a time to review their videotape with a member of the faculty and receive additional input about their performance. Students who do not do well in demonstrating baseline skills and competencies are required to meet with a faculty member, review their videotapes, and establish remediation plans to improve overall performance. Students are not given a grade for the OSCE, but faculty uses it to direct the students' learning and to give feedback to their respective clinical preceptor.

Summative Evaluation: CPX and CPX Administration

The Clinical Practice Exam (CPX) is a clinical practice exam that also utilizes SPs in a summative assessment of the student's skills, knowledge, and patient management of various case presentations. Most CPX exams are six to 10 stations in length, and the cases for this exam are complex and frequently measure more than one competency. This exam is usually administered in the last month of the program. Midway through the academic year, faculty begins to select case presentations from the CPX case bank that exists in the College of Medicine. These cases have been used in medical education over multiple sites and are fine-tuned each year before they are selected to be part of an exam. Item analysis has been completed on each checklist item and has an extremely high level of interrater reliability.

For this exam, faculty members select cases that will measure multiple competencies over several encounters with a mix of acute and chronic case presentations. Checklists are not modified for this exam, so it is critical that faculty members select cases that are frequently seen in their practices and that the checklists measure FNP competencies. Fewer FNP faculty members are required to participate in this exam because students do not receive feedback. Faculty presence offers students some consolation if they are feeling anxious. However, once a student completed a previous OSCE he or she feels more comfortable in taking the CPX exam. Most students experience some test anxiety because of the high-stakes nature of this exam. Students must pass this exam to receive a certificate of completion from the program and understand if they do extremely poorly, they will have to repeat the exam the following academic year.

SPs who participate in this exam receive between 10 and 14 hours of training to ensure they are calibrated at an extremely high level in terms of performance and checklist accuracy. SPs record the student's performance, either online or using a paper checklist, as "done," "not done," or "done incorrectly." They also complete a Patient/Physician Interaction rating form (PPI). This is a six-point Likert-type rating form that specifically rates the student's interpersonal communication skills with an area for the SP to write comments regarding the encounter with the student. Like the OSCE, the student-training center provides all the pre- and postexam support.

On the day of the exam, the students come to the student-training center and receive a standardized formal orientation to ensure that all students have the same information when taking the exam. The student-training center exam coordinator presents the orientation. Faculty may or may not be present for the orientation. Like the OSCE, the exam is timed (15 minutes per encounter), proctored, and videotaped. However, in the CPX, the students do not get feedback at each station but are

(continued)

required to complete a 7-minute postencounter exercise after each station. For the most part, these exercises relate to management of the patient they just saw. These exercises may be online or on paper. The exam is usually six to eight stations in length, so both students and SPs get a 15-minute break after four encounters. The faculty that is present for the exam observes student performance in the monitoring room. The instructors are particularly interested in observing any student who may have been in a remedial program because of poor performance during the OSCE, who is having some difficulty with a clinical rotation, or who is marginal in overall performance in the program. After students complete the exam, they are debriefed by a member of the faculty and again, case content or checklists are discussed. The cases and checklists are considered confidential test material. Like the debriefing session after the OSCE, faculty reassure students that they did well or if they did not do well, that they will meet with them to assist them to develop a plan to remediate before completing the program.

Support staff in medical education and/or faculty calculates the exam score. Students receive a pass or fail grade. Failure is defined as two standard deviations below the mean for the exam. To date, two students have failed this exam, and this exam proved to be the evaluation tool that reaffirmed all other assessments of these students in the program. It is difficult for the students to challenge the fairness of the evaluation because it is extremely objective and there is a video recording of their performance. The students can challenge other types of evaluations by saying they are very subjective, and everyone understands that this can be true in some situations.

Conclusions

UCICOMFNP faculty values the OSCE and the CPX as critical components of the evaluation process of the student and the program. They recognize that the OSCE is an invaluable formative evaluation tool to assess individual student progress and that the CPX is likewise valuable as a summative tool. The OSCE helped faculty to counsel students and guide their individual learning. The CPX performance helped faculty to focus on curriculum needs, which resulted in program enhancements. For example, in the first year of the program, several students had difficulty performing appropriate orthopedic exams of the shoulder and knee to assess for injury. At subsequent curriculum committee meetings, the course content on orthopedic exams was expanded. The following year the majority of the students performed the shoulder and knee exams appropriately.

The CPX, as a summative evaluation, is another method to identify the degree to which programmatic outcomes are achieved. At present, the UCICOMFNP program has both the OSCE and the CPX as mandatory components of the program and will continue these assessments with the expectation that students pass the CPX prior to completion of the program. As UCICOMFNP faculty continues to move into the future, the domains and core competencies, as defined by the National Organization of Nurse Practitioner Faculties (NONPF) in partnership with the American Association of Colleges of Nursing (AACN) in 2002, will guide case selection and checklist modification to ensure that these exams continue to be rich, formative, and summative evaluation processes (U.S Department of Health and Human Services Administration, 2002). The ultimate goal of the program is to ensure that graduates of the program achieve core competencies for safe practice as entry level FNPs and achieve national certification. To date, these goals have been achieved.

DISCUSSION QUESTIONS

1. Explain how a nursing education program could utilize its evaluation plan to demonstrate total quality management for nursing students or staff. To what extent is the educational evaluation plan similar to or different from total quality management in the practice setting?
2. To what extent could the simulated/standardized patient assessment format be applied to other clinical performance situations in nursing education? Give the pros and cons for its use for each situation.

SUGGESTED LEARNING ACTIVITIES

Student Activities

1. Select a curriculum evaluation model and identify how you would implement that model in a nursing curriculum. The curriculum you are interested in evaluating could be a nursing program or a portion of the curriculum.
2. Based on your knowledge of curriculum evaluation models, develop an evaluation model to evaluate a curriculum you choose. Specify how you would use the model.
3. Prepare a poster presentation on the use of a curriculum evaluation model. The poster should include a description of the model, a list of references and resources related to the model, the evaluation components to consider, and the expected outcomes from using the model.

Faculty Activities

1. Analyze your current evaluation plan for your program and curriculum for its components and emphasis on outcomes or processes. What model of evaluation is utilized, and how does it fit the program's mission, philosophy, goals, and objectives?
2. Compare the CIPP and Baldrige curriculum models by addressing the strengths and weaknesses of each. Apply them to your current evaluation plan and discuss how they apply or don't apply to your program and curriculum.

REFERENCES

Baldrige National Quality Program. (2000). *Criteria for performance excellence.* Malcolm Baldrige National Quality Award.

Barrows, H. S. (1987). *Simulated (standardized) patients and other human simulations: A comprehensive guide to their training and use in teaching and evaluation.* Chapel Hill, NC: Health Sciences Consortium.

Colliver, J. A., & Williams, R. G. (1993). Technical issues: Test application. *Academic Medicine, 68*(6), 454–460.

Gibbons, S., Adamo, G., Padden, D., Ricciardi, R., Graziano, M., Levine, E., et al. (2002). Clinical evaluation in advanced practice nursing education: Using standardized patients in health assessment. *Journal of Nursing Education, 41*(5), 215–221.

Harden, R. M., Crosby, J.R., & Davis, M. H. (1999). Outcome-based education: Part I—An introduction to outcome-based education. *AMEE Guide, 14*(Part I), 7–14.

Karlowicz, K. A. (2000). The value of student portfolios to evaluate undergraduate nursing programs. *Nursing Educator, 25*(2), 82–87.

Klass, D., Fletcher, E., King, A., Durinze, Nungster, R. J., Clauser, B., et al. (1992). Developing a standard patient test of clinical skills at the National Board of Medical Examiners. In: Harden, R.M., Hart, I.R., Mulholland, M., (eds). *Approaches to the assessment of clinical competence. Part 1.* Proceedings of the Fifth Ottawa International Conference, Centre for Medical Education, University of Dundee. Dundee, Scotland 1002: 58–70.

Lindeman, C. (2000). The future of nursing education. *Journal of Nursing Education, 39*(1), 5–12.

Miller, A. M., Wilbur, J., Montgomery, A. C., & Talashek, M. L. (1998). Standardizing faculty evaluation of nurse practitioner students by simulated patients. *Clinical Excellence Nurse Practitioner, 2*(2), 102–109.

Nagoshi, M. H. (2001). Role of standardized patients in medical education. *Hawaii Medical Journal, 6*(12), 323–324.

Nicol, M., & Freeth, D. (1998). Assessment of clinical skills: A new approach to an old problem. Nurse Education Today, 18(8), 601–609.

O'Connor, F. W., Albert, M. L., & Thomas, M. D. (1999). Incorporating standardized patients into a Psychosocial nurse practitioner program. *Archive Psychiatric Nursing, 13*(5), 240–247.

Prislin, M., Giglio, M., Lewis, E. M., Ahearn, S., & Radecki, S. (2000). Assessing the acquisition of core clinical skills through the use of serial standardized patient assessments. *Academic Medicine, 75*(5), 480–483.

Reznick, R., Blackmore, D., & Cohen, R. (1993). An objective structured clinical examination for the licentiate of the medical council of Canada: From research to reality. *Academic Medicine, 68*(Suppl. 10). S4–S6.

Samuel Merritt College. (1999). *The California governor's quality award program.* Application and WASC accreditation supplement, Oakland, CA.

Stroud, S. D., Smith, C. A., Edlund, B. J., & Erkel, E. A. (1999). Evaluating clinical decision-making skills of nurse practitioner students. *Clinical Excellence Nurse Practitioner, 3*(4), 230–237.

Stufflebeam, D. (1971). The relevance of the CIPP evaluation model for educational accountability. *Journal of Research and Development in Education, 5*(1), 1925.

Stufflebeam, D. (1983). The CIPP model for program evaluation. In G. Madaus, M. Scriven, & D. Stufflebeam, (Eds.), *Evaluation models: Viewpoints on educational and human services evaluation.* Boston: Kluwer-Nijhoff Publishing.

Stufflebeam, D. E. (2000). The CIPP model for evaluation. In D. L. Stufflebeam, G. F. Madaus, & T. Kellaghan. (Eds.), *Evaluation models: Viewpoints on education and human services evaluation* (2nd ed.). Boston: Kluwer Academic Publishers.

Swanson, D. B., Norman, G. R., & Linn, R. L. (1995). Performance-based assessment: Lessons learned from the health professions. *Educational Researcher, 24*(5), 5–35.

Tyler, R. W. (1942) General statement on evaluation. *Journal of Educational Research.* (35), 492–501.

U.S. Medical Licensing Examination. (2004). Home page. Retrieved June 10, 2004, from http://www.usmle.org

U. S. Department of Health and Human Services Administration. (2002). *Nurse practitioner primary care competencies in specialty areas: Adult, family, gerontological, pediatric, and women's health.* Washington, DC: Author.

Van der Vleuten, C. P. M., & Swanson, D. B. (1990). Assessment of clinical skills with standardized patients: State of the art. *Teaching and Learning in Medicine, 2,* 58–76, Mahwah, NJ. Lawrence Erlbaum Associates Publishing.

Vu, N. V., & Barrows, H. S. (1994). Use of standardized patients in clinical assessments: Recent developments and measurement findings. *Educational Researcher, 23,* 30.

Planning for Accreditation: Evaluating the Curriculum

Abby M. Heydman, PhD, RN

OBJECTIVES

Upon conclusion of Chapter 12, the reader will be able to:

1. Analyze the various forms of accreditation and typical accreditation processes that are used to indicate that a program meets specific standards and criteria.
2. Outline a plan for accreditation, developing a timeline, and providing for involvement of faculty, students, and other stakeholders in the self-study and site visit.
3. Apply principles of continuous quality improvement to accreditation activities.
4. Evaluate current issues in accreditation within higher education, particularly those related to the impact of technology and the development of a global marketplace in higher education.

12

▲ OVERVIEW

Accreditation is a process that educational programs and curricula undergo to receive recognition for meeting basis standards or criteria set by national, regional, or state organizations. Programs undergo accreditation to demonstrate their quality to the consumers of their products (students, alumni, and employers). Because programs such as nursing prepare students for the practice of a profession, which involves activities that have a direct impact on public health and safety, there are more rigorous standards and numerous types of accreditation reviews than for other academic programs. For this reason, it is important for faculty and program directors to have a broad understanding of accreditation and the various processes of quality improvement that are embraced by these processes.

Accreditation and certification of educational programs are important to the programs to gain legal status for offering the program and to validate the quality of the program. This chapter explores the world of accreditation and the external requirements that must be satisfied for a nursing program to operate successfully in the context of the state or province in which it exists, within its region, and within the larger boundaries of the country. This chapter also explores trends and issues in accreditation affecting nursing programs and the trend toward globalization of accreditation.

▲ NATIONAL ACCREDITING BODIES

The United States is distinctive in that historically, its accreditation efforts have been managed by private, voluntary organizations formed by peer institutions for the purpose of judging quality and setting standards to guide educational practice. Although the federal and state governments play a role, particularly relating to eligibility for federal or state financial aid, the private regional accrediting associations are key agencies in the accreditation of colleges, universities, and technical schools. There is no similar system of voluntary regional accreditation in any other country (Eaton, 2002). In Canada, as is generally true in the international community, institutions are granted the right to operate within their respective province according to statutes established by provincial legislatures. The provincial Minister of Education approves the mandate of each institution and the provincial Department of Education approves academic programs (Ministry of Education Ontario, 2004).

Although the structure of accreditation may differ from country to country, colleges and nursing education programs are generally required to be accredited or approved by regulatory bodies within the country, state, or province in which they operate. Other forms of accreditation, even regional accreditation in the United States, are voluntary; that is, the institution or nursing program may choose to seek accreditation to demonstrate that it has a particular commitment to meeting high standards. Some would argue that it is a euphemism to say that regional accreditation and specialized accreditation are voluntary today, because eligibility for student financial aid is tied to these approvals, but technically, most forms of accreditation remain voluntary in the United States.

Depending on their purposes, accreditation agencies evaluate institutions or specialized units within an institution. Thus, colleges or universities have institutional accreditation, and programs, departments, or schools within larger institutions have specialized accreditation.

A few specialized accreditation agencies accredit single-purpose institutions of higher education. (Single-purpose institutions are those schools with only one major or program of study.) Over the years, as the number of students enrolled in postsecondary institutions has increased dramatically, and as higher education received increased funding both for direct operations and for student financial aid, accreditation requirements and expectations for accountability have increased (Council for Higher Education Accreditation, 2002c).

Role of the U.S. Department of Education

Unlike many other countries, the United States does not have a central ministry of education that controls postsecondary institutions of higher education. Although the states assume a role in the approval and control of colleges and universities, these processes and regulations vary widely among them. Thus, American colleges and universities operate with a great deal of autonomy and independence (Eaton, 2002). A distinctive feature of American higher education, and one that may be considered both a strength and a weakness, is the diversity in types and kinds of institutions operating with variation in quality and reputation.

The U.S. Department of Education's (USDE) primary role is to ensure that federal student-aid funds are used to provide access for students enrolling in academic programs and courses of high quality (Glazer, 1997). The USDE's recognition process uses 10 standards that address recruitment and admission practices, fiscal and administrative capacity and facilities, curricula, faculty, student support programs, records of student complaints, and success in student achievement. Only those colleges and universities accredited by an USDE-recognized accrediting agency are eligible to receive federal financial aid for students. Accrediting agencies are periodically reviewed by the USDE or a private organization, the Council for Higher Education Accreditation (CHEA). The recognition process for institutional and specialized accrediting agencies is a part of the federal regulatory mandate (CHEA, 2002c).

The Council for Higher Education Accreditation

CHEA was formed in 1996 as a private, nonprofit, national organization designed to coordinate accreditation activities in the United States. CHEA accomplishes its purposes by providing formal recognition of regional, national, and specialized higher accreditation bodies. Various types of accreditation agencies have been developed to oversee the quality of the more than 6,500 degree- and nondegree-granting postsecondary institutions in the United States. For an accreditation agency to be recognized by CHEA, more than 50% of the institution's programs reviewed by the agency must be degree granting. The USDE and CHEA recognize many of the same accrediting organizations (Eaton, 2002).

▲ PURPOSES OF ACCREDITATION

The primary purpose of accreditation is to ensure that at least minimum standards of quality are met. Most voluntary accreditation agencies state that they aim to achieve higher-than-minimum standards as determined by peers in the field. A second purpose of accreditation is to provide recognition for funding and student financial aid. A third purpose for accreditation is to ensure consistency in quality across academic programs, thus facilitating transfer of academic credit from one institution to another and the acknowledgement of the comparability of one degree to another in the same field across institutions. Accreditation, licensure, and certification are the various means used to regulate the professions (Barnum, 1997).

In the United States, where voluntary accreditation is the norm, accreditation is distinguished by an emphasis on both self-regulation and peer evaluation. In this environment, accreditation processes tend to be both formative and summative, seeking continuous improvement rather than being oriented only to compliance. The establishment of accreditation standards requires institutions or programs to develop evaluation plans and to write comprehensive self-studies, which ensure self-regulation. These activities facilitate assessment and reflection on findings. Peer evaluation is also a core value in voluntary accreditation. Peers work collaboratively to set standards, assist staff with the conduct of site visits, and serve on review panels and appeal panels (Young, and others 1983).

In recent years, there has been some dissatisfaction with traditional accreditation processes and practices. Concern has been raised about whether quality is really ensured by the current process of voluntary accreditation in the United States. Some congressional leaders and educators have recommended that eligibility to award financial aid should be separated from regional or professional accreditation (Guerard, 2002; Morgan, 2002). Increasingly, institutions of higher education are asked to demonstrate to the USDE (through regulations imposed on regional and professional accreditation agencies) that they are tracking trends in key performance indicators, such as student graduation rates, graduates' loan default rates, and postgraduation employment (Bacon, 2003).

A major issue is the question of accrediting agencies keeping their standards and criteria up to date. With the expansion of technology-driven distance education programs and rapid changes in the health care system, it becomes difficult to make changes in the curriculum in response to the changes and at the same time ensure that the program continues to meet program approval standards and accreditation criteria. Many state boards of nursing and accreditation agencies require notification of any major (or even minor) changes in the existing program. While this ensures quality and maintenance of approval or accreditation, it can hamper creativity and a speedy response to external changes and demands on the program.

The advantage of notifying the program approval and accreditation agencies of pending changes is the preservation of quality; the disadvantage is a lowered motivation for creating change. In these cases, the wise strategy is to consult with the agencies when the idea for change begins to form and to continue the consultation throughout the planning stages so that the appropriate paperwork and visits, if necessary, are ready for timely approval processes. In addition, educators have a responsibility to participate in accreditation processes, including review of standards and criteria, becoming site visitors, and becoming members on review boards and committees of the agencies. These kinds of activities contribute to faculty's professional development and the ability of the approval and accrediting agencies to keep abreast of changes occurring in education and the profession that call for modifications of standards and criteria.

▲ PROS AND CONS OF ACCREDITATION

Faculty will undoubtedly engage in discussions about the pros and cons of accreditation, such discussions being particularly common when in the midst of a self-study or a site visit.

Accreditation certainly looms larger as a factor in faculty and staff workload than was the case some decades ago when accreditation was in its infancy. It should be remembered, however, that accreditation came about not just because of the public demand for accountability and quality, but because peers felt a responsibility to work collaboratively to establish standards that would guide their practice.

Perhaps the biggest complaint about accreditation is its cost. Staff and faculty time involved in planning for either institutional or specialized accreditation is significant and costly. Often institutions or programs must postpone major initiatives while they are working on a major accreditation review. This highlights the "opportunity cost" that may be attendant to accreditation. In a time where resources are perceived to be scarce, institutions and programs sometimes feel these resources should be used for more important activities or initiatives (O'Neil, 1997). The base prices for nursing program accreditation for 2003 and 2005 for both the Commission on Collegiate Nursing Education (CCNE) and the National League for Nursing Accrediting Commission (NLNAC) are listed in Table 12.1 (CCNE, 2004; NLNAC, 2004). These base prices do not include the costs for printing the report, postage, and the preparation of display rooms and resources for the site visitors.

While preparing the self-study report takes place over a year and the site visit is usually limited to 3 or 4 days with three or four visitors, the ongoing costs of an annual fee to maintain accreditation must be placed into the operating budget each year. Additional future

▲TABLE 12.1   2004 Fee Structure for Accreditation

Fee	CCNE		NLNAC	
	BSN *or* MSN	BSN *and* MSN	NLN Member	NLN Nonmember
New applicant fee/ Membership fee	$3,500	$5,500	0-50 graduates $850 51-100 graduates $1,050 101 and over $1,250	
Annual accreditation fee	$1,700	$2,100	$1,560 for one program and $560 per additional program	$2810 for one program and $560 per additional program
Process application initial fee			$1,000	$1,500
Process application continuing fee			$1,000	$1,000
Site visit/evaluator	$1,400		$835	

Sources: CCNE (2004); NLNAC (2004).

funds must be planned for preparing for accreditation renewal every 5 (new programs) to 8 or 10 years (continuing accreditation). If recommendations for an interim report to remedy noncompliance or warnings are issued to programs, additional costs to respond to them must be budgeted. It should be noted that specialty accreditation for advanced practice programs is in addition to the total program accreditation costs.

Table 12.1, which highlights the fee structure for the two major nursing education accreditation agencies, reveals that there are no adjustments in fees for smaller colleges, state-supported universities, or private colleges who may not have the resources to pay for accreditation. Thus, it becomes apparent that educational institutions, the profession, accrediting agencies, and even the USDE on the federal level need to address the cost issues related to accreditation. Strategies for cost savings should be explored for the benefit of the educational institutions and their stakeholders without compromising quality.

Duplication of effort with overlapping requirements in regional and specialized accreditation is yet another frequent complaint of current accreditation systems (The Center for Health Professions, University of California, San Franciso,1999). Ryan (2003) also raises a number of important issues and questions regarding accreditation practices, particularly the challenge of keeping faculty abreast of needed change and best practices. Accreditation is sometimes charged with being inflexible, being parochial, failing to take institutional diversity into account, stifling innovation, and being too focused on inputs. Some critics have expressed the viewpoint that accreditation standards do not ensure quality (Morgan, 2002).

The use of technology in higher education and the overt development of higher education as a market commodity have also created new issues and criticism surrounding accreditation. Technology permits institutions to offer programs outside of their traditional state, provincial, or regional boundaries. More institutions are offering programs through distance-learning strategies that provide global student access to degree programs. Thus, questions arise about which agency has jurisdiction in accreditation of these out-of-region programs (Council for Higher Education Accreditation, 2002a). The entry of for-profit colleges and universities into the realm of higher education brought attention to the vast financial and economic enterprise of higher education. Consider the case of the University of Phoenix (UOP), the largest independent college in the United States. UOP enrolls approximately 125,000 students in 38 campuses in 25 states, British Columbia, and Puerto Rico. Almost 45,000 of its students are enrolled in programs that are offered totally online (Morgan, 2002).

▲ CONTINUOUS QUALITY IMPROVEMENT

In recent years, concerns about the deficiencies in accreditation and the very episodic nature of accreditation led to consideration of alternative evaluation methods for educational programs. Higher education has begun to adopt concepts and processes of continuous quality improvement (CQI) from the corporate world in its evaluation systems. CQI calls on institutions or programs to identify customers clearly. Customers include students, alumni, clinical agencies, the profession, and consumers. Establishing key requirements for satisfaction of these stakeholders is an important step in the CQI process. Typically, evaluation strategies in

CQI include evaluating satisfaction of students and other customers, as well as establishing whether key requirements have been met (i.e., benchmarks for graduates' performance and learning outcomes). Cross-functional teams (staff and faculty) work to assess whether systems are optimal to produce best practices and results. A major advantage in the CQI process is that it is a continuous activity in which organizational data are evaluated regularly to target results needing improvement. Key performance indicators are established to provide a set of metrics that a program can monitor on a regular basis.

Regional and specialized accreditation standards and practices are incorporating concepts from CQI. As more and more clinical agencies adopt CQI processes, some faculty members have begun to recommend that CQI concepts and clinical experiences be incorporated into the curriculum (Volger and Ratcliffe, 1993; Taylor, 2001; Grant, Kelley, Northington, and Barlow, 2002). Collins (1997) makes a strong statement on the importance of ongoing program evaluation in preparation for accreditation:

> "Accreditation is needed. However, accreditation must become an integral part of the daily functioning of the program or school, not an episodic event. It is justifiable use of resources when it leads to overall continuous program improvement. By incorporating quality standards of nursing education into ongoing activities, a seamless, continuous development of the program or school exists" (p. 6).

▲ THE GLOBAL ENVIRONMENT

Developments in recent years have highlighted the growing competition for the international market of higher education, as evidenced by universities offering high-demand programs around the world. Increasingly, higher education is becoming a "commodity" with value added because of the opportunities presented to those who receive credentials through higher education. These developments lead many to believe that current accreditation structures are antiquated and inadequate for dealing with new realities of the global marketplace for higher education (Van Damme, 2002).

▲ POLITICAL REALITIES

A key question being asked today is whether all the money being spent on higher education is really worth the investment. Would this funding be better spent on health care, housing, or other pressing social needs? The accountability question is driving the federal appetite to become more directly involved in accreditation in the United States, particularly as it relates to an institution's eligibility to handle student financial aid awards. With the up-and-coming renewal of the Higher Education Act in 2003–2004, this debate is likely to become even more intense. As a result, regional and specialized accreditation agencies feel a sense of urgency about demonstrating that voluntary accreditation processes are effective. Regional accreditation agencies are responding to this threat with a number of new initiatives that focus on evidence of quality (Gose, 2002).

▲ ORGANIZATIONAL OVERVIEW OF THE STRUCTURE OF ACCREDITATION

As noted earlier in this chapter, legitimate accrediting agencies in the United States must be recognized by the USDE or CHEA. There are two major types of accreditation bodies: institutional and specialized. Institutional accreditation agencies include six regional associations and their separate commissions that accredit senior colleges, community (junior) colleges, technical schools, and secondary (high) schools. A regional accreditation agency in the United States is a voluntary organization comprised of member schools from a defined geographic region of the country. These include:

1. Middle States Association of Colleges and Schools
    Commission on Higher Education
2. New England Association of Schools and Colleges
    Commission on Institutions of Higher Education
    Commission on Technical and Career Institutions
3. North Central Association of Colleges and Schools
    Commission on Institutions of Higher Education
    Executive Board of the Commission on Schools
4. Northwest Association of Schools and Colleges
    Commission on Colleges
5. Southwest Association of Colleges and Schools
    Commission on Colleges
6. Western Association of Schools and Colleges
    Accrediting Commission for Community and Junior Colleges
    Accrediting Commission for Schools
    Accrediting Commission for Senior Colleges and Universities
                                                                (Burke, 2002)

Regional accreditation agencies offer institutional accreditation following a comprehensive review of the mission and goals, infrastructure, resources, and evidence of educational effectiveness of the institution seeking accreditation. A regional accreditation body in the United States usually accredits degree-granting institutions of postsecondary education. Some single-purpose professional schools and proprietary and/or technical schools are accredited by various national agencies that provide institutional accreditation. Nonetheless, regional accreditation is generally held to be the standard required to ensure transferability of academic credit from one postsecondary institution of higher education to another in the United States.

▲ INTERNATIONAL ACCREDITATION

In many countries, a centralized Ministry of Education governs postsecondary education, including quality standards and quality assurance. In Canada, the Constitution Act provides authority to each province to make laws and statues governing education, including higher education. Each of the provinces typically has its own Minister of Education or a comparable official who is charged with the oversight of universities and degree programs within the province. Institutions may not operate without the approval of the provincial Ministry or some other authority, such as an agency founded to accredit independent colleges or universities. An example of this type of agency is the Private Colleges Accreditation Board in Alberta, to which the provincial government has delegated accreditation authority (Ministry of Education Ontario, 2003).

Accrediting agencies in the United States are also involved in international accreditation. In many cases, this involves U.S. programs that are being offered overseas, but in some cases, agencies actually accredit programs from other countries upon request (Council for Higher Education Accreditation, 2002b).

The Commission on Graduates of Foreign Nursing Schools

The Commission on Graduates of Foreign Nursing Schools (CGFNS) is not an accreditation agency per se. However, this independent, nonprofit organization plays a key role in the certification of nursing credentials of nurses migrating into the United States. Faced with a growing rate of migration and the significant complexity in evaluating the educational preparation of nurses educated in foreign countries, a number of national and state nursing and professional associations held a conference in 1975 to address the problem of foreign nurse credentials. CGFNS was formed as an outgrowth of this conference and today, the organization operates to ensure that nurses educated in countries other than the United States are eligible and qualified to meet state licensure requirements. Eighty-five percent of state boards of nursing require foreign nurses to be screened through the CGFNS process. CGFNS offers a certification program in which a nurse must meet three requirements to be considered for licensure: a credentials review, successful passing of a standardized examination, and an English language proficiency examination. Nurses eligible for this program include those who are graduates of first-level general nursing education programs as defined by the International Council of Nurses. General nursing education includes didactic and clinical instruction across a broad spectrum of nursing practice (Commission on Graduates of Foreign Schools of Nursing, 1999).

Accreditation of Schools of Nursing in Canada

Specialized accreditation for nursing in Canada is under the auspices of the Canadian Association of Schools of Nursing (CASN). Schools of nursing meet the standards of practice that are set by the governing colleges of nurses through the College of Nurses of Ontario (CNO). These standards of practice are incorporated into the schools' outcomes as deemed by the Canadian Association of Schools of Nursing (CASN). The CASN Board on Accreditation is authorized to review and approve policies. It makes decisions on candidacy and accreditation reviews within established policies and procedures. CASN accreditation is conducted according to guiding principles of the Association of Accrediting Agencies of Canada (AAAC), of which it is a founding member. Accreditation policies were last revised in September 2002 and are available online at http://www.causn.org (Canadian Association of Schools of Nursing, 2004).

▲SPECIALIZED ACCREDITING AGENCIES

From 1952 to 1998, the National League for Nursing (NLN) was the only professional accrediting agency for nursing. The NLN operated its accreditation functions through four councils that established criteria for programs at various levels (vocational, diploma, associate, and baccalaureate and higher degree). In 1998, however, the American Association of Colleges of Nursing announced its intention to establish its own accreditation body, the Commission on Collegiate Nursing Education (CCNE), which would accredit baccalaureate and higher degree programs. An early study indicated that a significant number of baccalaureate and higher degree programs planned to seek CCNE accreditation or obtain approval by both agencies. At the time, the NLN was having difficulty with meeting new standards established by the USDE for accrediting agencies. Subsequently, the NLN reorganized its accreditation structures, founding the independent National League for Nursing Accrediting Commission (Bellack, O'Neil, & Thomsen, 1999).

Both the NLNAC and CCNE are accredited at the present time by CHEA and approved by the DOE. It is important to note that only those programs whose institutions are not part of a regionally accredited college or university may use NLNAC accreditation to establish eligibility for federal student financial aid assistance. NLNAC accredits LPN/LVN, diploma, associate degree, and baccalaureate and higher degree nursing programs. CCNE accredits only baccalaureate and higher degree programs. Overbay and Aaltonen (2001) have provided an interesting comparison of NLNAC and CCNE accreditation criteria and commissions for those considering which agency to choose for accreditation. See Table 12.2 for a comparison of NLNAC and CCNE.

▲ TABLE 12.2	National Nursing Accreditation Agencies in the United States			
Agency Name	**Type of Program Accredited**	**Year Accreditation of Schools Initiated**	**Approved by Department of Education****	**Approved by CHEA****
National League for Nursing Accreditation Agency	Vocational, Diploma, Associate Degree, Baccalaureate and Higher Degree	1998*	2002	2000
Commission on Collegiate Nursing Education	Baccalaureate and Higher Degree	2000	2001	

*The National League for Nursing originally engaged in accreditation in 1952. The independent NLNAC was established in 1998.
**Notes most recent approval

| ▲ TABLE 12.3 | Specialized Nursing Accreditation Agencies in the United States |

Agency Name	Type of Program Accredited	Year Established	Number of Programs Accredited	Year Last Approved by the Department of Education CHEA
Council on Accreditation of Nurse Anesthesia Educational Programs (AANA)*	Nurse anesthesia educational programs at the certificate, master's, and doctoral degree levels	1952	87	2002
Division of Accreditation American College of Nurse Midwives (ACNM)**	Precertification, basic certificate, and master's degree nurse-midwifery educational programs	1982	44	2001
Council on Accreditation National Association of Nurse Practitioners in Women's Health***	Women's health nurse practitioner programs	1982	5	2002

*American Association of Nurse Anesthetists (2004).
** American College of Nurse Midwives (2004).
*** National Association of Nurse Practitioners in Women's Health (2004).

There are a number of additional specialized nursing accreditation agencies for advanced-practice nursing programs. These include the Nurse Anesthesia, Midwifery, and Nurse Practitioners in Women's Health. Additional information on these agencies is provided in Table 12.3.

▲ THE ACCREDITATION PROCESS

According to CHEA (2002c), the accreditation process typically involves five major elements: institutional self-study, peer review, site visit, action by the accrediting association, and monitoring and oversight. The self-study is a self-analysis of performance completed by the school based on the standards of the accrediting association. Peer review occurs because of the broad involvement of the various stakeholders in the educational environment (i.e., faculty, administrators, key partners, and the public). Site visits are typically conducted to verify the results of the self-study and to provide additional clarification to the accrediting agency. The action of the accrediting agency occurs after the submission of the self-study and the site visit with consideration of the entire body of evidence by the review panel for the accrediting agency.

Programs or schools are normally reviewed in a cycle of 5 to 10 years, with monitoring and oversight occurring through the submission of annual reports by the schools and substantive change reports to the agency when major change occurs.

Curriculum Planning and Accreditation

Curriculum planning should take accreditation requirements and statements of essential competencies into account from the onset (AACN, 1998a, 1998b). A basic understanding of accreditation requirements enables faculty to develop a program that complies with the key requirements established by accreditation agencies. Although such agencies generally attempt to avoid being overly prescriptive, there may be specific criteria or standards that must be met by a program to be approved. Accreditation standards for professional programs, for example, will often outline a minimum set of academic and clinical requirements that must be included in the program. Thus, the minimum number of credits for the entire professional component of the program may be prescribed, and even the minimum number of credits or hours of clinical practice within a specialized clinical area may be indicated. These requirements have been established by the accreditation agency or regulatory board based on broad input from the profession as well as other constituents, including public consumers. Among the many considerations in developing a new or revised curriculum are the standards and criteria established by those agencies that accredit the college or university, as well as those required by nursing accrediting bodies (CCNE, 1998; NLN, 2004).

The development of the organizing curriculum framework also warrants consideration of accreditation standards. Daggett, Butts, and Smith (2002) describe the development of an updated organizing framework by one faculty in its long-term preparation for accreditation. Seager and Anema (2003) and Heinrich, Karner, Gaglione, and Lambert (2002) describe the benefits of using a matrix or audit process to ensure curriculum integrity in preparation for accreditation and as a part of continuous improvement efforts.

Planning for Accreditation

DEVELOPING AN EVALUATION PLAN

The previous chapters provided guidance on the development of a school or program evaluation plan. It is a good idea to formulate this plan early on in order to begin collecting baseline data when students first begin a nursing program. Thompson and Bartels (1999) review the literature on assessment and describe one school's response to the development of a systematic plan for outcomes assessment. It is important that this plan focus on learning outcomes and not just program outputs. Ewell (2001) describes this shift in emphasis to learning outcomes in a CHEA publication on accreditation and student learning outcomes. Ingersoll and Sauter (1998) describe how accreditation criteria can be integrated effectively into the evaluation plan. Accreditation standards, criteria, procedures, and policies are readily available from the accrediting associations and their websites.

THEORETICAL FRAMEWORKS FOR EVALUATION

Several evaluation theories are available to provide a framework for the evaluation plan. The use of a theoretical approach helps provide an organizing lens for identification and analysis of data. Refer to theories described in the previous two chapters for guidance in this area.

DEVELOPING A TIMELINE

Accreditation is like any major project. The scope and size of the work can be overwhelming. A way to deal with this effectively is to break this task up into manageable bits that can be delegated and timed over a lengthy preparation period. Often the accrediting agency will provide some useful directions about possible key dates in a planning timeline. A sample timeline is also provided in Figure 12.1. These are just general guides, however, that must be modified based on the particular situation for each program or school. Preparation time may need to be extended if it must include faculty development for the director and/or faculty who do not have prior experience with the accreditation process.

ROLE OF ADMINISTRATORS, FACULTY, STUDENTS, AND CONSUMERS

Everyone has a role in the accreditation process. Administrators provide leadership and direction, supporting the efforts of the taskforce or faculty committee assigned to conduct the self-study. Faculty aids the work of the team by becoming familiar with the accreditation standards, providing timely information needed for the self-study, providing critical feedback on the draft of the report, and preparing to participate in the site visit. Students participate by learning about accreditation, cooperating with the site visitors during visits to classes and clinical sites, and by participating in school committees engaged in continuous quality improvement. Other stakeholders include clinical partners and consumers who participate by responding to evaluation surveys and serving on advisory committees. One of the major recommendations of a national taskforce on accreditation of health professions (and a key principle in continuous quality improvement) is that programs should be required to establish effective linkages with their stakeholders, including the public, students, and professional organizations (The Center for Health Professions, University of California, San Francisco, 1999). When developing the evaluation plan, faculty should give thoughtful consideration to how these linkages can be effectively established.

PREPARING THE ACCREDITATION REPORT

Assignments should be given to teams or individuals to prepare drafts of the various sections of the self-study report. The drafts should be widely circulated for discussion among faculty. An open forum for faculty, students, and other stakeholders may be offered to provide maximum opportunity for constructive criticism and shaping of final recommendations. One person should do the final writing of the report to provide a coherent and consistent voice to the document. It is also recommended that someone be asked to do a final editing of the report before printing. The report should be candid and accurate. You do not want the site visitors to find that the report glossed over major issues or controversies.

PREPARING FOR THE SITE VISIT

The purpose of the site visit is to provide an opportunity for external reviewers (site visitors) to verify the information provided in the self-study and to provide supplemental information to aid the review panel in making the accreditation decision. Thus, planning for the site visit is a key part of the accreditation process. Faculty, students, and staff will need to be oriented to the site visit process and procedures. Careful attention to this aspect of the process can make a major difference in the success of the visit (Davidhizar & Vance, 1998).

Ongoing Activities

Implementation of continuous quality improvement evaluation plan with tracking of key performance indicators.

Documentation of continuous improvement efforts.

Encourage select leaders to train and serve as accreditation site visitors.

2 to 3 Years Before Visit

Curriculum Audit (if needed)

Review of evaluation plan.

Analysis of changes made due to evaluation evidence.

Begin faculty & staff development regarding accreditation workshops. Hire consultant if needed.

Obtain current accreditation standards & review with faculty.

2 Years Before Visit

Select a chair/leader for the accreditation process.

Develop a work plan and timeline for the self-study.

Establish an accreditation taskforce or designate a regular committee to take the accreditation lead.

18 Months Before Visit

Conduct self-study with broad participation of students, faculty, and staff.

Give notice to the college community, alumni, and clinical partners regarding accreditation and site visit.

Post information on your college website regarding accreditation activities.

Inform key college or university officers of visit and expectation of them.

Prepare a draft of the self-study report for broad distribution and comment.

3 Months Before Visit

Do final editing of self-study report.

Print and bind report as directed by the accreditation agency.

Provide copies of the self-study in key places (i.e. Library) for access by students.

Confirm travel plans and hotel arrangements for visitors.

2 Months Before Visit

Mail copies to accreditation agency as directed.

Distribute copies of self-study to full-time faculty and administrators.

Make self-study available for students, alumni, and other stakeholders on website or by providing copies in key locations such as the library.

Plan schedule for site visit with leader of visiting team.

Reserve a room for exhibits and team conferences.

Reserve a room for final oral report.

One Month Before Visit

Orient students to the self-study results; review key policies and curriculum conceptual framework.

Schedule final faculty review of self-study, key policies, and conceptual framework.

Prepare exhibits.

Confirm final schedule for site visit and local transportation arrangements.

Post invitations to the site visitors' oral report to be held at conclusion of visit.

One Week Before Visit

Confirm plans with site visitors.

Set up exhibit room and computers for site visitors' use.

F I G U R E   1 2 . 1 A timeline for accreditation.

Approximately 2 to 3 months before the site visit, planning begins to shift to the site visit phase of accreditation. The designated chair of the institution's accreditation process should follow the guidelines of the accreditation agency in making hotel accommodations for site visitors. This information is available on the agency's website (CCNE, 2004).

Faculty and support staff that have not been involved in the self-study process should be oriented to the accreditation process and procedures prior to the site visit. Davidhizar and Vance (1998) suggest that such sessions provide an opportunity to review the organizing framework of a curriculum and key policies (e.g., grievance procedures) with both students and faculty. It is also advisable to make an appointment with administrators such as the president, academic vice president, and dean of the division, if nursing is a part of a larger academic unit, to familiarize them with the date and purpose of the visit, providing a context for their involvement and likely interviews by the site visitors. It is very important to provide significant advanced notice of the site visit to these individuals to ensure they will be available at some point during the visit if requested by the site visitors.

Some programs have found that arranging a mock site visit a month or so before the actual site visit can be a valuable exercise if the majority of faculty have never experienced an accreditation visit previously. A mock site visit can be arranged by having one or two peers who have experience in accreditation visit the institution to conduct interviews and to make class and clinical visits just like the official site visitors will do. A mock visit is like a dress rehearsal and can be a real learning experience for less seasoned faculty as well as for students. Often this experience motivates faculty to read the self-study with more care than they might otherwise exercise!

It is highly recommended that accommodations that are not too far from the campus be provided to save travel time. Depending on the size of the team, it is often feasible that the chair of the team be provided with a larger hotel room or suite to accommodate team conferences and writing of the summative report. A meeting space at the hotel is important, because the team will often spend long evening hours discussing the materials and interviews scheduled for each day and writing the report.

An exhibit room on campus should be provided for displays of evidence and supplemental materials that the site visitors can use to verify information presented in the self-study report. It is helpful to provide a matrix of the display materials according to the standards and criteria so that the visitors can quickly find materials (Flannigan, Cluskey, & Gard, 2002). Typically, the materials in the exhibit room are those materials that are too large or too numerous to be included in the self-study report. These include the *Faculty Handbook*, samples of examinations or student work, institutional data such as *Fact Books*, institutional and departmental strategic plans, and so on. Application sketches may be developed by students and faculty prior to the visit to help capture learning outcomes for the site visitors (Myers & Schlapman, 2001). The exhibit room should provide a computer and printer for the site visitors' use on campus. A conference table for team meetings is also recommended to be available in the exhibit room.

Site visitors themselves usually make travel arrangements. Institutions and programs are discouraged from entertaining or providing gifts to site visitors other than small tokens such as items with the institution's logo (e.g., a mug or portfolio). Sometimes even this type of courtesy is prohibited, and site visitors may even be required by the agency to pay for their own meals to ensure that there is no perception of conflict of interest. It is important to remember that site visitors do not make the accreditation decision themselves. Typically, the site visitor describes findings and may note strengths or weaknesses in the program, but the review panel of the accrediting body will be the actual decision maker. For this reason, site visitors may recommend that supplemental materials be sent to the review panel if they find that information that may be important to demonstrating that an institution or program is meeting accreditation standards has not been included in the self-study.

Typically, the board or designated review panel of the accrediting agency or regulatory body meets at regular intervals to review the entire body of evidence provided by the institution and the site visitors. Three or four readers may be assigned as primary readers and reviewers of the materials. Following a summation of evidence, the review panel will make its decision. Review panels usually only meet a few times a year, so programs may not learn about the final outcomes of their accreditation report and site visit until several months after the team has left campus. Normally, programs will be given some indication by the site visitors on whether there are any major deficiencies or recommendations to address. It is often advantageous to begin work on these items shortly after the visit, because these items are very salient to faculty who are motivated to respond to the recommendations. It should be remembered, however, that the review panel makes the final recommendations and they may not come to the exact same conclusions as the site visitors. It is not uncommon to see that the review panel emphasizes certain issues and drops some recommendations made by the site visitors.

The program will receive a formal decision and set of recommendations from the accrediting agency. A copy of this report is usually sent to the president or chancellor of the institution as well as to the dean or director of the school. Follow-up activities may include a progress report after a defined period of time if deficiencies have been noted or if institutional capacity to sustain its present positive state is not clearly demonstrated.

▲ SUMMARY

Preparation for accreditation is a core activity for the current generation of nursing faculty. An effective way to build the collective expertise of faculty in accreditation is to plan for orientation and faculty development on this topic on a regular basis. Engagement in regular activities that demonstrate the principles of continuous quality improvement is recommended to ensure faculty and student appreciation and cooperation in accreditation activities. Development of an evaluation plan, which uses selected tools such as a curriculum matrix or audit, is identified as a best practice in preparation for accreditation. Student, alumni, and employer surveys to assess stakeholder key requirements and satisfaction are other elements that should be used regularly to enhance program improvement. Development of an accreditation timeline with definitive deadlines is strongly recommended as a tool to mange the accreditation task.

DISCUSSION QUESTIONS

1. To what extent do nursing faculty bear the responsibility for basing a curriculum on accreditation standards as well as the mission and goals of the program? Explain your rationale.

2. What are ways in which students and faculty can be motivated to participate actively in preparation for accreditation?
3. What strategies can be used to begin to imbed a culture of continuous quality improvement within a school of nursing?
4. What data provide credible evidence that a nursing program is succeeding in achieving its mission and stated learning outcomes?

LEARNING ACTIVITIES

Student Learning Activities

1. In a small group, explore the implications of accreditation for you as a student nurse. What difference would it make if your nursing school does not have accreditation?
2. Go to a website for specialized nursing accreditation and review the standards for accreditation. Describe how these standards focus on achievement of learning outcomes and educational effectiveness.
3. Pick one standard and write a draft report on how your program meets that standard. Indicate what information you would have to collect to provide evidence that your program meets that standard.

Faculty Development Activities

1. Take the evaluation plan for your nursing program or school and develop a timeline for the next accreditation visit.
2. Develop an orientation program for new faculty to accreditation and the accreditation process.
3. Describe the two issues and challenges facing accreditation in the rapidly changing environment of higher education today.

REFERENCES

American Association of Colleges of Nursing. (1998a). *The essentials of baccalaureate education for professional nursing practice.* Washington, DC: Author.

American Association of Colleges of Nursing. (1998b). *The essentials of master's education for advanced practice nursing.* Washington, DC: Author.

American Association of Nurse Anesthetists. *Standards for accreditation of nurse anesthesia educational programs revisions.* Retrieved June 11, 2004, from http://www.aana.com/accreditation/

American College of Nurse Midwives. (2004). *The division of accreditation.* Retrieved June 11, 2004, from, http://www.midwife.org/about/doa.cfm

Bacon, P. (2003, May 12). Don't know much about history: Congress debates bringing colleges to bear with academic standards [Electronic version]. *Time.* Retrieved May 6, 2003, from http://www.time.com.time/archive/preview

Barnum, B. S. (1997, August 13). Licensure, certification, and accreditation [Electronic version]. *Online Journal of Issues in Nursing.* Retrieved June 11, 2004, from http://www.nursingworld.org/ojin

Bellack, J. G. O'Neil, E., & Thomsen, C. (1999) Responses of baccalaureate and graduate programs to the emergence of choice in nursing accreditation. *Journal of Nursing Education, 38*(2), 53–61.

Burke, J. (Ed.). (2002). Accrediting agencies (pp. vii–xii). *The higher education directory* (2003 Edition). Falls Church: VA: Higher Education Publications.

Canadian Association of Schools of Nursing. Home page (2004). Retrieved June 10, 2004 from http://www.causn.org

Center for the Health Professions, University of California, San Francisco. (June 1999). *Strategies for change and improvement: Taskforce on accreditation of health professions education.* San Francisco, CA: Author. Retrieved June 11, 2004, from: http://futurehealth.ucsf.edu/pubs.html

Collins, M. S. (1997, August 13). Issues of accreditation: A dean's perspective. *Online Journal of Issues in Nursing.* Retrieved June 11, 2004, from http://www.nursingworld.org/ojin

Commission on Collegiate Nursing Education. (1998). *Standards for accreditation of baccalaureate and graduate nursing education programs.* Washington, DC: Author.

Commission on Collegiate Nursing Education. (2004). *CCNE accreditation.* Retrieved June 11, 2004, from http://www.aacn.nche.edu/Accreditation/index.htm

Commission on Graduates of Foreign Nursing Schools. (CGFNS). (1999). *History, mission, and frequently asked questions.* Retrieved June 11, 2004, from http://www.cgfns.org/cgfns/aboutcgfns/history.html

Council for Higher Education Accreditation. (2002a). *Accreditation and assuring quality in distance learning.* CHEA Monograph Series 2002 (1). Washington, DC: Author.

Council for Higher Education Accreditation. (2002b). *CHEA letter from the president: International quality review and accreditation: The role of U.S. recognized accrediting organizations.* Washington, DC: Author

Council for Higher Education Accreditation. (2002c). *The fundamentals of accreditation: What do you need to know?* Washington, DC: CHEA.

Daggett, L. M., Butts, J. B., & Smith K. K. (2002). The development of an organizing framework to implement AACN guidelines for nursing education. *Journal of Nursing Education, 41*(1), 34–37.

Davidhizar, R., & Vance, A. R. (1998). Preparing for a National League for Nursing Accreditation Commission site visit. *ABNF Journal, 9*(3), 65–68.

Eaton, J. S. (2002). *An overview of U.S. accreditation.* Washington, DC: Council for Higher Education Accreditation.

Ewell, P. T. (2001). *Accreditation and student learning outcomes: A proposed point of departure.* Council for Higher Education Accreditation Occasional Paper, Washington, DC.

Flannigan, P., Cluskey, M., & Gard, C. (2002). Accreditation strategies: Planning for an accreditation visit. *Nurse Educator, 27*(4), 157–158.

Glazer, G. (1997). Legislative background surrounding the accreditation process. *Online Journal of Issues in Nursing.* Retrieved June 11, 2004, from http://www.nursingworld.org/ojin

Gose, B. (2002, November 1). A radical approach to accreditation. *The Chronicle of Higher Education,* A25-A27.

Grant, L. E., Kelley, J. H., Northington, L., & Barlow, D. (2002) Using TQM/CQI processes to guide development of independent and collaborative learning in two levels of baccalaureate nursing students. *Journal of Nursing Education, 41*(12), 537–540.

Guerard, E. B. (2002, October 3). Lawmakers question role of college accrediting agencies. *Education Daily, 35*(187) 8–9. Elec. Coll.: A92801569.

Heinrich, C. R., Karner, K. J., Gaglione, B. H., & Lambert, L. J. (2002). Order out of chaos: The use of a matrix to validate curriculum integrity. *Nurse Educator, 27*(3), 136–140, 271–273.

Ingersoll, G. L., & Sauter, M. (1998). Integrating accreditation criteria into educational program evaluation. *Nursing and Health Care Perspectives, 19*(5), 224–229.

Ministry of Education Ontario. (2004). *The role of ministries.* Retrieved October 31, 2004, from http://www.edu.gov.on.ca/eng/general/general.html

Morgan, R. (2002). Lawmakers at hearing on college-accreditation system call for more accountability. Retrieved October 2, 2002, from the Chronicle of Higher Education's website http://chronicle.com/daily/2002/10/2002100204n.htm

Myers, N., & Schlapman, N. (2001). Accreditation: Enhancing accreditation visits with application sketches. *Nurse Educator, 26*(6), 271–273.

National Association of Nurse Practitioners in Women's Health. (2004). NPWH Program for Accreditation. Retrieved June 11, 2004, from http://www.npwh.org/accreditation1.htm

National League for Nursing Accrediting Commission. (2004). Standards and criteria. Retrieved June 11, 2004, from http://www.nlnac.org

O'Neil, E. (1997, June). Using accreditation for your purposes [Electronic version]. *AAHE Bulletin.* Retrieved November 11, 2002, from http://aahebulletin.com/public/archive

Overbay, J. D., & Aaltonen, P. M. (2001). A comparison of NLNAC and CCNE accreditation. *Nurse Educator, 26*(1), 17–27.

Ryan, S. (2003. August 20). Accreditation for the future. *Online Journal of Nursing Issues.* Retrieved June 11, 2004, from http://www.nursingworld.org/ojin

Seager, S. R., & Anema, M. G. (2003). A process for conducting a curriculum audit. *Nurse Educator, 28*(1), 5–6.

Taylor, K. (2001). Involving nursing students in continuous improvement projects. *Nurse Educator, 26*(4), 175–177.

Thompson, C., & Bartels, J. E. (1999). Outcomes assessment: implications for nursing education. *Journal of Professional Nursing, 15*(3): 170–178.

Van Damme, D. (2002, August). Quality assurance in an international environment: National and international interests and tensions. *International Quality Review: Values, Opportunities, and Issues.* Council for Higher Education Accreditation Occasional Paper.

Vogler, J., & Ratliffe, C. E. (1993). Quality improvement and managed care as curricular elements. *Nurse Educator, 18*(3), 29–33.

Young, and others (1983). *Understanding accreditation.* San Francisco, CA: Jossey Bass Publishers.

Curriculum Development and Evaluation in the Practice Setting

▼

Sarah B. Keating, EdD, RN, FAAN

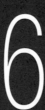

▲ OVERVIEW

This section describes the role of the nursing educator in staff development and health education services for clients. While this segment of nursing education differs in its target audiences, many of the same activities that relate to curriculum development and evaluation in the academic setting apply. Chapter 13 assists staff developers and health educators to adapt the information in the text to their area of nursing practice.

Although the major focus of the text is on curriculum development and evaluation for faculty in schools of nursing, many of the same components for curriculum planning apply to staff development and health education. Chapter 13 discusses the topics from the text thus far and how they apply to the practice setting. The process of conducting a needs assessment applies to the practice setting as well as to academe. The mission, philosophy, purpose, and goals for an education program in the practice setting must be in line with the health agency's mission and purpose. This applies to staff development programs within the agency and health education programs that meet the needs of the population that the health agency serves.

Section 5 topics on program evaluation and accreditation also apply to the practice setting. The Joint Commission of Accreditation of Healthcare Organizations' accreditation criteria and goals for patient education and the American Nurses Association's professional practice standards apply to staff development and health education programs. The processes for undergoing accreditation in schools of nursing are very similar to health care agency accreditation. Also, program evaluation theories, concepts, and models apply to the assessment of the effectiveness of health education and staff development programs.

The current role of educators in nursing practice settings, their qualifications, and their desired educational levels are discussed. Issues and trends that apply to staff development and health education are reviewed. Implications for the future and the potential for partnerships between practice and schools of nursing are included.

Adaptation of Curriculum Development and Evaluation to Staff Development and Client-Centered Health Education

Mary Ann Haw, PhD, RN, and Sarah B. Keating, EdD, RN, FAAN

OBJECTIVES

Upon completion of Chapter 13, the reader will be able to:

1. Adapt curriculum development principles and processes to nursing education in the practice setting for staff development and client-centered health education.
2. Conduct a needs assessment of internal and external frame factors as they relate to curriculum development for staff development and health education programs.
3. Evaluate selected learning theories for their application to staff development and health education programs.
4. Analyze the budgeting processes for staff development and health education programs.
5. Apply program evaluation concepts to staff development and health education programs.
6. Examine some of the issues facing nurse educators in the practice setting.

13

▲ OVERVIEW

The roles of nurse educators in the practice setting are two-fold and can focus on both or on only one. The two major roles are staff development and client-centered education. This chapter provides information on curriculum development and evaluation for staff development and client-centered health education programs in health care organizations and agencies. For the sake of brevity, the latter role is identified as "health education" throughout the chapter and implies education activities focused on individual patients, families, aggregates (groups at risk), or communities. Topics are divided into separate sections according to the two roles, or combined if the topic applies to both.

Overview: Staff Development

The staff development function involves the postlicensure education of nurses in health care organizations to ensure that members of the nursing staff have the most current knowledge and skills for nursing practice. In large health maintenance organizations (HMOs), university medical centers, and major county hospitals, the staff development function may be centralized with responsibilities for the training and professional development of all personnel, from custodial staff and unlicensed health care workers to nurses, physicians, managers, and administrators. Activities of staff development educators often include new graduate programs, orientation, competency assessment, cross training, new product and technology training, specialty practice education, research utilization, leadership and management development, and continuing education to encourage lifelong learning.

Nurse educators who focus on staff development can provide nurse faculties with their perspectives on the competencies and knowledge base of students and graduates of the programs. Their wisdom is valuable in helping faculty prepare new graduates for practice in the reality setting. Nursing faculty members, on the other hand, have the expertise in pedagogy and andragogy and can share these strategies with nurse educators in the practice settings. They also have clinical specialty knowledge and skills that can be offered as in-service opportunities for nursing staff in health agencies and used to educate nurse preceptors and mentors for students and new graduates. Research partnerships between nursing service and education benefit nursing faculty members as they earn promotion and tenure and keep abreast of changes in health care, while students can carry out their graduate theses or dissertations in the practice arena. All levels of students can apply the newest knowledge from research to evidence-based practice. This, in turn, is shared with nursing staff members who can reciprocate with their knowledge and clinical skills in the latest advances in health care.

There are increasing instances of industry and education partnerships with industry assisting schools of nursing with the costs for additional faculty members to help increase enrollments. Qualified staff members from the agencies serve as instructors while continuing in their practice roles in the agencies. The pitfalls of these arrangements include the temporary nature of the arrangement; pressure on the person who serves as faculty from both the education half and the service half of the contract; and salary and benefits arrangements. If these issues are worked out in advance and remedied, if necessary, during the contract, then it can be a short-term solution to the nursing shortage and faculty crises.

It is imperative that the integrity of the school of nursing curriculum be protected by ensuring that adjunct faculty from the service area is well oriented to the curriculum and its goals and objectives. There must be opportunities for new members' participation in faculty and curriculum meetings. Experienced faculty must act as mentors to impart the curriculum plan and the pedagogical and andragogical knowledge and skills necessary to the teaching and learning role. It is possible in these types of arrangements that the result is recruitment of clinical personnel into full-time faculty roles, which is a great advantage to schools of nursing and the profession.

A reminder to nurse educators in both settings comes from Kee and Ryser (2001), Kells and Koerner (2000), and "Bridging the Gap Between Academia and the Working World" (2000), who describe partnerships between schools of nursing and service to ease transition of the new graduate into the reality setting. One method is through work-study programs for senior nursing students assigned to agency preceptors. Through this method, students work part time in the clinical setting and continue studies, enabling them to earn income while earning credit toward the degree. Another method is to provide opportunities for students in the clinical setting to relate to expert nurses—for example, postclinical conferences to discuss reality-based experiences. Both of these types of experiences provide students with "real world" clinical practice, credit toward their courses, and in some cases, through the work-study programs, income. The key to success is partnership between the education program and the health care agency. Faculty members, clinical staff nurses, and advanced practice nurses collaborate to provide learning experiences for students about to enter practice.

The advantages for the health care agency are the abilities to have knowledgeable and skillful providers of nursing care at reasonable costs, to evaluate students as potential employees, to provide students with an orientation that will not be as extensive as with new employees who did not have the experience, and to build student loyalty to the agency. The advantages for the students are financial assistance, potential employment opportunities, close mentorship from experienced clinicians, and credit toward their nursing degrees. The advantages for the school of nursing are the provision of clinical experiences for students, the opportunity to work with experienced clinicians, and research and scholarship opportunities in the clinical setting.

Overview: Health Education

Nurse educators in academe and in the practice setting have much to offer each other. Nurses involved in health education are aware of the health needs of the population and the aggregates that make up the under- and unserved segments of the community. They can share this knowledge with nursing school faculties to integrate the knowledge into the curriculum and to arrange for student clinical experiences that prepare them for the real world of practice.

The health education function rose dramatically in importance in response to shorter hospital stays and the increasing complexity of care to be managed by the patient or family caregivers at home (Rankin & Stallings, 2001). Similarly, the national emphasis on primary care and prevention of diseases and injuries elevated the importance of health education and promotion in health care facilities for improving the nation's health.

Although primary care prevention and health teaching responsibilities are shared by all members of the health team, it is not unusual for health care organizations to have well-developed educational programs. These offerings can include the following topics:

1. Health recovery
2. Rehabilitation

3. Restoration after acute illness, injury, or major surgery
4. Health maintenance and health promotion programs to prevent disease, complications from existing disease, and injury
5. Health promotion across the lifespan

Issues of concern to nurse health educators include changes in population demographics; emerging health problems; an increasingly diverse patient population; the growing gap between the rich and the poor, with increasing health disparities among low-income and minority populations; keeping apace with advances in knowledge and technology; and declines in funding and resource development for education (Bailey, Hoeppner, Jeska, Schneller, & Wolohan, 1995; Lindeman, 2000; O'Neil & the Pew Health Commission, 1998).

▲ COMPONENTS OF CURRICULUM DEVELOPMENT IN THE PRACTICE SETTING

The same components of curriculum development discussed in Chapter 7 for schools of nursing apply to staff development and health education. It is essential that the educational program's mission or vision, philosophy, and overall goal or purpose are congruent with those of the sponsoring agency. A conceptual framework may be utilized to organize the knowledge and skills to be learned into a logical sequence. Many health care agencies or nursing services employ nursing theories or conceptual frameworks such as Benner's from-novice-to-expert model (Benner, 1984) or andragogy learning theories such as Knowles, Holton, and Swanson (1998). Table 13.1 summarizes the questions for data collection and the desired outcomes that relate to each component for nurse educators to use in these settings when assessing, revising, or developing educational programs.

Goals, Objectives, and Instructional Design for the Practice Setting

The overall goal(s) or purpose(s) can be viewed as macro objectives and reflect the overall intent of the program. They are the outcome expectations of the educational program for the staff or the patients, families, aggregates, and community. They should flow logically from the agency's mission, vision, and philosophy. (See Chapter 4 for detailed information on the development of goals and objectives.) Based on the overall purpose or goal of the educational program, objectives are developed to provide the implementation plan for the program.

While there is debate about the use of behaviorally stated goals and objectives, the overall goal and its objectives are usually stated in this format to facilitate the development of the instructional plan and the measurement of the success of the program. This is especially true for nurse educators practicing in health care agencies where productivity, quality assurance, and cost effectiveness can determine the continued existence of an educational program or initiation of a new program.

Many health agencies have preprogrammed educational materials and objectives that include all of the components of a teaching session. These materials are used to share knowledge and skills with staff and/or patients and families. While these programs may limit creativity for the nurse delivering the educational session, they ensure some quality control over the purpose, objectives, and content that is intended for the consumer.

▲ **TABLE 13.1**   **Adaptation of the Components of the Curriculum to Staff Development and Patient and Family Education**

Component of the Curriculum	Questions for Data Collection	Desired Outcome
Agency mission, vision, and/or philosophy statements	To what extent are the mission, vision, and/or philosophy statements visible to the agency's consumers?	The mission, vision, and/or philosophy statements are readily apparent and drive the type of health care services the agency provides to the public.
	To what extent are the mission, vision, and/or philosophy statements of the agency congruent with its educational programs' missions?	All educational programs in the institution have mission, vision, and/or philosophy statements and they are congruent with that of the agency.
Purpose or overall goal	To what extent does the overall goal or purpose of the agency flow from the mission, vision, and/or philosophy statements?	The agency's overall goal or purpose flows logically from the mission, vision, and/or philosophy statements.
	To what extent does the overall goal or purpose of the agency imply the need for educational programs?	The overall goal or purpose of the agency explicitly or implicitly includes educational programs as part of its service.
	What is the evidence of an overall goal or purpose for the agency's educational programs, and is it congruent with the agency goal or purpose?	All educational programs within the agency have statements relating to their overall purpose and goals that are congruent with the agency's goal or purpose.
Organizing or conceptual framework	To what extent is the framework (if it exists) congruent with the mission, vision, philosophy, and/or overall goal or purpose?	The organizing or conceptual framework is congruent with the agency's mission, vision, philosophy, and/or overall purpose or goal.
	If the agency or service unit of the agency utilizes an organizing or conceptual framework for its educational program, to what extent do the programs' curricula reflect that framework?	Educational programs within the agency integrate its organizing or conceptual framework into curriculum plans.
Program objectives	To what extent do the educational programs' objectives flow from the overall goal or purpose of the agency?	Program objectives within have specific goal statements that are congruent with the agency's overall goal or purpose statements.

(table continues on page 324)

▲ TABLE 13.1	Adaptation of the Components of the Curriculum to Staff Development and Patient and Family Education (continued)	

Component of the Curriculum	Questions for Data Collection	Desired Outcome
Program objectives (continued)	To what extent are the educational objectives in a format that allows for measurement of the learners' success and evaluation of the teaching session(s)?	Each objective is learner centered, and includes the content of the learning experience, how the learner will achieve the specified behavior, knowledge, or skill, at what level of competency, and when.
Implementation plan	To what extent does the agency demonstrate support for its educational programs through staff, resources, facilities, and materials?	There is a central place for educational programs, staff, resources, learning environment facilities with available instructional support, and a listing of all educational offerings.
	Is there a dedicated budget for the educational program, and under whose control is it?	There is a dedicated budget in place for educational programs with its control in the hands of the education manager.
	To what extent does each educational program include an overview, objectives, learner characteristics, content outline, teaching and learning methods, setting, and resources?	The implementation plan for each educational program in the agency includes an overview, objectives, learner characteristics, content outline, teaching and learning methods, setting, and resources.

The instructional design should include a brief description of the purpose of the class, characteristics and educational needs of the learner, teaching strategies, a content outline, the learning environment, teaching aids, necessary supplies and equipment, and an evaluation plan for measuring the success of the program. There are several staff development and patient and family education textbooks that provide detailed information for the development of educational programs; thus, a detailed description of these latter components for instructional design are not included in this chapter. Recommended texts are Bastable (2003), Gilbert and Sawyer (2000), Pender, Murdaugh, and Parsons (2002), and Rankin and Stallings (2001).

▲ NEEDS ASSESSMENT

Curriculum development for staff development and health education programs begins with a needs assessment, involving an examination of both external and internal frame factors to provide the foundation for developing and revising curricula (Johnson, 1977). Rarely does a nurse educator actually develop a new staff development or health education program from the ground up. In the case of new programs, a needs assessment is essential. A needs assessment is also appropriate for program revision based on the changing demographics and learning needs of the health agency staff, changes in the health status of the population served by the health care organization, and the response to emerging issues and threats to the health of the community.

External Frame Factors

The need for program revision is based on information from an updated community needs assessment, including the current and projected needs of the health populace and feedback from the recipients of previous staff development and health education offerings. Chapter 5 of this text goes into detail for assessing the external frame factors that affect a school of nursing, and many of these same factors apply to the practice setting. Guidelines for conducting a community needs assessment are found in Table 13.2. Questions for assessing the major external factors that apply to staff development and health education are presented in Table 13.3.

Internal Frame Factors

Internal frame factors to consider in developing staff development and health education curricula are the mission, philosophy, and goals of the institution and their match to the educational program. Additional internal frame factors affecting educational programs are characteristics of the health care setting such as organizational structure, including the decision-making structure, particularly as it applies to staff development and health education; institutional economics, including resources for staff development and health education; and the characteristics and learning needs of the staff and target learner populations.

▲ TABLE 13.2   Guidelines for a Community Needs Assessment

1. A description of the community, including size, community services such as transportation systems and communication mechanisms, major industries, educational and religious institutions, political parties, and local government
2. Population demographics—gender, race/ethnicity and age distribution across the life span
3. Employment information, income levels, percent with health insurance coverage, education and literacy levels, and languages spoken
4. Family and household characteristics
5. Percent in the population with health insurance
6. Health-promoting and/or health-damaging aspects of the community and environment
7. Health and wellness measures in the client population served by the clinical agency, including risk factors, health problems, and morbidity and mortality data
8. Health care and social service agencies, such as hospitals, clinics, home care agencies, long-term care agencies, public health services, voluntary health organizations, and other community-based organizations

▲ **TABLE 13.3**   **Guidelines for Assessing External Frame Factors**

Frame Factor	Questions for Data Collection	Desired Outcome
Description of the community	Is the community served by the health care facility urban, suburban, or rural? What community services are available to patients seeking health care and health information, such as transportation, libraries, childcare, and other health care and social service organizations?	Hospital staff and clients have access to the health care facility by public transportation. Other resources in the community can be tapped to support patients and families seeking health care and health education.
Demographics of the population	What are the characteristics of the population served by the health care facility, such as gender, race, ethnicity, and age distribution across the lifespan; family and household characteristics; employment data and income level; education, languages spoken, and literacy level?	Health education programs and learning methods are designed to fit the current demographics of the population. Staff development programs are developed or revised to address the current shift in population demographics.
Health needs of the populace	What are the measures of health and wellness in the population served by the health care facility? What are the risk factors and measures of morbidity and mortality in this population? What health problems are emerging in the population? What percent of the population live at or below poverty level? What percentage has health insurance?	Staff development and health education programs are developed or revised to address current and emerging major health risks, health problems, diseases, and injuries in the community; health education programs provide outreach to unserved and underserved populations in the community.
The health care system	What are the major health insurance programs and entitlement programs within the population served by the health care facility, such as HMOs, Medicare, Medicaid, Supplemental Security Income, General Assistance, and Veterans Administration benefits? What are other health care and social service resources in the community, such as hospitals, clinics, home care and long-term care agencies, public health services, and voluntary health organizations?	Clients have health insurance coverage to provide access to health care, including patient and family teaching, and community outreach health education. Entitlement programs support the basic prerequisites for health, such as income, housing, food, childcare and transportation.
The nursing workforce	What are the numbers of nurses in the region served by the health care facility? Is there a shortage of nurses, and if so, what are the specific areas of severe nursing shortages, such as ER, critical	Staff development programs are tailored to the educational level, job responsibilities, and learning needs of the nursing workforce. Creative staff development programming addresses the shortage of nurses.

▲ TABLE 13.3	Guidelines for Assessing External Frame Factors (continued)	
Frame Factor	**Questions for Data Collection**	**Desired Outcome**
The nursing workforce (continued)	care, gerontology, and long-term care? Among the nursing staff at the health care facility, what is the level of education? How many are prepared for and certified in advanced practice roles, such as nurse practitioner, clinical nurse specialist, nurse midwife, and nurse anesthetist?	
Regulations and accreditation	What are the state regulations governing approval of continuing education curricula and course offerings for nurses? What are the ANA standards for professional development of staff? What are the JCAHO standards for health education?	Staff development and continuing education programs offered in the health care facility meet state requirements for approval of continuing education offerings and ANA Standards for Nursing Professional Development programs. Patient and family education programs meet the JCAHO criteria for accreditation.
Need for development or revision of the program	Has there been a major shift in population demographics? Are there major changes in health risks, morbidity, and mortality in the population served by the health care facility?	Staff development and health education programs address changing demographics and emerging health risks, morbidity, and mortality.
	Do the external and/or internal program evaluation findings reveal areas for improvement?	Program revisions address areas identified for improvement from internal and external evaluations.
	Are staff and health education programs culturally, linguistically, and educationally appropriate for the intended recipients? Are staff and health education programs and teaching methods based on the latest research evidence? Are there newer technologies for delivery-effective staff and patient education?	Program revisions are based on current research findings on teaching methods and learning strategies, including effective use of advances in technology in delivering educational programs.

RELATIONSHIP OF THE INSTITUTIONAL MISSION PHILOSOPHY AND GOALS TO THE EDUCATIONAL PROGRAM

The health care facility's mission, philosophy, and goals provide the overall framework and direction for the organization. Therefore, the mission, philosophy, and goals of the staff development and health education programs should be closely aligned with those of the parent organization. Nurse educators should have a solid understanding of the organizational structure and decision-making process as they relate to education programs. Final decisions regarding program course offerings for education programs, including the commitment of resources to them, are made with consideration for the extent to which they will support the goals of the overall organization. Successful education programs are those that address the needs of the staff, community and population served, and the goals and priorities of the health care organization.

INSTITUTIONAL ECONOMICS AND RESOURCES FOR STAFF AND PATIENT EDUCATION

An analysis of the institutional economics and financial health of the health care organization provides information on fiscal resources for curriculum development in staff development and health education. A lack of resources for staff development and patient education programming is primary among the major issues faced by nursing educators in health care agencies. In lean financial times, the education function is often the first to be downsized. Nursing educators need to develop collaborative relationships with fiscal officers and agency administrators to build the case for financial investment in staff development and patient education programs. Showing the relationship between educational programs and the achievement of organizational goals is an effective strategy for securing support and material resources for education, particularly if there is program evaluation and/or cost-effectiveness data to support the positive returns on investment in education.

CHARACTERISTICS AND LEARNING NEEDS OF STAFF AND CLIENTS

The characteristics and needs of the learners, whether staff or clients, need to be considered in developing and revising curricula. Because the target learner groups vary, the following discussion addresses the two learner groups separately.

Staff Learning Needs Assessment

The characteristics of staff members include prior education; work experience; present level of knowledge and skill, particularly in relationship to new or changing job responsibilities; and clinical practice expectations. Staff members may have additional needs and skills arising from other demands and situations in their lives. For example, they may have family responsibilities that at times take priority over the employment setting. Some may have multilingual skills and represent various cultural and ethnic groups and, thus, have additional knowledge to contribute to the care of clients. The availability of staff for professional development programs outside of scheduled work shifts may be limited among those with family responsibilities or those who live a long distance from the health care organization. Using advanced technology, such as distance-education technology, can ameliorate some of the problems with staff access to professional development programs.

There are a number of methods for assessing learning needs of staff. Sources of data include nursing audits and quality improvement reports, performance evaluations of staff, incident reports, input from nursing staff, interviews with nursing managers, and position analysis vis-à-vis the level of desired performance. Collecting data from multiple sources is highly recommended in that similar themes may emerge from a number of sources, increasing the validity of the needs assessment findings (Abruzzese, 1996).

Client Learning Needs Assessment

Among the characteristics to consider about individual patients, families, groups, and communities are gender, race, ethnicity, age, education, language(s) spoken, and literacy. Health beliefs, health values, present knowledge of health condition and expectations, and preferences for treatment need to be explored. These characteristics form the basis for developing patient and family education programs that are age- and gender-appropriate and tailored to the specific patient, family, community, culture, language, and educational level (Huff & Kline, 1999). See Table 13.4 for guidelines for assessing internal frame factors affecting educational programs in the practice setting.

▲ TABLE 13.4	Guidelines for Assessing Internal Frame Factors	
Frame Factor	**Questions for Data Collection**	**Desired Outcomes**
Mission, philosophy, and goals of the health care organization	Do the mission, philosophy, and goals of the institution speak to staff development and health education curricula?	The mission, philosophy, and goals of the institution address the professional development of staff and health education needs.
	Is the mission, philosophy, and goals of the staff development and health education programs congruent with the institution's?	The mission, philosophy, and goals of the staff development and health education programs are congruent with those of the health care organization.
Characteristics and learning needs of staff and clients	What are the learning needs of staff? What are the learning needs of clients?	Learning needs of staff and patients are assessed using multiple sources of information.
	What are important characteristics of staff and/or clients to consider in developing appropriate and effective educational programs?	Characteristics of staff and clients affecting access to education and having an impact on learning are taken into consideration in developing educational programs.
Institutional economics and resources for staff development and health education	What are creative strategies for increasing resources for educational programs?	Creative strategies, such as partnering with other experts from nearby health and social service organizations in the community and recruiting course faculty from among the in-house professional staff, are implemented.
	What is the present financial health of the institution? What are the existing and potential resources for staff and health education programs?	Financial health and resources are sufficient for developing and implementing needed staff and patient education programs.

Analysis of Data and Program Decisions

Analyzing the data from the external and internal frame factors assessment often reveals multiple learning needs, more than can be addressed simultaneously. Reasoned choices are imperative regarding the educational programs to be developed. The analyses and decisions may differ according to the type of program (i.e., staff development or health education). Thus, the discussion to follow is divided accordingly.

ANALYSIS OF DATA AND PROGRAM DECISIONS: STAFF DEVELOPMENT

As a framework for making program decisions related to staff development, discrepancy analysis, developed by Mager and Pipe (1970) and later modified by Abruzzese (1996), is useful. It involves a series of questions determining if there is a discrepancy (a difference between present and desired staff performance), its cause and importance, how frequently the task is performed, and if the person once knew how to perform it. If the task is a critical skill and frequently used, it should have high priority. If the task is a critical skill and infrequently used, such as CPR, it also should have high priority. If it is not critical and not frequently used, it should have low priority.

If the cause is a *knowledge discrepancy*, it needs to be determined if the person once knew how to perform the task. If yes, the educator decides if a class is needed or if a quick review or written procedure might suffice. If it is a *performance discrepancy*, it may arise from performance needs other than lack or knowledge or skill. Among the possibilities for lack of optimal performance in the work setting is lack of rewards, supplies, or time. Under these circumstances, developing a class will not solve the problem (Abruzzese, 1996).

ANALYSIS OF DATA AND PROGRAM DECISIONS: HEALTH EDUCATION

In addition to following the guidelines listed in Tables 13.2, 13.3, and 13.4, health care organizations with limited resources for conducting in-depth needs assessments can use the following four questions (McKenzie & Smeltzer 1997, pp. 52–53):

1. "What is the most pressing problem?
2. Are resources adequate to deal with the problem?
3. Can it best be solved by a health education program or could it be handled better through administration, politics, or changes in the economy?
4. Can it be resolved in a reasonable amount of time?"

The answers to these questions can help educators establish program priorities and determine the best use of patient education resources.

▲ LEARNING THEORIES

Chapter 3 describes in detail classic and postmodernistic learning theories applied to nursing education. For the health agency setting, adult learning theories usually prevail in educational programs, especially for staff development. However, for health education programs, some developmental learning theories are appropriate when the target audience is composed of children and early adolescents. The terms andragogy and pedagogy are especially relevant to these practice-setting situations. Andragogy is the science of adult learning (Robles, 1998). Pedagogy is "the art, science, or profession of teaching" (Merriam-Webster Collegiate Dictionary, 2004). While the root of pedagogy (*ped*) implies education of children, its use in the United States became more generic and applied to all ages of learners. However, as continuing education needs became apparent, and especially after World War II with the return of America's war veterans, the andragogy term became popular to differentiate between the learning needs of students of different ages and to develop strategies that were consistent with adult learning theories.

Robles (1998) uses Ingalls' (1972) work to compare andragogy and pedagogy by contrasting four major characteristics of adult learners to those of children and youth: self-concept, experience, readiness to learn, and time perspective and orientation to learning. In thinking about these characteristics, it becomes obvious that adult learners have more mature self-concepts and life experiences that add to their knowledge base as compared to children and youth. As to readiness to learn, most pedagogical strategies are set in preplanned sequential order to relay the knowledge and skills desired in the learner, and adults are more likely to indicate their own learning needs and interests and work with the teacher to identify the methods for acquiring the knowledge and skills they desire.

The time perspective and orientation to learning differ for the two types of learners, with children and youth participating in structured educational experiences that focus on subjects and "end" in graduation. Adult learning experiences, on the other hand, focus on problem-centered experiences within a reality context. Robles (1998) notes that some of the adult learning strategies such as "experiential, collaborative and interactive learning" (p.3) are becoming more common in elementary and secondary schools as well as in adult learning situations. The favorite learning theorist for andragogy or adult education is Knowles (Knowles et al., 1998).

Nurse educators in practice settings assume responsibility for the education of adults (of varying ages, diversity, education, and experience) and for patients and families ranging from the newborn to senescence with varying cultures, ethnic groups, and socioeconomic status. Thus, nurse educators need an arsenal of learning theories applied across the lifespan and teaching strategies that are specific to learner targets.

▲ TEACHING AND LEARNING METHODS

The following articles from the literature describe some models of teaching and learning methods that are useful in designing instruction for staff development and health education programs. In planning programs, it is useful to have a variety of teaching and learning methods to meet the diverse learning needs of the target audience.

Sparling (2001) presents specific suggestions for enhancing learning such as building confidence through a supportive learning environment, accommodating a variety of learning styles, and providing opportunities to practice new skills. Learners gain control of the learning situation by formulating learning objectives, completing problem-solving activities, participating in discussion groups, and submitting a self-evaluation at the program's end. As with traditional learning strategies, effective components of self-directed learning involve a needs assessment of the learner, identifying goals and objectives, obtaining feedback from learners, and evaluating program outcomes.

Wolford and Hughes (2001) describe the use of computer-based training (CBT) provided through the hospital intranet, which can provide 24-hours-a-day, 7-days-a-week accessibility to staff, using a multimedia and interactive approach. Approval ratings are presented along with a discussion of complaints from the intranet's users.

Using the case method and case study as problem-based methods of teaching and learning, Tomey (2003) discusses a transformation process from a focus on teaching to learning. The case method can be used with small groups of students who may have little knowledge of the subject matter, whereas the case study method can be used with more sophisticated learners. The article concludes with guidelines for writing cases.

▲ DISTANCE EDUCATION AND CONTINUING EDUCATION

Chapter 14 discusses distance education from the point of view of nursing education (i.e., schools of nursing); however, staff development and health education programs use distance education technology and strategies for the delivery of educational programs as well. There are many examples of education and practice partnerships that lead to degrees or certificates for staff in health agencies, some of which are cited in Chapter 14. This discussion focuses on distance education as it applies to staff development and health education.

Havice and Knowles (1995) discuss two-way interactive video distance education in detail and its advantages, such as cost issues and the efficacy of distance learning in nursing. Some of the uses for this technology include conferences, in-service sessions, risk management discussions, research exchanges, and other continuing education opportunities. They cite several references that support the use of this technology to bring about positive learner outcomes. Delivery of health education programs are open to this type of education, facilitating the ability of the nurse educator to reach groups of clients with the same health care needs at a distance and providing them with interactive situations for clarification of health information.

An overview of the use of the World Wide Web as a continuing education strategy is discussed by Billings and Rowles (2001). Their article is very useful for educators who plan to develop web-based programs and includes an analysis of the various tools that can be employed on the web. They add considerations for developing a business plan, marketing strategies, and the application of various evaluation methods such as formative and summative evaluation, benchmarking, and continuous quality improvement.

Sproat (2002) has an excellent article on how to design and develop website educational programs. She provides easy-to-understand terminology, an overview of software that can be utilized for authoring web-based education programs, a list of related recommended readings, and five basic rules in the development of web-based programs.

Hayes, Huckstadt, and Gibson (2000) describe the application of a web-based interactive format for a continuing education program for nurse practitioners. They developed three online courses for advanced-practice nurses that include current information on case management and its application to practice. They observed that it takes the developers much time and money to develop the program initially. Additionally, it requires monitoring and periodic updates as well as communication with the learners. They are studying the amount of time these maintenance activities take. Web-based technology can be a useful tool for providing continuing education for nurses in advanced practice. Some of the issues raised by the authors are the recognition of continuing education credits by licensing and certification boards and student learning outcomes.

▲ EDUCATION PROGRAMS IN THE PRACTICE SETTING

The two major roles of nurse educators in the practice setting are staff development and client-centered health education programs. The following discussion reviews the common types of staff development programs in health care agencies and presents an overview of general principles that apply to client-centered education programs.

Staff Development Programs

Most health agencies have departments of education for the purpose of staff orientation, employee training programs, new graduate programs, continuing education (in-service), competency assessment, and preparing staff for specialty roles such as the operating room, intensive care units, home care intravenous therapy programs, and so forth. The following are overviews of the essential curriculum components for each type of program; do recognize, however, that smaller agencies may not have the resources to offer all of the programs mentioned.

ORIENTATION, EMPLOYEE TRAINING PROGRAMS, AND NEW GRADUATE PROGRAMS

Orientation, employee training, and new graduate programs have much in common with the development and evaluation of nursing educational programs. The major differences are the characteristics of the target learning audiences and the length of the program according to the learning needs of the participants. Orientation programs are geared to new employees who have the educational and experiential qualifications to assume a specified position in the health care agency. These programs can be scheduled for an initial in-depth, intensive period of time where critical pieces of information are presented, such as the agency's mission, purpose, policies, procedures, and specific job functions and expectations. These sessions are followed up periodically to add important information and to answer any questions that arise as the new staff members adjust to the health care agency. The sessions also provide an opportunity for the agency to evaluate the members' performance prior to making a permanent appointment.

New graduate nurse programs are usually at least 6 weeks long and preferably 6 months to 1 year with periodic follow-up sessions to reinforce learning and introduce new knowledge. Previous studies demonstrate that the length of time for a new graduate to reach the competent or proficient level of a beginning level staff nurse is at least 6 months (Hom, 2003; Krozak, 2001; Pearson, 2003).

Orientation content includes an in-depth review of the agency's mission, policies, procedures, and the physical plant, including the assigned unit(s). The program should be planned around the results of an assessment of the graduates' experience in health care and clinical experiences in the school of nursing, levels of competency in nursing skills, the application of critical-thinking skills to clinical decision making, and professionalism. A core part of these programs is assigning new graduates to experienced staff preceptors/mentors who assist them throughout the orientation program and continue to provide guidance as needed after the "probationary" period. It is helpful to differentiate between the roles of mentors and preceptors. A preceptor is a person officially assigned to a new employee as the individual (teacher) who provides knowledge regarding nursing science, clinical skills, agency policies and procedures, and professional behaviors. Objectives and learning activities are planned for a specified period of time, during which the new employee has opportunities to apply knowledge and refine clinical skills within the prescribed time of the preceptorship. It is expected that the new employee increasingly gains independence and by the end of the period is ready to assume the responsibilities of a full-time position.

A mentor, on the other hand, is an experienced clinician who is either assigned formally or selected informally by mutual agreement between the new employee and the mentor. The mentor acts as a counselor and teacher for the new employee and as an advocate for that person in the health care arena. If the relationship is formal, a certain time period is usually set. However, the relationship may continue periodically as the mentor and the new employee experience episodes they wish to share. For informal mentoring relationships, the time may last as long as the two people feel the need for sharing knowledge. Whatever the relationship, it is to the advantage of the agency's program and the new employees to include classes for preceptors/mentors on their role and functions in guiding new employees.

A competency-based orientation program for new graduates was instituted in a large metropolitan hospital where, prior to the nursing shortage, there was no need for this type of program (Fey & Miltner, 2000). Although the program was expensive, its outcomes in nurse retention, cross-service use of resources, and other quality-related activities were positive and realized in cost-savings. The article presents a nursing practice competency model ranging from core competencies to patient care management and describes in detail the performance criteria that were set. It is very useful for nurse educators planning new graduate programs that include competency assessment and attainment.

Employee technician training programs target new staff members in the health agency who may not have the education or experience for the positions for which they were hired. These include such people as those who staff janitorial services, food services, plant maintenance, transportation, and laboratories. Depending on state regulations and accreditation issues, some support staff including those under the supervision of nursing, such as nursing assistants, orderlies, home health aides, clerical assistants, and outreach workers. DeOnna (2002) describes her experience in using a "Develop A CurriculUM" (DACUM) analysis in developing a nurse aide training program. DACUM is a form of a job analysis and the development of skills profiles by gathering information from experienced workers in the field. The skill profile is then used for program planning, curriculum development, and development of learning materials.

New employee education programs include orientation to the health care agency and content related to specific knowledge, skills, behaviors (professionalism), and attitudes (such as valuing customer satisfaction) that accompany the positions they fill. The initial training programs can last as long as a period of 1 to 2 months, with later reinforcement and additional sessions, to as short as 1 to 2 weeks. Again, the length of the program depends on the nature of the position and the material to be learned. The complexity of the programs will depend on the job's description and performance expectations. It is important for the nurse educator to be aware of state regulations or accreditation standards that require approval of these types of programs. Standardized curriculum plans from regulatory agencies or professional organizations can be tailored to the health care agency's education needs.

COMPETENCY ASSESSMENT

Competency assessment programs are essential to the delivery of quality care and risk management in health care agencies. They are an integral part of new staff, employee training, and new graduate programs as well as other educational programs that prepare staff members for specialized tasks in their health care provider roles and the maintenance of current staff's skills. It is the nurse educator's role to identify the required skills for each specific job description and the level of competency expected for them.

Lundgren and Houseman (2002) reviewed the continued competence expectations of several health care professions, including nursing. Their survey of the literature found few conclusions, if any, as to the connection between continuing education programs and the maintenance of professional competence. For nursing, they refer to the National Council of State Boards of Nursing (NCSBN) (1996) and the American Nurses Association standards of practice as nursing's contribution to maintaining competence within the profession (ANA) (2004). The NCSBN recommends that nurses build a portfolio to demonstrate their continued competence. They identify nursing academe as sharing in some of the responsibility for maintenance of competence by including standards of practice in nursing curricula and promoting a commitment to lifelong learning by students. The authors observe that in addition to individual responsibilities, institutions and the health care system must be part of a program to ensure continuing competence in health professionals.

As skills become more complex, experience and additional education may become necessary to reach higher levels of performance. The majority of agencies have specific skills that are expected in their job descriptions, and many times, these are part of clinical ladder classifications or requirements for promotions. There is a plethora of job descriptions in the literature and public domain that include clinical competencies, clinical ladder classifications, and competency-based role differentiation models that can be used as guidelines for developing educational programs.

SPECIALTY EDUCATION

Specialty education in staff development is the preparation of staff for functioning knowledgeably and competently in specialty areas of patient care. Many times these programs are linked to orientation or new graduate programs to ensure the delivery of quality care for clients. Other situations calling for specialty education include personnel shortages in certain areas, the need for flexibility of staff assignments, newly opened patient care services within the agency, and career development and promotion opportunities for current staff. While there are packaged teaching plans for specialty education from many of the professional and specialty organizations, it is important that the instructor who delivers the program has clinical expertise related to the specialty as well as andragogical skills.

Client-Centered Health Education Programs

A cardinal rule in client-centered education is the formation of a partnership between the client and educator in identifying and prioritizing learning needs and planning education interventions that are in line with the client's values, beliefs, and motivation to learn. The same principles utilized in the development of staff development programs apply to health education. A major difference in the programs is the target audience that encompasses the health needs of clients across the lifespan, various cultures, ethnic groups, languages, educational background, occupations, and socioeconomic status. Another feature of health education is the fact that nurse educators frequently work with a variety of clients, including individuals and/or their care providers, small groups, or even aggregates (at-risk populations). These "targets" of education require the educator to have an in-depth knowledge of their characteristics to match teaching and learning strategies to their specific needs. Four nursing textbooks that are especially useful to patient and family educators for assessment of learner characteristics, teaching strategies, disease prevention and health promotion interventions, behavioral change, or motivation strategies are: Gilbert and Sawyer (2000), Murray and Zentner (2001), Pender et al.(2002), and Rankin and Stallings (2001). These texts refer the reader to additional references regarding teaching and learning behaviors and health belief models.

Additional theories that are especially applicable to generating motivation for behavioral changes in patients, families, and groups are Pender's Health Promotion Model (Pender et al., 2002) and Bandura's Self-Efficacy model (1997). An individual patient, family, or group's health problem or crisis situation creates an immediate opportunity for health teaching; however, it is important to follow up on these types of learning situations because the problem or crisis of the moment can interfere with assimilation of the information into behavioral change. Societal norms, peer pressure, family and significant others' influence, financial resources, self-image and concept, health beliefs, and values contribute to people's motivation to assume healthy behaviors and are included in the nurse educator's repertoire of educational strategies.

Generation of fear based on the possible consequences of unhealthy behaviors and coercion on the part of health care providers are the least desirable strategies and do not result in a long-term commitment on the part of the client to healthy behaviors (Saarmann, Daugherty, & Riegel, 2000). Roter, Stashefsky-Margalit, and Rudd (2001) discuss health education as it applies to the empowerment of the person, family, or community. They reiterate the fact that past medical or health education activities did not involve the patient and focused on the medical model as compared to newer emphasis on health promotion and health maintenance. Involving the learners in the process of identifying the problems or health needs is an important factor in empowering them to change their behaviors toward a more healthy living style. Some of the methods to enhance empowerment include disclosure, storytelling, problem posing and solution, negotiation, autonomous and thoughtful action, reinforcement, and social support. The authors argue that client empowerment and quality-of-life issues must be of priority in measuring health education outcomes in addition to those emphasized currently that measure cognitive or behavioral change outcomes.

Saarman, Daugherty, and Riegel (2000) point out that knowledge alone is not enough to create patient health behavior change. Traditional teaching and learning situations between nurses and their clients focused on presenting information related to health care; however, in the process, nurses neglected to assess the person's perception of the need or his or her motivation to change behavior. The authors discuss the process of creating change in behavior that includes knowledge of the condition, motivation, the resources to change, making the change, and maintaining that behavior. Their article provides detailed explanations and strategies for nurses to use in effective patient and family teaching.

▲ EVALUATION OF STAFF DEVELOPMENT AND HEALTH EDUCATION PROGRAMS

The evaluation of education programs in health agencies is an important activity on the part of nurse educators for several reasons. Positive evaluations provide justification for the education program's place in the agency and the value of the service to the agency, clients, and community.

Evaluation activities such as continuous quality assessment lead to improvement of the program and the achievement of excellence.

The principles of total quality management (TQM) in staff development and health education programs are the same as those applied to evaluation strategies in schools of nursing. Section 5 and Chapter 11 of this text offers an overview of definitions, concepts, theories, and models that are relevant to educational programs in health agencies. For an overview of TQM applied to education, an excellent resource is Sallis (2002). There are two major components of evaluation in staff development and health education. On the micro level are the individual teaching and learning sessions provided to the target audience and on the macro level is program evaluation to assess the effectiveness and worth of the total education program and its services for the health agency.

Micro-Level of Evaluation: Individual Teaching and Learning Sessions

Developing and implementing individual teaching and learning sessions are ongoing processes, and it is advised that plans for evaluation of the sessions occur during the initial development. Carefully stated learning objectives serve as one method for measuring the success of the session. If the objectives are learner-centered, include in the teaching plan a time frame, an action on the part of the learner that can be measured, how it can be measured, and the level of competency expected. If this is done, the evaluation becomes quite simple; that is, the teacher needs only to check to what extent the learner accomplished each objective. This can be accomplished through teacher observation, self-report on the part of the learner, and quizzes based on the objectives.

In addition to learner achievement, there are other aspects to the teaching session that the evaluator assesses. They include the effectiveness of the teacher and his or her strategies, the learning environment and materials, and the students' and teacher's satisfaction with the session. These latter assessments can be measured through surveys completed by the learners and teachers, with rating scale responses to questions or open-ended questions that are subjected to content analysis. There are many tools in the literature to measure learners' satisfaction, and several texts are especially helpful for the development of evaluation tools (Bastable, 2003; Linn & Gronlund, 2000; Rankin & Stallings, 2001). The evaluation of individual sessions is an essential link to total program evaluation and helps to demonstrate the value of the program to health agencies and their clients.

Macro-Level of Evaluation: Program Evaluation

The elements of program evaluation in staff development and health education are similar to those found in schools of nursing. The first items to assess are the congruence of the health agency's mission, philosophy, and conceptual framework to the education program. They should be in alignment, and if not, a rationale for why there is a difference should be prominent in the description of the program or the components of the education program should be adjusted to those of the parent agency. The next step is to determine to what extent the outcomes of the educational program are measured by its goals and objectives, its overall impact on the staff/clients and the community it serves, its cost effectiveness, its measure of quality compared to other staff development and community education programs, its achievement of benchmarks that the agency and program set for it, and its accreditation, licensure, or certification status. Table 13.5 summarizes the elements according to evaluation elements and the desired outcomes. As with nursing education programs, a master plan of evaluation is recommended so that evaluation becomes an ongoing process and guides the activities of the participants for total quality management.

The pyramid model of evaluation for continuing education programs described by Hawkins and Sherwood (1999) is an excellent model as a comprehensive tool for the evaluation of education programs in health care agencies. The pyramid model is based on Donabedian's (1966) structure, process, and outcome model of evaluation and the social science evaluation model developed by Rossi and Freeman (1993). It incorporates all of the elements of program and curriculum development discussed thus far in this chapter, including a look at the internal and external frame factors that impact educational programs. In addition to assessing the program design, implementation, outcomes, and impact, it addresses cost-effectiveness issues. It is a highly recommended reading for nurse educators considering the use of a master plan of evaluation for staff development and patient and family education.

Regulations and Accreditation Requirements and Standards for Practice

As an integral part of educational program development or revision, the most current regulations, standards of practice, and accreditation criteria for staff development and health education are reviewed to ensure that new and revised programs are in compliance. Moreover, it is far easier to build in mechanisms at the ground level for collecting evidence to document adherence to regulations, standards, and accreditation criteria than to retrospectively attempt to do so under the deadline of an approaching accreditation visit.

Nurse educators in states with mandatory continuing education for nurses need to review their state regulations for receiving approval for continuing education offerings in their agencies. Awarding continuing education credit is a perk that nursing staff appreciates on the part of their employers.

The current standards for staff development, *Scope and Standards of Practice for Nursing Professional Development*, were published by the ANA in 2000 (ANA, 2004). In addition, the American Nurses Association has standards of practice for many nursing specialties and settings for practice that include elements of education to apply to staff development and health education. Information on the standards is located at their website: http://nursingworld.org/anp/pdescr.cfm?CNum=15. Additional information and resources may be found at the National Nursing Staff Development Organization (NNSDO) (2004) website: http://nnsdo.org/Index.htm.

Staff educators have the responsibility for ensuring that nursing staff members are skilled teachers who can demonstrate learning outcomes and facilitate a change in client health behavior. Additionally, evaluation activities and reports contribute to the accreditation, licensure, or certification of the program and the health agency. The Joint Commission on the Accreditation of Healthcare Organizations (JCAHO) (2004) has specific goals and standards of care for patient education. Specific and additional information can be located at the JCAHO website: http://www.jcaho.org/htba/index.htm.

▲ TABLE 13.5	The Elements of an Evaluation Plan for Staff Development and Health Education	
Evaluation Element	**Questions for Data Collection**	**Desired Outcome**
Mission and overall purpose	To what extent are the mission and overall purpose of the agency and its educational program congruent?	The mission and overall purpose of the educational program are congruent with that of the agency.
Philosophy and conceptual framework	To what extent are the philosophy and conceptual framework statements congruent with the agency and program missions and purposes?	The philosophy and conceptual framework are congruent with the agency and program missions and purposes.
	To what extent is there evidence of the philosophy and conceptual framework in the objectives and implementation plan of the educational program?	The philosophy and conceptual framework are evident in the objectives and implementation plan of the educational program.
Goals (long term)	Is it evident that the overall or long-term goal(s) flow from the mission, purpose, philosophy, and conceptual framework?	The overall or long-term goal(s) flow from the mission, purpose, philosophy, and conceptual framework.
Objectives (short term) and implementation plan	Is it evident that the objectives for the program and each learning session flow from the overall goal(s) and are congruent with the mission, philosophy, and conceptual framework?	The objectives for the program and each learning session flow from the overall goal(s) and are congruent with the mission, philosophy, and conceptual framework.
	To what extent do the objectives include specification of the learner, the learning content, behavior of the learner, expected outcome, and timeframe?	The objectives are stated in such a way that they can be measured for their outcomes.
	Is there evidence that the implementation plan flows from the mission, conceptual framework, goal(s), and objectives?	The implementation plan flows from the mission, conceptual framework, goal(s), and objectives.
Cost effectiveness	What are the major sources of financial support for the program?	
	To what extent is the education program self-sufficient?	The education program is self-sufficient.
	Have other possible funding resources been identified, and are they part of a plan to secure funds?	
	To what extent does the education program contribute to the financial stability of the agency?	The education program contributes to the quality and financial stability of the agency.
	Is there a plan for either maintaining or reaching financial stability?	

(table continues on page 340)

▲ **TABLE 13.5** The Elements of an Evaluation Plan for Staff Development and Health Education (continued)

Evaluation Element	Questions for Data Collection	Desired Outcomes
Outcomes (clients and community)	To what extent do data from the assessment of the outcomes from the education program indicate achievement of its goal and objectives?	Outcomes from the education program indicate achievement of its goal and objectives.
	To what extent do clients report a high level of satisfaction with the program?	Clients report a high level of satisfaction with the program.
	Is there a plan in place to either maintain or improve outcomes?	There is a plan to maintain or improve outcomes.
	To what extent is the community aware of the agency's education program?	The community is aware of the agency's education program and holds it in high regard.
	Is there a plan in place for raising the public's awareness of the education program and its contributions to the community?	
Comparison to similar programs and benchmarks	To what extent is the education program superior to or on par with similar education programs?	The education program is superior to or on par with similar education programs.
	Does the program costs meet budget limits? To what extent does the program meets its goals and objectives each year?	The program costs meet budget limits.
	Are there plans in place to improve the program or set higher benchmarks?	The program meets its goals and objectives each year.
Accreditation, licensure, and certification	Has the program received accreditation, licensure, or certification?	
	If the program is an integral part of the health agency, to what extent does it contribute to accreditation, licensure, or certification?	Depending on the nature of the program, the education program has accreditation, licensure, or certification.
	Is there a plan in place to continually assess the program for maintenance of accreditation, licensure, or certification?	
	To what extent is there a record keeping system in place for accreditation, licensure, or certification?	

▲ BUDGET PLANNING FOR STAFF DEVELOPMENT AND PATIENT AND FAMILY EDUCATION

Nurse educators have a responsibility for planning, managing, and reporting budgets to the administration of the sponsoring health agency. It is an essential task to justify the existence of the educational program and its relevance to the mission of the agency and its service. It demonstrates cost effectiveness as well as cost recovery over the long term. For example, well-oriented new staff members and well-prepared new graduates are more apt to become long-term employees rather than entering and exiting through a revolving door. An example of cost effectiveness for health education programs is teaching the patient's lay (or family) care provider how to provide activities of daily living at home for a recovering stroke patient. This results in the need for intermittent professional services rather than frequent and costly physical therapy and skilled nursing care in the home or health care agency.

Welch, Fisher, and Dayhoff (2002) developed a worksheet for their clinical nurse specialist students to evaluate the cost effectiveness of patient education programs. It has a comprehensive cost analysis worksheet that includes the major components of patient education programs, such as community needs, indirect costs, program development, staff training, coordination activities, administrative overhead, and evaluation, and other categories such as in-kind contributions.

When preparing a budget, the first item to assess is the source of revenues. These include the income generated by the health agency through general funds (if government sponsored), patient fees, insurance programs, and Medicare and Medicaid. These sources are fairly stable but cannot always be depended upon owing to changing patient care demands and the ever-changing reimbursement or prospective pay systems. Thus, it is important for nurse educators to investigate other possible sources of income for the program, such as grants from other health-related organizations federal, state, or regional grants, benefactor gifts, or fees for services. The type of revenue will determine how it will be spent; that is, established, long-term income and resources maintain the ongoing programs, while new program development, or one-time-only programs, may be funded through short-term grants and other gift monies.

The two largest items on the debit or cost side of the budget are capital expenditures and personnel. Capital expenditures include office, classroom, and laboratory facilities that are usually shared spaces and can be calculated according to the percentage of use by the educational program. Other capital expenditures include "big ticket items," such as instructional support systems (videoconferencing, telecommunications, and web-based technology), computers, audio-visual hardware, mannequins, and large software teaching packages (e.g., a physical assessment series). While these items are usually considered on the debit side, their value can also be considered as assets with only their depreciation added to the costs each year. If the educational program expects to undergo accreditation or certification, the expenses for preparing a self-study and site visits are included.

Personnel expenses include the salaries and benefits of the educators, staff, and administrators, and, in some instances, the costs for released time of staff to attend educational programs. Each year, the budget must build in salary increases and concomitant benefit increases for the staff. The time staff members put in to mentor new employees is an additional personnel cost to be calculated.

Other expenses for the program include office supplies, books, journal subscriptions, teaching supplies, software, pamphlets, travel expenses for staff and students, continuing education and professional meetings for the educator staff members, and meals or refreshments for students or clients when attending classes.

The budget should be prepared at least 6 months in advance of its submission for approval by the administration, though the timing can differ from agency to agency. A budget prepared in advance gives administration time to review it and make decisions for the next fiscal year. It is wise to build in a contingency fund to cover any unexpected costs that the program encounters during the year. When submitting the budget, it is advisable to include an attachment with brief justifications for each item.

▲ **TABLE 13.6**   **Educational Program Budgeting**

Major Budget Item	Income or (Debit)	Items Included
Program maintenance	Income	Agency funds from fees, insurance, reimbursements, general revenues
Program development or enhancement	Income	Grants, contributions, gifts, endowments
Personnel	(Debit)	Salaries, benefits, released time
Capital expenditures	Assets and (Debit: Depreciation)	Offices, labs, classrooms, conference rooms, furniture, equipment, utilities, contracts for maintenance of equipment, major software packages
Supplies and services	(Debit)	Office and teaching supplies, texts, journal subscriptions, travel, food, and refreshments

In the ideal health education setting, the chief nurse educator manages the budget and has administrative assistance for tracking expenditures, preparing purchase orders, receiving, cataloging, inventorying equipment and supplies, and managing the payroll. Careful records are kept so that quarterly and end-of-year reports are easily assembled and provide the agency with the program's accountability as well as trends in income generation and expenditures for future planning.

While each agency has its own budget format, the items in the previous discussion can be adapted to the agency's specific format. Table 13.6 summarizes the discussion and can be applied to both staff development and health education programs.

▲ ISSUES AND TRENDS IN STAFF DEVELOPMENT AND PATIENT AND FAMILY EDUCATION

The major issues and trends in staff development and patient education are categorized as follows: the justification and funding for them; the qualifications, responsibilities, and functions of nurse educators in health agencies; and the maintenance of quality and plans for the future. With the growth of health maintenance organizations and managed care systems, educational programs play an important part in the delivery of services to their clients and to the maintenance of an adequately prepared and competent staff to serve the clients.

Nursing shortages and the growing demand for health care services result in an ever-expanding need for staff development programs. There are increasing instances of the health care delivery system entering into partnerships with schools of nursing. The nurse educator in the health agency or health care delivery system has a key role in fostering these partnerships and establishing internship programs for new graduates as well as course, certificate, or degree programs for the continuing education and career opportunities of the current staff in the agency.

Health education plays an equally important role in the services of the health care agency for the clients and community they serve. Informing the public about the health care services provided by the agency, teaching patients and families about care for rehabilitation and health maintenance, and providing health promotion and prevention of disease education programs as a community service are critical parts of the services of health care agencies. Nurse educators have an important role in planning, implementing, and evaluating these programs because they have the clinical knowledge and the pedagogical/andragogical skills that are complementary to the community's learning needs.

Justification and Funding for Educational Programs in Health Agencies

It is not unusual for health agencies experiencing budget crises to think of cutting personnel and programs associated with "nonessential" services. Educational programs are frequently the targets of such cuts in spite of the impact they have on cost savings and the delivery of quality care to the agency's staff and its clients. Earlier in the discussion on the budget for education programs, there was mention of the need to demonstrate cost effectiveness and related cost-savings from the educational program to the administration of the health agency as well as to the public or consumers of the program.

JUSTIFICATION FOR STAFF DEVELOPMENT FUNDING

The nurse educator in the health care agency can compare the major costs of bringing in traveling RNs to staff the agency to the lesser cost of providing incentives for staff retention derived from the support of new graduates through mentorship programs, continuing education programs, and in-service opportunities. As to the value of the program, the health care agency that has a satisfied staff soon sees gains in the quality of the care delivered, which, in turn, translates into patient or customer satisfaction. Magnet hospitals are excellent examples of quality care, and part of their success are staff development and educational program achievements. Information on magnet hospitals can be found at: http://www.jcaho.org/news+room/press+kits/facts+ about+ magnet+hospitals.htm (Joint Commission of Accreditation of Healthcare Organization, 2004).

JUSTIFICATION FOR HEALTH EDUCATION FUNDING

Health education programs in agencies can demonstrate cost effectiveness and, in many cases, cost-savings. Teaching staff to seize opportunities for education while caring for the patient and the family can result in the fostering of client self-care during the episode of illness and after discharge from the facility. Reinforcing the knowledge and skills gained by them throughout the stay decreases the amount of follow-up care required to ensure positive patient outcomes, thereby saving in costs and increasing the quality of care and client satisfaction.

Educational programs for aggregates save the agency the cost of individual learning sessions and enhances the experience for patients and families who have the opportunity to share their concerns with others experiencing similar health problems. These are only a few examples of how the nurse educator can demonstrate to administration and the community the value of the program and the contribution it makes to quality of care and cost effectiveness.

Qualifications, Responsibilities, and Functions of Nursing Educators

The role of the nurse educator in the practice setting is complex. Bailey et al. (1995) describe the vital role that nurse educators will play in the future in educating patients and personnel in health care systems. To support their thesis, they cite growing interest in the empowerment of clients to improve and maintain health, an increased need for management of chronic diseases, an expansion of medical technology, and an interest in cost containment by health care systems. They offer a curriculum for preparing nurse educators through a stepwise program, from a beginning pathway for the nurse to assimilate theories and principles of teaching and learning, to the implementation of instructional methods and preceptorships, to advanced teaching and learning strategies that apply critical-thinking skills and serve clients and health care staff.

As a follow-up to Bailey et al.'s recommended curriculum for nurse educators, Johnson (2002) reported on the use of an evaluation tool to assess the competencies of nurse educators to promote their professional development to reach higher levels of performance in delivering educational programs. Johnson describes a professional review process for nurse educators that includes peer review, self-evaluation, and the development of a portfolio. The process provided the desired professional development information for the nurse educators, and an added benefit was the increased services for the staff of the health care system. These services ultimately improved services for clients served by the system.

It is apparent that the educator must have a wide range of clinical knowledge and skills or the ability to identify specialists within the practice setting who can provide that knowledge for staff and clients. In addition to nursing and health care knowledge, the nurse educator needs knowledge and skills in program or curriculum development, learning theories, instructional design, teaching strategies, program evaluation, and budget management. Excellence in communications is key to building support for the program, dealing with the public and vendors, and building relationships with administrators, advisory boards, staff, school of nursing faculty and students, other agency personnel, patients, families, and the community. While many of these qualifications come with experience, additional education is recommended, preferably at the master's or doctorate level. The trend in staff development and patient education is for the nurses in these positions to have a master's degree in nursing education, a clinical specialty, or related discipline such as health education or education. The nursing degree is preferable because it combines the functions of clinical nursing, management, and education.

Maintaining Quality Programs and Planning for the Future

Heller, Oros, and Durney-Crowley (2000) discuss 10 trends in health care and nursing that have an impact on nursing education, including staff development and health education. While the article was published in 2000, it continues to be relevant to the current and future health care system and provides 10 major trends to watch as they influence education. The 10 trends are:

1. Changing demographics and increasing diversity
2. The technological explosion

3. Globalization of the world's economy and society
4. Educated consumers, alternative therapies, genomics, and palliative care
5. Shift to population-based care and increasing complexity of patient care
6. Cost of health care and challenge of managed care
7. Impact of health policy and regulation
8. Growing need for interdisciplinary education for collaborative practice
9. Workforce development
10. Advances in nursing science and research

Their reflections on these trends are helpful in planning for the future and provide guidelines for factors to assess within each trend.

The growing need for interdisciplinary collaboration and the role that education plays in fostering it is described by Parker, Thurber, and Asselin (2001). They describe a hospital-based department of nursing education that experienced a major change in its functions to become congruent with the agency's vision and mission. From their review of the literature, there was agreement that nurse educators need to widen their scope of services and include other health disciplines and services in line with the agency's vision and mission. Some of the strategies they suggest for changing the education program to meet the needs of a wider and more diverse population are: providing leadership for a network of educators throughout the institution; helping to change managers' roles from supervisors to mentors, teachers, and coaches; changing the role of nurse educators to resource persons and coordinators; promoting train-the-trainer programs; and focusing on multidisciplinary educational programs. As managed care and large health care agencies predominate the health care delivery system, these types of models of staff development and health services should increase.

In the recommendations and implications of the Pew Health Professions Commission's final report, *Recreating Nursing Practice for a New Century*, Bellack and O'Neil (2000) pose 21 competencies for the 21st century. Among those especially applicable to the role of nurse educators in staff development and health education are:

▲ "Apply knowledge of the new sciences.
▲ Demonstrate critical thinking, reflection, and problem solving skills.
▲ Integrate population-based care and services into practice.
▲ Provide culturally-sensitive care to a diverse society.
▲ Use communication and information technology effectively and appropriately.
▲ Contribute to continuous improvement of the health care system.
▲ Continue to learn and help others learn" (p.16).

These competencies serve nurse educators well in setting goals for the future. If they are integrated into the role of nurse educators, they will demonstrate to health care systems how the development of staff and the education of consumers meet the mission and purpose of health agencies.

As society places increasing value on wellness and the maintenance and promotion of health, the role of nurse educators in the practice setting will expand. Health care delivery systems view health promotion and prevention of disease as essential elements of their services to the public, and nursing is a profession that has the credentials for initiating these programs. Nurse educators are found in all manners of settings, such as schools, industry, acute-care facilities, nursing homes, extended care, home care, public health, and other health-related community agencies. Their services provide quality health care education for the clients of the agencies and, in the long term, promote the health of the population. Nurse educators as a group should examine the issues in nursing education and practice and health care for the future and join forces to promote the important role of nurse educators in shaping public policy to improve health care and reach optimal health for all people.

▲ SUMMARY

The two major roles of nurse educators in the practice setting for staff development and client-centered health education were reviewed. The adaptation of a needs assessment and the curriculum's components to the development of staff and health education programs were summarized and compared to those in the development of nursing education programs. Learning theories applied to staff development and health education and to teaching strategies in the practice setting were reviewed. Evaluation methodologies in staff development and health education, including regulation, accreditation, standard of practice, and total quality management, were discussed. Cost effectiveness, an important aspect to educational programs in health care systems, and guidelines for developing budgets were outlined in a table. Major issues facing education in the practice setting were examined and trends for the future were analyzed.

DISCUSSION QUESTIONS

1. In what way(s) do you believe nursing shortages have an effect on the delivery of staff development and health education programs in the practice setting? Explain your answer and offer solutions to any problems you identify.
2. Is it or is it not important for a nurse educator to be able to prepare, manage, and evaluate the budget of an education program? Explain your answer.

LEARNING ACTIVITIES

1. Select an education program in a health agency and assess it for its recognition of the impact of the external and internal frame factors on the program. Evaluate the program according to the classic components of curriculum development and evaluation. Include an analysis of the evaluation plan in place for individual sessions and the program as a whole. Is there evidence that the data collected for evaluation are used to revise the program and improve quality? Analyze the budget of the program for its relationship to the mission and goals of the agency and the education program. Based upon your analyses, how would you revise the program?

REFERENCES

Abruzzese, R. S. (1996). *Nursing staff development: Strategies for success* (2nd ed.). St. Louis: Mosby.
American Nurses Association's Nursing Standards (2004). *ANA nursing standards.* Retrieved June 17, 2004, from, http://nursingworld.org/books/pdescr.cfm?CNum=15
Bailey, K., Hoeppner, M., Jeska, S., Schneller, S., & Wolohan, C. (1995). The nurse as educator. *Journal of Nursing Staff Development, 11*(4), 205–209.

Bandura, A. (1997). *Self-efficacy. The exercise of control.* New York: W.H. Freeman.

Bastable, S. B. (2003). *Nurse as educator. Principles of teaching and learning for nursing practice* (2nd ed). Boston: Jones and Bartlett.

Bellack, J. P., & O'Neil, E. H. (2000). Recreating nursing practice for a new century. Recommendations and implications. *Nursing and Health Care Perspectives, 21*(1), 14–21.

Benner, P. (1984). *From novice to expert: Excellence and power in clinical practice.* Menlo Park: CA: Addison-Wesley.

Billings, D. M., & Rowles, C. J. (2001). Development of continuing nursing education offerings for the world wide web. *The Journal of Continuing Education in Nursing, 32*(3), 107–133.

DeOnna, J. (2002). DACUM: A versatile competency-based framework for Staff Development. *Journal for Nurses in Staff Development, 18*(1), 5–13.

Donabedian, A. (1966). Evaluating the quality of medical care. *Milbank Memorial Fund Quarterly, 44*(Part 2), 166–206.

Fey, M. K., & Miltner, R. S. (2000). A competency-based orientation program for new graduate nurses. *Journal of Nursing Administration, 30*(3), 126–132.

Gilbert, G. G., & Sawyer, R. G. (2000). *Health education creating strategies for school and community health* (2nd ed). Boston: Jones and Bartlett.

Havice, P.A., & Knowles, M. H. (1995). Two-way interactive video: Maximizing distance learning. *The Journal of Continuing Education in Nursing, 26*(1), 28–30.

Hawkins, V. E., & Sherwood, G. D. (1999). The Pyramid model: An integrated approach for evaluation continuing education programs and outcomes. *The Journal of Continuing Education in Nursing, 30*(5), 203–212.

Hayes, K., Huckstadt, A., & Gibson, R. (2000). Developing interactive continuing education on the web. *The Journal of Continuing Education in Nursing, 31*(5), 199–203.

Heller, B. R., Oros, M. T., & Durney-Crowley, J. (2000). The future of nursing education. Ten trends to watch. *Nursing and Health Care Perspectives, 21*(1), 9–13.

Hom, E. M. (2003). Coaching and mentoring new graduates entering perinatal nursing practice. *Journal of Perinatal & Neonatal Nursing, 17*(1), 35–49.

Huff, R. M., & Kline, M. V. (1999). *Promoting health in multicultural populations: A handbook for practitioners.* Thousand Oaks, CA: Sage Publications.

Ingalls, J. D. (1972). *A trainer's guide to andragogy* (rev. ed) (017-061-00033-0). Washington, DC: U.S. Department of Health, Education and Welfare.

Johnson, M. (1977). *Intentionality in education.* (Distributed by the Center for Curriculum Research and Services, Albany, N.Y.). Troy, NY: Walter Snyder, Printer, Inc.

Johnson, S. (2002). Development of educator competencies and the professional review process. *Journal for Nurses in Staff Development, 18*(2), 92–102.

Joint Commission of Accreditation of Healthcare Organizations. (2004). *Facts about American Nurses Credentialing Center magnet recognition program.* Retrieved June 17, 2004, from http://www.jcaho.org/news+room/press+kits/facts+about+magnet+hospitals.htm

Joint Commission of the Accreditation of Healthcare Organizations. (2004). *Setting the standard for care. How to become accredited.* Retrieved June 17, 2004, from http://www.jcaho.org/htba/index.htm

Kee, G., & Ryser, F. (2001). Work-study-scholarship program for undergraduate nursing students: A win-win service education partnership. *Nursing Administration Quarterly, 26*(1), 29–34.

Kells, K., & Koerner, D. K. (2000). Supporting the new nurse in practice. *Kansas State Nurses Association, 75*(7), 1–2.

Knowles, M. S., Holton, E. F., & Swanson, R. A. (1998). *The adult learner: The definitive classic in adult education and human resource development.* (5th ed.). Houston, TX: Gulf Publishing.

Krozak, C. (2001). Implementing a nursing new graduate mentoring program (Number 2002117989). *CINAHL Information Systems,* 1–8. Glendale, CA: CINAHL.

Lindeman, C. A. (2000). The future of nursing education. *Journal of Nursing Education, 39*(1), 5–12.

Linn, R. L., & Gronlund, N. E. (2000). *Measurement and Assessment in Teaching* (8th ed.). Upper Saddle River, NJ: Prentice Hall.

Lundgren, B. S., & Houseman, C. A. (2002). Continuing competence in selected health professions. *Journal of Allied Health, 31*(4), 233–240.

Mager, R. F., & Pipe, P. (1970). *Analyzing performance problems.* Beaumont, CA: Fearon.

McKenzie, J. F., & Smeltzer, J. L. (1997). *Planning, implementing and evaluating health promotion programs* (2nd ed.). Boston: Allyn and Bacon.

Merriam-Webster Collegiate Dictionary. Merriam-Webster Online (2004). Retrieved November 2, 2004, from http://80-search.eb.com.hokhmah .stmarysca.edu:2048/dictionary

Murray, R. B., & Zentner, J. P. (2001). *Health promotion strategies through the life span* (7th ed.). Upper Saddle River, NJ: Prentice Hall.

National Council of State Boards of Nursing. (1996). *Assuring competence.* A regulatory responsibility National Council Position Paper. Retrieved June 17, 2004, from http://www.ncsbn.org/public/about/reports/pospapers96.htm

National Nursing Staff Development Organization (NNSDO). Home Page (2004). Retrieved June 18, 2004, from http://nnsdo.org/

Bridging the gap between academia and the working world. (2000). *Nebraska Nurse., 33*(2), 26.

O'Neil, E. H., & the Pew Health Commission. (1998). *Recreating health professional practice for the new century.* San Francisco: Pew Health Professions Commission.

Parker, E. D., Thurber, R. F., & Asselin, M. E. (2001). Making the transition to a hospital-wide department of education: Strategies for success. *Journal for Nurses in Staff Development, 17*(4), 175–181.

Pearson, J. (2003). How nurse preceptors influence new graduates. *Critical Care Nurse, 23*(1), 26–28.

Pender, N. J., Murdaugh, C. L., & Parsons, M. A. (2002). *Health promotion in nursing Practice* (4th ed.). Upper Saddle River, NJ: Prentice Hall.

Rankin, S. H., & Stallings, K. D. (2001). *Patient education principles and practice* (4th ed.). Philadelphia: Lippincott.

Robles, H. J. (1998, March 28). Andragogy. The adult learner and faculty as learners. US Department of Education. Educational Resources Information (ERIC document Reproduction Service No. ED426740).

Rossi, P. H., & Freeman, H. E. (1993). *Evaluation: A systematic approach.* Thousand Oaks, CA: Sage Publications.

Roter, D. L., Stashefsky-Margalit, R., & Rudd, R. (2001). Current perspectives on patient education in the US. *Patient Education and Counseling, 44,* 79–86.

Saarmann, L., Daugherty, J., & Riegel, B. (2000). Patient teaching to promote behavioral change. *Nursing Outlook, 48*(6), 281–287.

Sallis, E. (2002). *Total quality management in education* (3rd ed.). London: Kogan Page, Ltd.

Sparling, L. A. (2001). Enhancing the learning in self-directed learning modules. *Journal for Nurses in Staff Development, 17*(4), 199–205.

Sproat, S. B. (2002). Principles of web site development and design. *Journal for Nurses in Staff Development, 18*(2), 72.

Tomey, A. M. (2003). Learning with cases. *The Journal of Continuing Education in Nursing, 34*(1), 34–38.

Welch, J. L., Fisher, M. L., & Dayhoff, N. E. (2002). A cost-effectiveness worksheet for patient-education programs. *Clinical Nurse Specialist, 16*(4), 187–192.

Wolford, R. A., & Hughes, L. K. (2001). Using the hospital intranet to meet competency standards for nurses. *Journal for Nurses in Staff Development, 17*(4), 182–189.

Issues and Trends in Curriculum Development and Evaluation

▼

Sarah B. Keating, EdD, RN, FAAN

7

▲ OVERVIEW

Section 7 reviews current trends and issues in nursing education for their effects on curricula and the imperatives derived from them that should influence curriculum development and evaluation activities now and in the future. This section addresses a specific trend in nursing education (i.e., the growth of technology-driven distance education programs) that had a dramatic influence on the delivery of education in the late twentieth and early twenty-first centuries.

Chapter 14 examines distance education and its influence on nursing education. It traces the history of distance education from the early home study programs to today's high technology–based programs delivered from home campuses to distant satellite campuses as well as virtual campuses in cyberspace. The various methods for delivery of educational programs and their advantages and disadvantages are reviewed.

Through the rapid growth of technology and the development of user-friendly instructional packages, nursing programs developed both undergraduate and graduate programs that favor students who have limited access to education, owing to distance problems, and who lack available time to attend on-campus classes. Studies to measure the number of available distance education programs, their quality, and cost effectiveness are few or outdated because programs have multiplied so rapidly that the literature cannot keep pace with the growth. However, the trend to develop these types of programs remains high, and feedback from existing programs lends itself to the development of curricula that include the use of technology and evaluation methodologies specific to distance education.

Chapter 15 reexamines some of the issues raised in the text and offers some solutions for them that could affect the future of nursing education. A look at nursing education in hindsight leads to a forecast of the future, including several scenarios for education and their impact on the profession. Members of the nursing profession are asked to discard old prohibitive ways of thinking about nursing education and to move into the future with innovative and creative nursing programs that continue to educate nurses who are knowledgeable, competent, and caring professionals ready for the challenges of meeting the population's health care needs and demands of the health care system. At the same, nursing education programs must eliminate past barriers to nursing education that prohibited nurses from returning to school for higher education so that nurses are prepared to meet current and future complex health care system needs.

Several curricula are proposed with new ways to embrace the traditional career ladder feature of nursing and at the same time facilitate a nonstop quality education ending in a doctorate that produces nurse researchers, theorists, clinicians, and educators. The proposed curricula are not meant as templates, but rather as stimulants for discussion among nurse educators and those in practice to bring about the needed changes for nursing education now and in the future.

The issues and challenges raised throughout the text can change the face of nursing education and the profession, or they can be ignored and old, traditional ways of curriculum development and evaluation can continue to dominate the education scene. Unfortunately, if changes are not made, the profession may find itself outdated, unable to keep up with changes in the health care system and meet the needs of the populations it purports to serve, and out of sync with other health care disciplines. Chapters 14 and 15 begin the discussion for nurse educators and their plans for the future.

Distance Learning

▼

Sarah B. Keating, EdD, RN, FAAN

OBJECTIVES

Upon completion of Chapter 14, the reader will be able to:

1. Compare the various types of distance education programs that are utilized in the delivery of nursing education programs.
2. Analyze the role of faculty and administrators in the development of distance education programs.
3. Apply curriculum development and evaluation strategies to the development of distance education programs.
4. Analyze the trends in delivering nursing education through distance education modalities.
5. Examine the issues facing nurse educators that relate to distance education programs.

14

▲ OVERVIEW

Distance education is defined as any learning experience that takes place a distance away from the parent institution's home campus or central headquarters. It can be as close as a few blocks away in an urban center to as far away as another nation(s). It implements the curriculum through a planned strategy for the delivery of courses or classes that include off-site satellite classes managed by the home faculty or credentialed off-site faculty, broadcast of classes through videoconferencing and teleconferencing to off-campus sites, Web-based instruction, and faculty-supervised clinical experiences including preceptorships and internships. Distance education offers continuing education programs, degree programs, single academic courses, or a mixture of on-campus and off-campus course offerings.

The history of early education programs that still play a major role today in the delivery of curricula to distant sites from the parent institution is traced. A discussion of the types of distance education programs and details on teleconferencing and Web-based instruction follows. A needs assessment and the adaptation of the components of the curriculum to distance education programs are reviewed. Table 14.1 summarizes the guidelines for the development of distance education programs. Faculty's role in developing online courses along with a review of the research findings on the efficacy of the programs is presented. The chapter closes with a case study that exemplifies planning for the development of a distance education program based on the case study presented in Chapters 5, 6, and 7.

▲ HISTORY OF DISTANCE EDUCATION

Armstrong, Gessner, and Cooper (2000) provide a history of the use of distance education strategies, including those adapted by nursing starting from 1873 with home-based studies to the delivery of classes via radio in the 1920s, multiuser telephone communications in the 1950s, television and two-way televised communications in the 1960s, and, finally, to Web-based education in the 1990s. Armstrong et al. present an overview of the major types of methods utilized for distance education and advice on how to create a humanistic learning environment for distance education programs. The authors conclude with a look ahead at societal and technological changes that will influence nursing and education and the challenges that nurse educators face in developing education programs that meet the needs of learners.

To place the growth of distance education programs into perspective, the U.S. Department of Education stated that during the years 2000–2001, 56% of the 2- and 4-year institutions in the United States offered distance education, and another 12% planned to start courses within the next 3 years. During the same time period, 90% of public 2-year institutions and 89% of public 4-year institutions offered distance education courses, compared to 16% of private 2-year and 40% of private 4-year institutions. Fifty-two percent of undergraduate programs offered courses for credit, while 52% of the graduate and first-professional degree programs offered credit-granting courses (U.S. Department of Education Institute of Education Sciences, 2004).

The survey identified 127,400 different distance education courses compared to the 54,470 courses identified in 1999. In 2000–2001, there was a total of 3,007,000 enrollments compared "an estimated 1,661,100 enrollments in all distance education courses and 1.363,670 enrollments in college-level credit-granting distance education courses with most of those at the undergraduate level" in 1999 (U.S. Department of Education Institute of Education Sciences, 2004).

▲ TYPES OF DISTANCE EDUCATION PROGRAMS

There are a variety of distance education programs. For an overview of the types, Sackett, Dickerson, McCartney, and Erdley (2001) describe multiple technology-supported strategies for nursing education used in New York. The strategies include Web-based instruction, video-conferencing, the use of Internet resources, and computer-controlled mannequins that are utilized by undergraduate and graduate programs alike. The article gives examples of the use of each type of strategy and presents ideas for faculty who are considering technology-supported instructional designs.

This author has experience with the delivery of off-campus satellite theory and clinical courses, videoconferencing, satellite broadcasting, and Web-based courses. To follow are descriptions of each type and the pros and cons for them from the author's personal perspective as well as from the literature.

Satellite Campuses

For the purposes of this discussion, satellite campuses are defined as those programs that offer the curriculum in whole or in part in off-campus sites from the parent institution. While they can incorporate technology methods such as videoconferencing and Web-based instruction, the majority of the teaching and learning takes place in classrooms and involves in-person interactions between the faculty and students. Faculty members who teach in the parent institution serve as on-site faculty or act as consultants to off-site faculty who teach the same curriculum. For those faculty members on the home campus who actually teach in the satellite, travel costs and the related time it takes for travel are included in the costs. These costs are weighed against the cost of hiring on-site faculty and part-time versus full-time faculty and their impact on the quality of the program.

There are challenges to finding off-site faculty members who are qualified to teach the subject matter, and they must be oriented to the curriculum to ensure its integrity. Thus, it is not unusual for the parent institution to have an academic manager for the satellite program(s) who can serve as the curriculum and academic services coordinator. In the instances of off-site satellite campuses, the course content and materials for both theory and clinical are identical to that of the home campus. Special events to link the off-site and home campuses are often planned to foster the socialization process for students and faculty so that there is a milieu of all people belonging to the same institution.

Additional resources are needed to implement the satellite campus, such as students' access to texts either through the home bookstore or other resources (e.g., online book companies); library access; online access if it is part of the curriculum; and student services including academic, financial aid, and personal counseling usually through the on-site coordinator and his or her staff. Recruitment, admission, and enrollment services are additional resources that are served by on-site personnel if the program is large or, if small, by home-campus staff that travel periodically to the satellite campus.

Some of the arguments against these types of programs are the loss of students on the home campus; possible incongruence between the implementation of the courses in the curriculum owing to a loss of interaction among students and faculty with the home campus; a danger that the majority of the faculty and staff are part time and, therefore, some of the commitment to the institution is lost; and the possibility that the program is too costly and cannot become self-sufficient. Some of the arguments for these types of distance education programs include the interpersonal communications and relationships between faculty and students, a sense of belonging to the parent institution through face-to-face encounters on campus or other locations, and proximity of classes to the students' home communities.

Videoconferencing and Broadcasting Through Teleconferencing

Videoconferencing and teleconferencing require an infrastructure for cable television or closed-circuit television, dedicated classrooms that can both broadcast and receive communications, and technological support staff who manage the broadcasting and hardware and software for instructional support purposes. Unless the sessions are taped and can be shown after the session for independent viewing, the scheduling of the classes is time-certain and cannot be changed owing to the demand for the services by other entities. Yeaworth (1996) discusses the advantages to educational programs that work through consortia for videoconferencing. These consortia allow experienced faculty in the technology to share their expertise with less experienced faculty from other institutions. Advantages to these arrangements include quality control and lessening of conflicts of interest among the participating programs. The article describes several satellite networks and their operation, which can serve as models for persons interested in forming consortia.

Allen and Nero (1999) describe a partnership between two types of nursing educational programs: a community college and a baccalaureate program. In this instance, an Associate Degree in Nursing (ADN) to a Bachelor of Science in Nursing (BSN) program offered courses for nurses through videoconferencing. To supplement the video broadcasting, each interactive classroom gave access to students by telephone, fax, e-mail, and conference calls. The program was very successful, and the article provides many ideas for the development of partnerships between both levels of education. It discusses the added bonus of communication and collaboration between the faculties of both the ADN and BSN programs.

As with all delivery modes, the courses and/or classes offered through videoconferencing must be congruent with the curriculum and follow its goals and objectives. Videoconferencing includes all of the usual teaching methods and resources, such as lectures and the use of overhead projectors, slides, videotapes, movies, and PowerPoint presentations. Students and faculty can interact in real time through exchanges on-camera, telephone, or Web-based live chat rooms. These types of interactions require telecommunication and Web-based systems as well as satellite broadcasting systems.

Negative aspects to this type of delivery of distance education programs are the expenses related to it, such as the hardware and technical staffing, inflexible time frames, and the need for faculty expertise in a variety of teaching media. Positive aspects include real-time, live interactions between faculty and students; a wide array of available resources; delivery of the same subject matter to more than one audience and, therefore, to more students; and the likelihood that the integrity of the curriculum is maintained.

Online and Web-based Course Development

Online and Web-based instruction had their beginnings through faculty and student use of communication tools such as list-serves and e-mails and access to resources and references on the World Wide Web. In the 1990s and early 21st century, the use of Web-based instruction through learning management systems became more prevalent. They proved so popular with students that some courses are offered as a combination of Web-based and on-campus instruction classes for home campus students as well as for off-campus students. Web-based instruction is usually delivered through the use of learning management systems for which the institution has a contract. As the popularity of this method of teaching and learning increased, the systems grew in complexity but at the same time became more user-friendly. Thus, there are many products on the market that meet most of the needs of both novice and experienced faculty and students.

Web-based teaching and learning requires a learning management system, computer access to the web by faculty and students, technological support through the use of instructional support staff, and training sessions for faculty and students who are not familiar with the system. Some institutions of higher learning have experienced technical and instructional support staff and faculty who actually develop and manage courses for teachers who only have responsibility for the actual teaching or implementation of the course. This method provides technical support for teaching faculty; however, it may remove some of the academic freedom from the teacher-of-record. For example, the teacher does not have the ability to change course assignments or formats without going through the support staff that makes the changes. It can also prove to be expensive because the institution is paying for several staff members when only one may be required.

The initial time spent in converting a traditional course to a Web-based course is great and, as with all courses, requires updating and revisions each subsequent time it is taught. Multiple learning activities are available through the Internet, such as real-time chat rooms when students and faculty meet at a prearranged time and discuss topics or review questions about course assignments. Asynchronous entries (occurring at various times) about selected topics provide the students and faculty with opportunities to discuss topics and present their ideas and views on them. Another form of asynchronous communication is "threaded discussions." Threaded discussions allow students and faculty to interact on one topic within the course and to track the interactions related to that topic or thread. The discussion assignments usually require reading assignments or a review of the literature so that the exchanges are scholarly treatises on the subjects.

Faculty can post a lecture through an essay or PowerPoint presentation that includes notes, illustrations, references to URLs, videotapes, movies, and other audio-visual media and pose thought questions for discussions related to the "lecture." Group work assignments are possible through the use of chat rooms, threaded discussions, and e-mail communications. Many of the learning management systems have programs that give faculty the ability to develop surveys and examinations that are secure and provide statistical analyses of the results.

Larsen, Logan, and Pryor (2003) describe a statewide program for master's level courses, specifically clinical specialists. This article is very useful for faculty who plan to use learning management systems to develop online courses. The article describes a consortium of Louisiana schools that developed online courses for preparing advanced-practice nurses. It includes a literature review, background of the schools (equivalent to a needs assessment of the external and internal frame factors), the planning stage (including examining the curriculum to ensure its integrity), and the redesign of courses to fit the distance education modality. The authors describe the courses, including the use of Web-based technology to supplement the preceptor course for clinical experiences. They offer ideas for evaluating the success of the program and ways in which they will use the experience to continue to develop the program.

Pinch and Graves (2000) describe the use of a specific Web-based discussion learning management system. It was applied to the delivery of a course in bioethics. The authors found it to be a very satisfactory method for stimulating class discussion and remark that even reticent students participated in the discussion. They report that for the most part, students and faculty were satisfied with this method of teaching and learning; however, they believe that owing to the nature of the course, it could be enriched through interdisciplinary experiences.

Some of the disadvantages of online systems are the need for technological support; initial and ongoing costs related to contracts for learning management systems and computers; the lack of face-to-face encounters between faculty and students; the large amount of faculty time consumed in preparing the course; the possible loss of nursing values such as visible and tactile communications; and a sense of belonging to the home campus. Advantages include flexible times for students and faculty, multiple learning and teaching strategies, active participation on the part of all students, moderate maintenance times for managing and updating the course once it is developed, and assurance of curriculum integrity.

Clinical Courses and Distance Education

It is possible to provide quality clinical experiences for students through distance education modalities. For example, an off-site satellite campus with on-site faculty usually provides clinical experiences in the "traditional" mode. Faculty develops the clinical courses, including skills laboratory courses, according to the implementation plan of the curriculum. Students are assigned to clinical laboratories for the acquisition of assessment and clinical skills as well as to health care agencies for supervised clinical experiences. The latter are under the supervision of faculty members who either directly supervise a group of students in the clinical setting or coordinate student preceptorships, where students are assigned to qualified staff nurse preceptors.

With careful planning, it is possible to provide clinical experiences for students enrolled in courses through videoconferencing or teleconferencing and Web-based instruction. Keeping in mind that course objectives must remain the same to ensure the integrity of the curriculum, faculty responsible for clinical courses designs the courses so that their didactic and discussion components are delivered through the selected distance education technology. Assignments, logs, or journals describing the clinical experiences, examinations, pre- and postconferences can also take place through technology and can be asynchronous (occurring at various times) or synchronous (simultaneous). The actual clinical experiences occur through faculty-coordinated preceptorships, local faculty hired by the institution for clinical supervision of students, or faculty traveling to clinical sites to supervise groups of students.

When faculty members serve as coordinators for precepted clinical experiences, they must secure agreements and contracts between the educational program and the health care agency and preceptor. Other responsibilities include:

1. Setting standards for the qualifications of the preceptors
2. Orienting the preceptors to the curriculum, the course, and the role of preceptors
3. Providing guidance throughout the experience to the preceptors and students

4. Developing a communications network for participants that provides immediate or short-term turnaround time
5. Participating with preceptors and students in the assignment of grades
6. Supervising preceptors and students
7. Evaluating and revising the program based on achievement of the goals and feedback from all participants

A review of the literature provided a few articles that discuss distance education and clinical experiences. DeBourgh (2001) describes the integration of web technology into a clinical nursing course. This strategy involves students, faculty, and clinical staff in accessing and applying knowledge from the Internet, electronic resources, and references to clinical situations. It is an apprenticeship of sorts that includes stimulating the cognitive domain of knowledge (i.e., the what and how applied to clinical settings); communication by interactions between the students and professionals through the use of coaching by the instructor and threaded discussions between students and faculty; and a reflective journal by the student that helps him or her identify relationships among clinical experiences and personal and professional philosophies. The latter leads to critical thinking and, eventually, to clinical judgment.

Ndiwane (2001) reported on an international exchange program between nursing programs in Finland and the United States. Students in a community health nursing course from the United States spent 10 weeks in Finland for a clinical experience. Through this experience, they learned about a different culture and language. While the number of students was small, this experience serves as a model for international exchange programs in nursing and the use of Web-based technology in support of clinical experiences.

Johnson (1999) studied clinical preceptorships for registered nurse (RN) students enrolled in distance education programs in California. The advantages, such as students' gain in leadership and management skills through the preceptorships and the fostering of collaboration between educational institutions and health care settings, are discussed. There were several articles related to clinical experiences at the graduate level. Treistman and Fullerton (1996) describe a computer-mediated clinical experience for nurse midwife students who are supervised and evaluated by community-based faculty in their areas. They discuss advantages such as student access to current clinical science, increased numbers of students, and cost effectiveness. Sobralske and Naegele (2001) discuss nurse practitioner clinical experiences, including aspects of distance education preceptorships. The article is especially helpful in describing the important role that clinical coordinators play in the placement, coordination, and evaluation of nurse practitioner education programs.

▲ NEEDS ASSESSMENT ADAPTED TO DISTANCE EDUCATION

When planning for a distance education program, nurse educators must have supporting data from an assessment of the external and internal frame factors that document the need for a distance education program. Included is the projected success of the program based on a cost analysis, business plan, and assured applicant pool. The following discussion reviews the assessment of external and internal frame factors that can influence the development of distance education programs.

External Frame Factors

Assessment of the external frame factors contributes to the feasibility of developing a distance education program. The external frame factors include an assessment of the community where the off-site courses or classes will take place, with such factors as community location and receptivity to distance education, the population's characteristics and its sophistication in technology, the delivery of education away from the home campus, and the ability to create an academic setting away from the home campus being explored. Additional external frame factor considerations include the political climate and body politic—that is, the openness to off-site educational programs and possible competitive issues from vendors of distance education programs and other nursing education programs that serve the region. The health care system and health needs of the populace have an influence on the program as to how graduates of the program can serve them. It is necessary to learn if there are potential collaborative opportunities to supply the program with potential students from the staff of the health care agencies who are interested in furthering their education.

A demonstrated need for an academic distance education program includes an adequate potential student body that will continue for at least 5 years, support from the members of the nursing profession in the region that is to be served, and national, regional, and state regulations and accreditation agencies' approvals. Usually, the sponsoring educational program must notify all accrediting and approval agencies of its plans to offer the distance education program with each of these agencies requiring specific descriptions of the program, including the potential student body, faculty, curriculum plan, academic and capital infrastructure support systems, timelines, plans for evaluation, and, most important, financial feasibility with a business plan.

Internal Frame Factors

Much like the external frame factors, a review of the internal frame factors provides additional information in the planning for a distance education program. Of prime concern is the support of the parent academic institution and its experience with distance education programs. If the institution has a history of managing these types of programs, it is more apt to be supportive of the nursing program. Even more advantageous is an established distance education program that exists in the proposed delivery site, including cyberspace.

A check with the mission and purpose, philosophy, and goals of the parent institution and the nursing program is needed to ensure that the distance education program is in congruence. The internal economic situation and its influence on distance education programs are critical to the financial feasibility of the program. If prior distance education programs have demonstrated success in bringing revenues to the program or are, at the least, self-sufficient, it is more likely that new programs will be supported. Otherwise, a rationale with plans for initial grant support, start-up finds, and eventual self-sufficiency is required and should be submitted to the administration for its review and approval. The plans should include the resources that are required from the parent institution, some of which follow:

1. Off-site offices, laboratories, and classrooms
2. Clinical experience facilities
3. Technological support systems for videoconferencing, teleconferencing, and Web-based instruction

4. Administrative, faculty, and staff expenses
5. Academic support systems such as library, academic, and student services
6. A list of potential administrators, staff, and faculty and the proposed program's student body characteristics

Economic Feasibility and Cost Issues

If the recommendations from the needs assessment demonstrate that the distance education program is viable, the school of nursing or parent institution's chief financial officer develops a detailed business plan. The first and foremost cost issue to address is the economic feasibility of the distance education program based on an analysis of expected start-up costs, administrative costs, required number of faculty and staff, capital expenses (on-site facilities and technology support systems), and academic support (recruitment, admission, records, library access, and student support systems). The expected start-up costs include administrative, staff, and faculty costs in time and associated expenses incurred when conducting the needs assessment. Many times this becomes a write-off at the expense of the nursing program and is financed through contingency funds or program development support funds generated from grant overhead costs.

The administration's role and costs include supervisory or management functions to implement the program, such as budget and personnel management, liaison activities with regional stakeholders, public relations, coordination, marketing plans, and preparation of reports to seek approval and accreditation of the distance education program from relevant agencies. Some of the staff and/or faculty cost considerations are the required full-time and part-time equivalents, benefits, travel and other expenses, supplies, and equipment. Indirect costs should be calculated and include infrastructure support (e.g., physical facilities and their maintenance and administrative and staff services).

These expenses vary according to the selected method of delivery of the educational program. For example, off-site offices, classrooms, and lab facilities are necessary for satellite courses or classes conducted by on-site faculty or traveling faculty from the home campus. Expenses for this type of program are rent; telephones; computer support for faculty, staff, and students; and the usual office and classroom teaching supplies, hardware, and software, such as computers, printers, audio-visual hardware and software, laboratory supplies, paper, correspondence materials, desks, chairs, laboratory clinical equipment and supplies, etc.

An additional example of administrative costs applies to distance education programs that choose to deliver the program through videoconferencing and/or telecommunications. Videoconferencing requires dedicated classrooms that can send and receive satellite broadcasting both on-site at the home campus and off-site at the distant campus(es). The ideal videoconferencing system has classrooms located on all sites with the ability to send and receive, thus facilitating live interactive teaching and learning experiences among students and faculty. However, some off-site campuses might have only reception ability, therefore limiting live interactions with other students and faculty except, perhaps, by telephoning in to facilitate audio communication or communicating by computer using chat rooms, e-mail messages, or list-serve systems.

While the videoconferencing method of distance education is expensive, the success rate is high for state- and regionally supported academic programs with satellite capabilities among the various levels of higher education (e.g., community colleges and state university systems). Additionally, partnerships between educational institutions and health care organizations that use satellite videoconferencing for staff development and patient and family education services benefit both partners.

The advantage to academic nursing programs for entering into these types of arrangements with established health care systems is the tremendous cost savings for initiating and maintaining the program. The disadvantage is that unless nursing was an early pioneer in the delivery system and has a major role in it, it may face implementation problems, such as least desirable times for broadcasting and possible displacement of class times owing to the priority rights of the sponsoring agency.

Web-based delivery of distance education programs has its associated costs as well, such as contracts with learning management systems. Some examples of these systems are Blackboard (2004), eCollege (2004), IBM Lotus (2004), and WebCT (2004). Other related costs include instructional support professional and technical staff; hardware, such as computers, for faculty and student use; costs for students and faculty to access courses, the library, and other remote resources; and computer classrooms and labs for training purposes. As the programs become more prevalent, it is likely that costs will decrease, owing to the larger and more competitive market for these types of products.

There are interesting combinations of all of these delivery methods to include both technology and more traditional methods such as facsimiles, telephone conferences, videotapes, and hard copy learning materials.

Congruence With the Components of the Curriculum

Once the needs assessment of the external and internal frame factors is completed and an analysis of the costs of the program demonstrates financial feasibility, a decision to offer the program is made. A timeframe for launching the program is set. Faculty, administrators, and staff initiate the planning process for the curriculum. Faculty, in particular, reviews the components of the curriculum to ensure congruence with the originating educational program (i.e., mission, philosophy, organizational framework, goals, and objectives).

▲ DEVELOPMENT OF DISTANCE EDUCATION PROGRAMS

The following presents an overview of the faculty role in the development of distance education programs. Selection of the delivery model for the curriculum follows, with a look at the application of teaching and learning theories and the integration of nursing values into the curriculum.

Faculty Role

The role of faculty in distance education programs is to adapt portions of the curriculum, such as individual classes and courses, both theory and clinical, to distance-learning modalities. To accomplish this task, faculty with experience in these modalities may choose to develop the courses independently, much the same as in traditional teaching–learning situations. However, faculty without experience need the support of administration to work with experienced faculty or instructional support staff, who can provide the academic and technical aspects of adapting the curriculum to distance education designs.

As Care and Scanlon (2000) point out, faculty choose how they will convert traditional classes to distance education methods. They studied how faculty in one baccalaureate and graduate program went about converting their courses. Eleven faculty members were interviewed about their experiences, and based on the interviews, they identified many issues that should be addressed before and during the development of distance education programs. These issues include the need for faculty expertise in distance education, including technology, workload, ownership of course materials, copyright issues, unexpected costs, and distance education concerns related to its application to scholarship and promotion and tenure concerns.

Koeckeritz, Malkiewicz, and Henderson (2002) list seven principles of good teaching practice for teachers to apply to nursing education in the online format. They reiterate that successful online programs result from the faculty's careful planning, development, implementation, communication, and interest in the students and their learning. The seven principles are as follows:

1. Encourages student and faculty contact
2. Encourages cooperation among students
3. Encourages active learning
4. Gives prompt feedback
5. Emphasizes time on task
6. Communicates high expectations
7. Respects diverse talents and ways of learning

Cravener (1999) reviewed the literature for faculty perspectives on advantages and disadvantages of computer-mediated distance education programs compared to traditional methods of teaching. Faculty listed both challenges and benefits to online teaching, which Cravener classified into four major categories: faculty workload, access to education, adapting to technology, and instructional quality. Challenges were predominantly in the workload, technology, and course management categories, while benefits mostly related to expanding students' access to resources, individualized instruction, and the promotion of active learning among students located in various geographic regions.

Delivery Model Selection and Implementation

Though course objectives remain the same in distance education programs, faculty members are free to utilize multiple teaching and learning strategies in the delivery of the programs. Videoconferencing and telecommunications allow for live visual and audio contact. Sending digital photographs on the web provides some visual contacts for students and faculty in Web-based courses. Periodic meetings on campus or at other sites during the semester for distance education courses give students and faculty Web-based face-to-face encounters they sometimes desire. An overriding principle when designing courses for distance education is that the integrity of the curriculum is protected; for example, the course objectives, level objectives, and their relationship to the program goal(s) do not change.

An excellent resource for faculty to design distance education courses is available at http://www.ihets.org. It consists of *Guiding Principles for Faculty in Distance Education* and was developed by the Working Group of the Indiana Partnership for Statewide Education (Indiana Higher Education Telecommunication System, 2004). An additional resource for faculty in designing and evaluating Web-based courses may be found at http://www.adec.edu/admin/papers/distance-teaching_principles.html (American Distance Education Consortium, 2004).

Teaching and Learning Theories and Principles Applied to Distance Education

Most distance education programs employ andragogy strategies for the delivery of courses and classes through off-campus satellite sites, videoconferencing, telecommunications, and online and Web-based technology. The majority of teaching and learning strategies offered in these formats is learner centered and facilitates active student participation in the process rather than the traditional pedagogical methods for presenting information to the student.

Huang (2002) discusses the constructivism learning theory as it applies to adult learners who participate in online education programs. Huang states that the adult learner constructs new knowledge based on existing knowledge and that it is the role of the educator to shape the acquisition of new knowledge by providing experiences that facilitate the learner's ability to actively search for new knowledge, find resources to build upon the new knowledge, and solve problems. Constructivism theorists believe that social interaction is a critical part of adding new knowledge and, therefore, distance education programs including Web-based formats need to build in opportunities for students and faculty to interact. As described previously, this is possible through the use of chat rooms, threaded discussions, e-mail, and so forth.

Osciak and Milheim (2001) discuss Gardner's (2000) theory of multiple intelligences as it applies to Web-based Web-based instruction. They believe that all eight of the intelligences—musical, linguistic, logical–mathematical, spatial, bodily kinesthetic, interpersonal, intrapersonal, and naturalist—can be stimulated through Web-based instruction. They describe the many tools within Web-based Web-based programs and other Internet modalities that apply to the stimulation of the eight intelligences. The Osciak and Milheim article is useful to educators as they develop Web-based Web-based courses and seek various strategies for developing learning processes.

There are several websites that list learning principles especially relevant to distance education. They are as follows: Principles of Adult Learning (Lieb, 2004), http://honolulu.hawaii.edu/intranet/committees/FacDevCom/activity/news0403.htm; 30 Things We Know for Sure About Adult Learning (Zemke & Zemke, 1984), http://www.hcc.hawaii.edu/intranet/committees/FacDevCom/guidebk/teachtip/adults-3.htm; and The Technology Source: The Brain, Technology, and Education: An Interview with Robert Sylwester by H. Marcinkiewicz (Michigan Virtual University, 2004), http://ts.mivu.org.

▲ NURSING VALUES

Nursing values should receive special attention when considering distance education programs. These values include caring, communication, professional socialization, moral and ethical values, humanistic teaching and learning theories, and interdisciplinary communication.

With the growing trend toward distance education and programs that utilize technological support systems, primarily videoconferencing and Web-based Web-based instruction, there continues to be a debate over the loss of face-to-face interactions between students and the faculty and over issues related to clinical experience and supervision at a distance issues.

Watson (2002) presents a persuasive, philosophical argument in support of learning modes that go beyond the physical world of learning to a metaphysical sphere of interactions. It is her contention that virtual, transformative learning experiences foster caring communities of learners, faculty, and leaders. She believes that the reality and virtual realms of understanding are merging and that it is possible to communicate with all of the senses in both the virtual world of space and the "real world." She links transformative learning through a metaphysical perspective to the science of caring and opens new vistas of thought regarding approaches to nursing practice and education.

▲ EVALUATION OF DISTANCE LEARNING PROGRAMS AND RESEARCH FINDINGS

While developing a distance education program and planning for its implementation, it is wise to include an evaluation plan to measure its effectiveness. Like the other components of the curriculum plan, an evaluation plan should be in place and congruent with the master plan of the existing program. Table 14.1 summarizes the discussion thus far on the planning for a distance education program and its curriculum. It provides further details and guidelines for the development and evaluation of the program.

When distance education programs first came into use by nursing educators, many issues were raised regarding the expense of technology, the need for retooling of faculty and students to utilize the technology, the loss of face-to-face interpersonal communications between faculty and students, the question of how many students can be accommodated in one course, and the loss of a sense of belonging to the home institution. As Web-basedWeb-based learning management systems became more prevalent and user-friendly and many of the technical glitches were smoothed out, the programs became more popular. Some of the advantages to the programs were the ability to reach out to students some distance away from the campus, an increase in enrollments by the use of videoconferencing and telecommunications at multiple sites, and an increase for potential applicants in the competitive market for students. Advantages to students meant less expense and time for traveling to campus, flexible schedules to allow for working nurses to continue their education, and the ability to interact with students from regions other than the home community. For faculty who like technology and enjoy the challenges of creative designs for teaching and learning experiences, distance education offers opportunities to develop new strategies for their repertoire of instructional tools.

A review of the current literature demonstrates more positive outcomes in distance education strategies than previously reported when technology-based instructional designs were in their infancy. The following review of the literature directs the reader to some of the findings related to outcomes from distance education programs.

Wambach, Boyle, Hagemaster, Teel, et al. (1999) describe the development of Web-based courses for master's programs in Kansas. They discuss the development phases and the use of technology support personnel to assist faculty in developing courses. In addition,

▲ **TABLE 14.1** Guidelines for the Development of a Distance Education Program

Guideline	Questions for Data Collection and Analysis	Desired Outcome
Needs assessment: External frame factors	To what extent are the distant sites supportive of the program and sophisticated in the use of technology?	The community is receptive to distance education programs, open to the technology of distance education, and has a health care system supportive of the program, the nursing profession, and student clinical experiences, if indicated.
	To what extent has the health care system demonstrated support for the program and the nursing profession?	
	To what extent is the health care system open to student clinical experiences, and what resources do they have available for the experiences?	
	To what extent is the program competitive with other educational programs at the site(s)?	The program is competitive with other programs.
	To what extent is there a potential student body at the site(s), and is there an indication that it will continue for at least 5 years?	There is a potential student body that will continue at least 5 years.
	Have program approval and accreditation bodies been notified of the program, and do they approve or is there an indication that they will approve the program in the future?	Relevant program approval and accrediting agencies have been notified and approve the program, or there are indications for approval in the future.
Needs assessment: Internal frame factors	To what extent does the distance education program's mission, philosophy, organizing framework, goals, and objectives reflect those of the parent institution?	The mission, purpose, philosophy, organizing framework, goals, and objectives of the distance education program are congruent with those of the parent institution.
	To what extent does the parent institution have experience in the selected modality(ies) of distance education and/or have the resources to support it?	The parent institution has experience with and/or the resources to support the program.
	Are there plans in place that indicate adequate resources for the program, including infrastructure, human resources, and academic program support?	Plans are in place and resources are adequate for academic infrastructure, human resources, and academic program support.

▲ **TABLE 14.1**   **Guidelines for the Development of a Distance Education Program** (continued)

Guideline	Questions for Data Collection and Analysis	Desired Outcome
Economic feasibility	To what extent will the parent institution support a needs assessment for the distance education program? If there are no funds from the institution, are there other possible resources?	There is support from the parent institution or other sources for a needs assessment.
	Are there start-up funds available from the institution or are there other sources such as funds from partner health care or educational institutions?	There are start-up funds from the parent institution or other sources.
	Has the business plan accounted for personnel costs (staff, technicians, and faculty); administrative costs; facilities (if indicated); academic support systems, (library, enrollment services, financial aid, etc.); and the required technology system(s)?	The business plan includes funds for the required personnel, administrative costs, facilities (if indicated), academic support systems, and the required technology system.
	To what extent are there plans for self-sufficiency? Are there projections for the size of the student body and other resources necessary to maintain the program?	There are financial plans in place for self-sufficiency and maintenance of the program.
Congruence with the components of the curriculum	To what extent does the curriculum plan for the distance education program reflect that of the parent institution (e.g., course descriptions, credits, objectives, and content)?	The distance education program's curriculum plan is congruent with that of the parent institution.
Delivery model options: Options	Have all modalities been considered, including off-site, on-land satellite campuses, videoconferencing and/or teleconferencing, and online or Web-based methods?	All modalities for the delivery method are reviewed to lead to a rationale for the selected model or combination of several.
Delivery model options: Selection and its rationale	To what extent does the selected model fit the learning needs of the students?	The selected model fits the learning needs of the students.
	To what extent is there faculty who can utilize the model(s)? If not, are there	The selected model is within the scope of the faculty's expertise or

(table continues on page 366)

▲ **TABLE 14.1** Guidelines for the Development of a Distance Education Program (continued)

Guideline	Questions for Data Collection and Analysis	Desired Outcome
Delivery model options: Selection and its rationale (continued)	faculty development plans and technical support in place?	there are faculty development plans in place.
	To what extent is the selected model "user- friendly" for students and faculty?	The selected model is "user-friendly" for students and faculty.
Teaching and learning theories and nursing values	To what extent does the program reinforce caring behaviors, foster professional socialization, promote communications (verbal, written, and interpersonal), analyze moral and ethical issues, apply humanistic teaching and learning theories, and include interdisciplinary communication?	The selected distance education program preserves nursing values such as caring, communications, professional socialization, moral and ethical values, humanistic teaching and learning theories, and interdisciplinary communications.
Delivery model: Implementation plan	To what extent is the selected model(s) congruent with the curriculum plan?	The selected model is congruent with the curriculum plan.
	Does the selected model fit the implementation plan of the curriculum (i.e., is it possible to deliver theory, lab, and clinical experiences)?	The curriculum plan can be implemented through utilization of the selected model(s).
Delivery model: Evaluation	Is there an evaluation plan in place and to what extent is it congruent with the master plan of the parent institution?	There is an evaluation plan in place and it is congruent with the master plan of evaluation for the parent institution.
	Does the evaluation plan include both formative and summative evaluation measures?	The evaluation plan includes both formative and summative measures.
	To what extent does the evaluation plan include strategies for follow-up and revisions if necessary based on the data analyses and recommendations from the evaluation plan?	The evaluation plan has mechanisms in place to revise the program according to data analyses and recommendations from evaluation activities.
	Is the selected delivery model(s) relevant to current education practices? To what extent is the selected model adaptable to future changes in the profession and education and health care systems?	The selected delivery model is relevant to current education practices and adaptable to future changes in the profession and education and health care systems.

they describe several of the courses that were developed and implemented for the master's program. They found no differences in the quality between the courses on campus and online. They reported positive outcomes for students and faculty alike, including student– faculty interactions, independent student learning activities, and the creativity experiences of faculty in developing the courses.

Billings (1999) provides an overview of assessment for distance education programs. She aptly points out that initially, programs were evaluated according to technology and its related issues. However, as distance education becomes more prevalent and technology is refined and adds newer innovations, there is a need to assess pedagogy and andragogy methods to evaluate the programs as well as to meet educational objectives. Some of the sources for assessment activities she mentions include faculty, students, technicians, and other stakeholders. She points out that the purpose of assessment is to improve the program and that it provides feedback to students and others as to the quality of the program. Additionally, results can be used as part of the teaching portfolio for faculty as part of the evaluation process.

Billings, Connors, and Skiba (2001) describe a benchmarking survey to measure outcomes from distance education programs. They used the tool to survey students in three nursing programs, and from analyses of the data, they concluded that the survey is useful for faculty to evaluate Web-based Web-based courses. Online courses facilitate more active learning on the part of students, and if this is not occurring, the authors advise faculty to seek out the reasons why this is not occurring and how to improve the course. In addition to student perspectives and the application of their feedback to quality improvement of courses, the benchmarking method provides information for instructional designers and administrators on how to better support these types of courses. This article is extremely helpful for its application to program evaluation of Web-based courses.

Kennedy (2002) discusses distance education not only in terms of geographic distance but also in terms of cognitive development and role. He compared a classroom experience with a virtual learning classroom and found that for the latter, students participated far more than those in the traditional classroom setting. Atack and Rankin (2002) surveyed RNs enrolled in a Web-based course and found that, overall, they were highly satisfied with the method. Some of the challenges raised were the need for computer-based skills, lack of access to the course from work compared to open access at home, and a misconception of the workload associated with the course on the part of the students.

Wills and Stommel (2002) conducted pre- and posttests on graduate students enrolled in a research course and a course on aging to measure students' perceptions and preferences for Web-based courses. The article includes a review of the literature and uses a conceptual model for measuring Web-based course outcomes that adds to Billings' (2000) assessment framework for Web-based courses. They found that students' perceptions and preferences for this modality of learning were positive; however, the students were more positive about the aging course than the research course. The authors attributed this possibility to the fact that the research course is required and is early in the program, while the aging course is an elective and is later in the program, and students had experience with Web-based courses. Both faculty members for the courses were rated highly by the students; thus, it was felt that teaching effectiveness did not contribute to the differences. Although the sample was small and confined to one university, this article offers ideas for measuring the success of Web-based courses.

Oehlkers and Gibson (2001) conducted a phenomenological study of RNs enrolled in a Web-based distance education program to identify their support systems. Although the sample was small and involved one university's distance education program, some interesting and useful points were raised based on the feedback from the students. Students seek information and support from their academic advisors, who serve as liaisons between the student and the institution. Students' families are helpful to them in working with the technology and finding resources for course assignments. Students who were near the university used its library for reference work, while those at a distance had to rely on health care agencies' libraries, which were not as useful as those in the university. (This reiterates the need for library access for distance education courses whether online and Web-based or on-site.) The students were aware of the support of the staff technology person and were appreciative of the help from that person. The instructor for the course played a major role in support of the students, although they complained about the long turnaround time for the return of their papers. As the authors point out, faculty should advise students how long it will take grade papers. Another challenge is the need for students to either renew or learn writing skills for formal papers, including format, organization, citations, etc. The article contains several other ideas for developingWeb-based courses that recognize the importance of support systems for students.

Waddell, Hayes, Horne, and Camann (2000) conducted a literature review on the outcomes of distance education through various modalities, including videoconferencing, Web-based classes, and clinical experiences enhanced by technology. Their review focused on RN students and found that while the course outcomes in terms of meeting objectives were much the same between those on and off campus, there were other issues raised that related to the loss of face-to-face encounters between students and faculty and students and students. Some of the issues related to role modeling and mentoring, the ability to foster caring and professional socialization, the lack of visual cues for interpersonal responses, and the additional faculty time necessary to develop online courses and respond to individual students. However, the overall impression was that working RN students who are at a distance from the home campus, while they prefer face-to-face meetings, find technology-supported distance education compatible with their work and lifestyles.

Shomaker and Fairbanks (1997), on the other hand, reported positive outcomes in their study of a telecommunications program to reach RNs in rural New Mexico and southern Colorado. They followed graduates of the program, which had been in existence for 6 years, and found that the great majority of students completed the program within an average of 2-1/2 years; that the percentage of underrepresented minorities was higher than on campus, with over one-third of the students being non-White; and that the students remained employed in their home communities, achieved the same academic ratings as students on campus (if not a little better), rated the program highly according to depth of material and faculty skills, and according to their employers, performed at higher levels of leadership and clinical practice upon completion of the program.

The development of professional socialization for students participating in nontraditional courses is one of the major issues facing educators who develop distance education programs. Nesler, Hanner, Melburg, and McGowan (2001) compared the professional socialization scores of students participating in distance education programs to nursing students in on-campus courses and also to non-nursing students in on-campus courses. They utilized two instruments for measuring professional socialization, and through the results of the studies and reliability and validity studies, found one that is a better measure of professional socialization. (Readers interested in these measures should refer to the article.) Students participating in distance education courses received higher professional socialization scores than on-campus nursing students who, in turn, measured higher than on-campus non-nursing students. While they were initially surprised at their findings, Nesler et al. found that, when compared to on-campus nursing students, the distance education students had more health care experience and many were licensed as nurses. Thus, a combination of health care and educational experiences seemed to contribute to professional socialization.

Cragg, Plotnikoff, Hugo, and Casey (2001) conducted a similar study at a university in Canada. They compared on-campus RN–to-baccalaureate graduates and graduating senior students to those enrolled in an audio-teleconferencing program or those in a combination of the two methods. They found that the distance education graduates scored higher on a professional-values measure than those on campus or a combination of the two. Again, experience in health care was a major contributing factor. The authors reported some difficulty with the tool to measure professional values. However, they concluded that participation in distance education programs promotes some of the desired changes in students related to the development of professional values.

MacIntosh (2001) surveyed RN students enrolled in a baccalaureate program based on videoconferencing. The survey was composed of open-ended questions, interviews, and focus groups. Based on the students' comments, MacIntosh recommends that instructional designs fit the technology, foster student interactions, and engage students in the process. Upvall, Decker, and Wilkerson (2000) used a questionnaire and focus groups with 25 RN-to-baccalaureate students enrolled in a two-way audio-video interactive television program. The authors found three major categories related to this type of distance education that included learning, teaching, and support for both.

Based on the studies reviewed and others, it becomes evident that telecommunications and videoconferencing are similar to the traditional classroom, lecture-type class. However, according to teaching and learning theories, efforts must be made to involve students in the process to meet their andragogy learning needs and for faculty and student satisfaction.

▲ ISSUES AND CHALLENGES IN DISTANCE EDUCATION

Pond (2004) presents a brief history of formal education in the 20th century and the impact of distributed education in the 21st century on past education formats. He discusses some of the contemporary issues that the newer modalities of instruction raise for quality assurance and accreditation of programs. He points out that these newer ways of teaching and learning are opening higher education to populations previously denied access. An interesting new paradigm for accreditation is proposed by Pond for accrediting the learner rather than the institution; faculty would certify students who meet certain defined benchmarks.

Pond's challenge leads to an emphasis on educational outcomes and their market value. The table in his manuscript titled "Old Versus New Paradigms for Accreditation and Quality Assurance" poignantly illustrates the very different educational paradigms of the formal

20th century and the learner-centered 21st century. He further points out that educational delivery models are outpacing the criteria and standards for accreditation. He recommends nine universal standards for educational quality and for accreditation agencies to consider in meeting the challenges of the 21st century. His last point is the need for educational institutions to open themselves to other stakeholders in the educational process, including the community, industry, professional organizations, peer institutions, and the students.

A persuasive article by Jones (2003) discusses the predicted growth for college enrollments over the next 10 years (2003–2013), the economic downturn of the early 21st century, and their effect on higher education. Distance education could solve this crisis by providing cost-effective, quality programs that do not require the addition of costly classrooms and other learning facilities. In addition to the growth of college-age students, there are increasing numbers of experienced learners looking for advanced education that favors distance education programs. Jones points out the continued need for distance education courses to include socialization, motivation, information exchanges, and access to resources—the same as traditional teaching and learning methods. He lists the costs associated with the development of distance education courses and argues that these costs are also associated with traditional development costs minus the larger capital expenses for classrooms and facilities. He does not target nontraditional students alone but includes on-campus traditional students. He recommends that courses could be in both formats, which would maintain quality and benefit students and faculty.

Cuellar (2002) discusses the changes and challenges that online modalities bring to nursing education programs and their faculty. Several of the changes she discusses include the use of andragogical principles of teaching and learning in contrast to pedagogical principles. Past methods of teaching change when developing online courses, which emphasize the development of cognitive strategies for learning as opposed to the behaviorist methodologies of the past. Newer platforms for the delivery of instruction mean that faculty must incorporate different ways to present content that was once in lecture format and now can be found in PowerPoint presentations (with notes) and questions that lead the student into the content through inquiry and exploration of the body of knowledge related to the subject. Faculty becomes facilitators and partners with students in the learning process. Cuellar reviews the process for transferring traditional course content into the online format, for example, syllabi, student technology needs, references for student access, and links to audiovisual materials and other resources that enhance learning. Newer ways or different formats for assessing learning are part of the course materials in technology-based methods.

Cuellar lists some implications for the future as they apply to online learning. They include evaluation and research related to online courses, collaborative relationships with other faculty in the home institution, strategic planning for the development of distance education, built-in versatility and flexibility in the programs, the effects on faculty promotion and tenure, a balance of online and on-campus courses, and technical training for student and faculty alike.

In 1999, the American Association of Colleges of Nursing (AACN) published a white paper on distance education and the use of technology in delivering courses and classes (AACN, 2003). At that time (1999), AACN listed issues related to distance education that needed to be addressed. Among the issues that continue to this day are those that relate to:

1. Funding for the development, support, and evaluation of programs.
2. Programs that are within the context of the mission and strategic plans.

3. Faculty development.
4. Legal and ethical issues such as intellectual property and privacy issues.
5. Quality education that meets the standards of higher education.
6. Increased student access to education through technology.

To remain competitive and current in the higher education market, nursing programs need to determine how they will expand their programs to meet the needs of students who may live and work some distance away from the home campus. While entry-level programs, especially undergraduate programs, will continue to take place on traditional home campuses, there is a need to offer higher-education programs for licensed personnel and other experienced learners. The majority of the U.S. nursing workforce received its entry-level education at the diploma or associate degree level (Bureau of Health Professions, 2004); yet, the health care industry prefers nurses prepared at the baccalaureate or higher degree level (Sechrist, Lewis, & Rutledge, 1999). Distance learning through technology offers the best opportunity for working nurses to continue their education and as described earlier in the chapter, has been successful. Through consortia of varying levels of education, regional collaboratives, and the health care industry, these programs can be cost effective and reach many more nurses than ever imagined.

The increasing market for learning management systems provides cost-effective, quality educational delivery programs through Web-based technology, and in many ways is proving to be an effective modality for engaging students in transformative learning experiences. These types of programs are far less expensive than videoconferencing and telecommunications; however, they require the technology, staffing, and faculty development programs to realize their full potential.

No matter the modality, the program must be within the context of the program's mission, philosophy, organizational framework, and goals and objectives. As with all curriculum development projects, faculty must examine the purpose of the distance education program in light of these components. In some cases, the program may not be compatible with the mission and, therefore, not an option. For those programs that are compatible, the usual formative evaluation strategies should take place to ensure that the planning and implementation phases of the program are congruent with the overall curriculum plan. An evaluation plan to measure outcomes must be in place to maintain quality, meet program approval and accreditation standards, and ensure a quality program for its stakeholders, including students, consumers, and faculty.

The majority of distance education programs have copyright and intellectual property policies in place that are congruent with the parent institution. For new programs, along with faculty development and implementation support, it is advised that these policies be developed early in the process. The ideal policy is one that gives the individual faculty member the rights to the course syllabus and learning activities; however, the course description and objectives remain the property of the institution.

Privacy issues are addressed through the maintenance of the same policies of the parent institution. For Web-based courses, owing to identification theft and computer hackers, many institutions issue identification numbers for students, staff, and faculty rather than social security numbers. Most learning management systems have built-in privacy safety mechanisms allowing only students and faculty access to courses through personal identification numbers (PINs).

Often, videoconferencing is delivered through closed circuit television or public broadcasting system and, thus, open to public access. However, only students officially enrolled in the courses can receive academic credit and have access to supplemental material necessary for the course such as library services, course resources, e-mail, list serves, and chat rooms.

An issue not addressed frequently in the literature is the matter of faculty-to-student ratios in distance education programs and their effect on quality of education, faculty workload, and method of instruction. Videoconferencing leads other technologies in reaching the greatest numbers of students while Web-based courses are limited in size per faculty member, usually to a maximum of 20 students and preferably less. Web-based instruction requires high intensity interactions between students and faculty for effective learning to take place. Videoconferencing can reach many students in multiple sites, but as with all lecture-type classes, fosters minimal student participation unless active learning assignments are included. All of these factors must be taken into consideration when planning the delivery choice.

As the number of distance education programs increases in the future, new issues and challenges face faculty and institutions of higher learning. Less attention will be needed on the actual technology of the delivery systems, and more attention will be necessary on the quality of the programs as they match the mission and purposes of the educational programs. Outcomes from distance education programs will be measured by increased opportunities for nurses to continue their education and the continued partnerships between education and service that result in a nursing workforce ready to meet the challenges of an ever-changing health care system and the health promotion and disease prevention needs of the populace.

▲ SUMMARY

Chapter 14 reviewed the various types of distance education programs and their relationship to curriculum development and evaluation. Some of the issues facing these types of programs were discussed, including cost effectiveness, faculty workload, the application of teaching and learning principles, and student and faculty satisfaction.

C A S E   S T U D Y

▼

Chapters 5, 6, and 7 presented a case study with a needs assessment and a proposed curriculum for an outreach program. The following continues the case study and describes the distance education methods for delivery of the curriculum. It utilizes the guidelines found in Table 14.1.

Needs Assessment

External Frame Factors

The needs assessment for the outreach program indicates support from the community, nursing profession, and health care system. The parent institution's extended education program has facilities that can be shared with the program, which include Web-based and videoconferencing facilities. The health care system indicated support for the program by agreeing to have students in its agencies for clinical experiences, and there are potential qualified nurses who can act as mentors and preceptors for the students. While other nursing programs exist in the area, the outreach program is unique and will draw from a different applicant pool, specifically that of non-nursing college graduates. The nursing faculty, in collaboration with enrollment services, held several focus groups of potential college graduates and academic counselors from the area's institutions of higher learning in the proposed site. Results from the focus groups indicated that there is an enthusiasm for the program and an adequate applicant pool that will exist for some time to come.

While conducting the needs assessment, records of the activities and results from the findings were kept. These records were compiled into reports that will meet the Board of Nursing requirements for outreach program approval and the regional and national accrediting bodies. Major items in the report include the specific program, target student body, financial feasibility and business plan, the program's congruence with the existing curriculum, academic and student support systems, administrative support, and faculty qualifications. Preliminary indications are that the program will receive approval.

Internal Frame Factors

The mission, philosophy, organizing framework, goals, and objectives will remain intact for the outreach program. The videoconferencing and Web-based systems of the extended education program are available. Because that program utilizes the videoconferencing system during the evening and weekend hours, the nursing outreach program must plan around those times.

The parent institution agreed to a business plan for the program, supported the needs assessment, and agreed to support start-up funds. An experienced faculty member was appointed as the director of the outreach program and met with the stakeholders of the program to develop a strategic plan for its initiation. He is in the process of interviewing potential faculty in the outreach

(case study continues on page 374)

program site and is working with key members of the faculty on campus for the delivery of the courses in the entry-level master's program. Additional activities on his part include working with the director of extended education to negotiate the use of classrooms, conference rooms, office space, staffing and enrollment services, academic and student support services, and technology support systems. He is also meeting with local health care agencies' personnel to arrange for students' clinical experiences.

Economic Feasibility

The comptroller of the parent institution drew up a business plan that includes costs for the director; administrative services; faculty; staff; rental of the facilities; videoconferencing and Web-based instructional systems; academic, enrollment, and student services; library access; and program approval and accreditation reports. The needs assessment and start-up funds are included in the debit side of the budget. On the income side are calculations of student fees and tuition for several proposed student aggregates, contracts with health care agencies that will provide learning lab space at no cost and scholarships for students, and the potential funding from a program development grant that seems assured. Projections for the future exist and are based on a 3-year self-sufficiency plan that includes enrollment targets for the future and the maintenance of the program after the initial 3 years.

Congruence With the Components of the Curriculum

The total curriculum plan for the entry-level master's program will be used for the outreach program; thus, congruence is guaranteed. The only difference will be in the way that it is delivered to students.

Selected Delivery Model and Rationale

Based on the existing curriculum plan, the availability of qualified potential clinical faculty in the outreach site, and the existing videoconferencing and Web-based systems, the selected delivery model is an eclectic model. On-campus faculty will deliver theory courses by lecture and discussion through videoconferencing and Web-based instruction. Clinical and laboratory courses will be delivered on-site by the outreach program's clinical faculty under the supervision and mentorship of the distance education program director and home campus faculty members. The selection of these various models are cost effective because they utilize existing faculty and can increase theory classes' faculty-to-student ratios, allow for active student participation in Web-based theory courses that foster independent learning and critical thinking, and preserve the close supervision and mentorship support of students through on-site faculty and preceptors during skills laboratories and clinical laboratory systems.

Implementation Plan

The selected models for the outreach program are congruent with the curriculum plan. See Chapter 7's case study for a complete description of each course and how it fits into the Knowledge, Skills, Values, Meanings, and Experience (KSVME) organizing framework (Webber, 2002).

(continued)

Teaching and Learning Theories and Nursing Values

Before detailing the curriculum plan and its implementation, faculty reviews the total nursing program's curriculum components and their application to the existing on-campus entry-level master's program. The mission and philosophy specify the preparation of "intellectually and socially responsible, competent and compassionate nurses and nurse leaders to meet the health care needs of their communities and societies." This weighty statement encompasses nursing values that include caring behaviors, professional socialization, moral and ethical issues, and interdisciplinary communication. The communications thread is apparent in the prerequisite communications courses and their application to client care and interdisciplinary collaboration.

The philosophy states that "students and faculty interact in teaching and learning processes that empower students to build upon a strong liberal arts and sciences foundation and assimilate the nursing knowledge and skills that lead to the provision of competent and compassionate nursing care and leadership for multicultural and ethnic persons, families, aggregates, and communities." This statement provides guidance to the faculty as it examines a variety of distance education delivery systems, especially in the selection of systems that meet humanistic teaching and learning theories. Thus far, the faculty determines that the mission and philosophy are explicit and help to direct the development of the outreach program.

Curriculum Implementation Plan for the Outreach Program: Entry-Level Master of Science in Nursing

Prerequisites

A baccalaureate with a 3.0 or higher cumulative grade point average in the last 60 credits
One semester Anatomy with a lab
One semester Physiology with a lab
  (or two semesters of a combined Anatomy and Physiology course with labs)
One semester Microbiology with a lab
One semester Statistics
One semester Chemistry
Two semesters of Communications, written and oral
One semester of a Social Sciences course
One semester Human Development across the Lifespan

Level 1

SEMESTER 1

Nursing and Health Care
3 units theory

Description
Introduces the student to the nursing profession, its history, the science of nursing, current issues, and ethics. Discusses the role of the multidisciplinary health care team. Reviews the definitions of health and the health and illness continuum across the lifespan.

(*case study continues on page 376*)

Selected Teaching Method
Videoconferencing interactive lecture and discussion broadcast from the home campus and supported by e-mail submission of course materials and assignments.

Pathophysiology
3 units theory

Description
Focuses on alterations and responses of the human body to altered states of health, environmental stresses, and the aging process.

Selected Teaching Method
Videoconferencing interactive lecture and discussion broadcast from the home campus and supported by e-mail submission of course materials and assignments.

Health Assessment
2 units: 1 unit theory and 1 unit lab (2-hour lab on campus)

Description
Introduces the nursing process. Applies communication skills and knowledge from the biologic and social sciences to the subjective and objective assessment of multicultural and ethnic individuals across the lifespan to identify deviations from normal.

Selected Teaching Methods
Videoconferencing interactive lecture and discussion broadcast from the home campus and supported by e-mail submission of course materials and assignments. On-site health assessment lab held in an outpatient clinic after hours in a cooperating health agency taught by onsite clinical faculty.

Basic Skills I
1 unit (2-hour lab on campus)

Description
Introduces fundamental nursing skills, including oral administration of drugs, activities of daily living, transfer techniques, and documentation of nursing care.

Selected Teaching Method
On-site skills lab held in an outpatient clinic after hours in a cooperating health agency under the supervision of on-site clinical faculty.

Care of the Older Adult
3 units (1 unit theory and 2 units lab with 6 hours clinical experience in elder care settings)

Description
Provides theories and concepts in geriatric nursing and opportunities for students to practice nursing care for multicultural and ethnic elders in community settings, assisted living, and skilled nursing facilities.

(continued)

Selected Teaching Methods

Videoconferencing interactive lecture and discussion broadcast from the home campus and supported by e-mail submission of course materials and assignments. On-site experiences in clients' homes, assisted living, and skilled nursing facilities under the supervision of on-site clinical faculty.

SEMESTER 2

Nursing Care of Reproductive Families

5 units (2 theory and 3 clinical hours for 9 clinical hours per week in reproductive health care settings)

Description

Reviews theories and concepts related to health promotion strategies for multicultural and ethnic reproductive families. Introduces nursing care for well families and those who are experiencing deviations from normal or major health problems. Applies health assessment and nursing skills to the care of reproductive families in a variety of multidiscipline health care settings.

Selected Teaching Methods

Videoconferencing interactive lecture and discussion broadcast from the home campus and supported by e-mail submission of course materials and assignments. On-site experiences in reproductive health care settings under the supervision of on-site clinical faculty.

Nursing Care of Children and Adolescents

5 units (2 theory and 3 clinical hours for 9 clinical hours per week in pediatric and well child/adolescent health care settings)

Description

Reviews theories and concepts related to health promotion strategies for children and adolescents and nursing care for those who are experiencing deviations from normal and major health problems. Applies health assessment and nursing skills to the care of multicultural and ethnic children and adolescents in a variety of multidiscipline health care settings.

Selected Teaching Methods

Videoconferencing interactive lecture and discussion broadcast from the home campus and supported by e-mail submission of course materials and assignments. On-site experiences in pediatric and well child/adolescent health care settings under the supervision of on-site clinical faculty.

Pharmacology

3 units theory

Description

Introduces the student to Pharmacology and its role in health care. Differentiates among prescribed drugs, over-the-counter drugs, and substance abuse. Reviews the pharmacology and the major classifications of drugs, their actions, interactions, and side effects.

(case study continues on page 378)

Selected Teaching Method

Videoconferencing interactive lecture and discussion broadcast from the home campus and supported by e-mail submission of course materials and assignments.

Basic Skills II

1 unit (2-hour lab on campus)

Description

Continues nursing skills including all routes of administration of medications, immunizations, treatments, and documentation.

Selected Teaching Method

On-site skills lab held in an outpatient clinic after hours in a cooperating health agency under the supervision of on-site clinical faculty.

SEMESTER 3

Nursing Care of Adults

5 units (2 theory and 3 clinical hours for 9 clinical hours per week in acute care settings)

Description

Reviews theories and concepts of health promotion strategies for adults and nursing care for adults experiencing acute episodes of illness. Applies nursing management and leadership skills to the care of adults in acute care settings and coordinates care with other disciplines.

Selected Teaching Methods

Videoconferencing interactive lecture and discussion broadcast from the home campus and supported by e-mail submission of course materials and assignments. On-site experiences in acute care settings under the supervision of on-site clinical faculty.

Mental Health and Psychiatric Nursing Care

5 units (2 theory and 3 clinical hours for 9 clinical hours per week in pediatric and well child/adolescent health care settings)

Description

Reviews theories and concepts of mental health promotion strategies across the lifespan. Provides opportunities for nursing care practice for multicultural and ethnic individuals and families who are experiencing episodes of psychiatric illness. Reviews coordination of care and provides opportunities for practice with other mental health and psychiatric care providers.

Selected Teaching Methods

Videoconferencing interactive lecture and discussion broadcast from the home campus and supported by e-mail submission of course materials and assignments. On-site experiences in mental health and psychiatric care settings under the supervision of on-site clinical faculty.

Nursing Management and Leadership

3 units theory

(continued)

Description

Introduces organizational behavior in health care settings. Provides the theory and concepts for nursing management and leadership, including the supervision of nursing staff and collaboration with other health care providers. Analyzes the role of nursing in leadership and management in health care settings.

Selected Teaching Methods

Web-based utilizing a variety of teaching and learning strategies by home-campus faculty. Application of theory supported in the clinical experience by on-site clinical faculty and preceptors.

Introduction to Nursing Research

2 units theory

Description

Introduces nursing research and theories and their application to practice. Includes the research process and how to critique research studies.

Selected Teaching Method

Web-based utilizing a variety of teaching and learning strategies by home-campus faculty.

Level 2

SEMESTER 4

Community Health Nursing

5 units (2 theory and 3 clinical hours for 9 clinical hours per week in community health settings)

Description

Reviews theories and concepts of public health and community health nursing. Examines the roles of health care team members in community settings. Applies disease prevention and health promotion strategies for multicultural and ethnic families, aggregates, and communities in community health care settings.

Selected Teaching Methods

Videoconferencing interactive lecture and discussion broadcast from the home campus and supported by e-mail submission of course materials and assignments. On-site experiences in community health care settings under the supervision of on-site clinical faculty.

Epidemiology

3 units of theory

Description

Presents theories and models of Epidemiology and their application to nursing and health care interventions. Reviews environmental health, ecology, and their contributions to Epidemiology. Utilizes Biostatistics as it applies to the analysis of health data and Epidemiology models.

(case study continues on page 380)

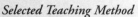

Selected Teaching Method
Videoconferencing interactive lecture and discussion broadcast from the home campus and supported by e-mail submission of course materials and assignments.

Health Care Policy and Social Justice
3 units theory

Description
Examines local, regional, national, and international health care systems and the social policy issues related to them. Describes strategies for shaping public policy in the health and social political arenas.

Selected Teaching Method
Web-based utilizing a variety of teaching and learning strategies by home-campus faculty.

Theoretical Foundations of Nursing Science
3 units theory

Description
Discusses concepts, theories, and models for building bodies of knowledge, disciplines, and professions. Reviews the nursing metaparadigm and leading nurse theorists as they apply to the science and practice of nursing.

Selected Teaching Method
Videoconferencing interactive lecture and discussion broadcast from the home campus faculty and supported by e-mail submission of course materials and assignments.

SEMESTER 5

Nursing Management of Acute Disease With Internship in a Clinical Specialty
6 units (2 theory units and 4 clinical units for 12 clinical hours per week in select health care settings)

Description
Reviews the diagnosis and treatment of major acute diseases and traumatic injuries and their impact on multicultural and ethnic client systems in a clinical specialty. In collaboration with other disciplines, applies the nursing process to the care of select client systems in acute, emergency, and/or intensive care settings.

Selected Teaching Methods
Videoconferencing interactive lecture and discussion broadcast from the home campus and supported by e-mail submission of course materials and assignments. On-site experiences in selected acute care settings under the supervision of on-site clinical faculty and preceptors.

Advanced Health Assessment
2 units (1 unit theory and 1 hour lab for 3 hours in the clinical setting)

Description
Reviews theories and skills for the advanced health assessment of multicultural and ethnic individuals and families with acute health problems and major traumatic injuries and interventions for their

(continued)

management. Applies advanced health assessment skills and interventions for major acute health problems or major traumatic injuries in the specialty clinical setting.

Selected Teaching Methods
Videoconferencing interactive lecture and discussion broadcast from the home campus and supported by e-mail submission of course materials and assignments. On-site health assessment lab held in an outpatient clinic in a cooperating health agency under the supervision of on-site clinical faculty.

Advanced Pharmacology
3 units theory

Description
Builds upon previous knowledge of drug classifications, effects, interactions, and side effects for the pharmacologic therapeutics for the management of chronic and acute illnesses.

Selected Teaching Method
Videoconferencing interactive lecture and discussion broadcast from the home campus and supported by e-mail submission of course materials and assignments.

Research Methods
3 units theory

Description
Reviews quantitative and qualitative research and the methodology for various types of research inquiries. Includes review of the literature and research processes and leads to a research (thesis) or special project proposal.

Selected Teaching Method
Videoconferencing interactive lecture and discussion broadcast from the home campus and supported by e-mail submission of course materials and assignments.

SEMESTER 6

Nursing Management of Chronic Disease With Internship in a Clinical Specialty
6 units (2 theory units and 4 clinical units for 12 clinical hours per week in select health care settings)

Description
Reviews major chronic diseases, their diagnosis and treatment, and their impact on client systems in a selected clinical specialty. Reviews the effectiveness of the health care system in providing chronic disease services. In collaboration with other disciplines, applies the nursing process to the care of client systems in select health care settings.

Selected Teaching Methods
Videoconferencing interactive lecture and discussion broadcast from the home campus and supported by e-mail submission of course materials and assignments. On-site experiences in selected chronic care settings under the supervision of on-site clinical faculty and preceptors.

(case study continues on page 382)

Leadership and Role Development in Nursing
3 units theory

Description
Discusses theories, concepts, and models of health care economics, organization, and quality assurance as they apply to nurse leader, manager, educator, and consultant roles. Reviews teaching and learning theories for application to staff development and patient education.

Selected Teaching Method
Web-based course utilizing a variety of teaching and learning strategies by home-campus faculty.

Research Project or Thesis
3 units theory

Description
This is the capstone experience for the master's graduate program. The student completes a research project based on a literature review and an original proposal that applies to nursing practice or health care innovation OR the student completes a master's thesis that is an original study and the product of the research process. Both the project and the thesis are under the guidance and approval of three faculty members.

Selected Teaching Methods
On-site or home campus meetings with faculty committee chair and communications through teleconferencing and e-mail with the chair and faculty committee members. Videoconference to present the final product.

Evaluation

The evaluation plan is the same as that of the home-campus plan and includes input, process, and outcome strategies for collecting data. There are specific follow-up directives within the evaluation plan to ensure quality and revise the program as needed. The plan is current and has built-in mechanisms for revisions based on recommendations from evaluation activities and changes in the health care and education systems. There is a plan to review the outreach program every 2 years for its relevancy to the health care system demands and the health care needs of the populace as well as the size of the applicant pool for economic feasibility purposes.

DISCUSSION QUESTIONS

1. To what extent do you believe that technology-supported distance education programs changed nursing education for the 21st century?
2. Of the multiple technology-supported distance education programs, which do you believe is:
   a. Most cost effective?
   b. Meets desired outcomes?
   c. Reaches the highest number of students?
   d. Fosters faculty development?
   Explain your rationale.

3. Discuss the pros and cons for the delivery of clinical courses through distance education strategies.

LEARNING ACTIVITIES

Student Learning Activities

1. Search the current literature (last 5 years) for research articles on distance education programs. Analyze at least three of them for a description of the outcomes for specific distance education modalities. Compare the modalities according to the outcomes that relate to teaching and learning effectiveness.

Faculty Development Activities

1. Select one course that you teach and adapt it to either videoconferencing or Web-based technology. Explain your rationale for selecting one or the other as it applies to the course.

REFERENCES

Allen, P., & Nero, L. (1999). Community partnerships in nursing education. *ABNF Journal, 10*(2), 54–55.

American Association of Colleges of Nursing. (2003). *AACN white paper: Distance technology in nursing education. Assessing a new frontier.* Retrieved June 21, 2004, from http://www.aacn.nche.edu?publications/positions/whitepaper.htm.

American Distance Education Consortium. (2004). *ADEC guiding principles for distance teaching and learning.* Retrieved June 21, 2004, from http://www.adec.edu/admin/papers/distance-teaching_principles.html.

Armstrong, M. L., Gessner, B. A., & Cooper, S. S. (2000). Posts, pans, and pearls: The nursing profession's rich history with distance education for a new century of nursing. *The Journal of Continuing Education in Nursing, 31*(2), 63–70.

Atack, L., & Rankin, J. (2002). A descriptive study of registered nurses' experiences with web-based learning. *Journal of Advanced Nursing, 40*(4), 457–465.

Billings, D. M. (1999). Program assessment and distance education in nursing. *Journal of Nursing Education, 38*(7), 292–293.

Billings, D. M. (2000). A framework for assessing outcomes and practices in Web-based courses in nursing. *Journal of Nursing Education, 39*, 60–67.

Billings, D. M., Connors, H. R., & Skiba, D. J. (2001). Benchmarking best practices in Web-based nursing courses. *Advances in Nursing Science, 23*(3), 41–52.

Blackboard. (2004). *About Blackboard.* Retrieved June 22, 2004, from http://company.blackboard.com

Bureau of Health Professions. (2004). *National center for health workforce analysis. The Registered Nurse population: Findings from the National Sample Survey of Registered Nurses.* Retrieved June 22, 2004, from http://bhpr.hrsa.gov/healthworkforce/reports/rnsurvey/default.htm.

Care, W. D., & Scanlon, J. M. (2000). Meeting the challenge of developing courses for distance delivery: Two different models for course development. *The Journal of Continuing Education in Nursing, 31*(3), 121–128.

Cragg, C. E., Plotnikoff, R. C., Hugo, K., & Casey, A. (2001). Perspective transformation in RN-to-BSN distance education. *Journal of Nursing Education, 40*(7), 317–322.

Cravener, P. A. (1999). Faculty experiences with providing online courses: Thorns among the roses. *Computers in Nursing, 17*(1), 42–47.

Cuellar, N. (2002). The transition from classroom to online teaching. *Nursing Forum, 37*(3), 5–13.

DeBourgh, G. A. (2001). Using web technology in a clinical nursing course. *Nurse Educator, 26*(5), 227–233.

eCollege. (2004). *eCollege. Supporting your success.* Retrieved June 22, 2004, from http://www.ecollege.com/indexstat.learn.

Gardner, H. (2000). *Intelligence reframed: Multiple intelligences for the 21st century.* Boulder, CO: Basic Books: Perseus.

Huang, H. M. (2002). Toward constructivism for adult learners in online learning environments. *British Journal of Educational Technology, 33*(1), 27–37.

IBM Lotus. (2004). *IBM Lotus.* Retrieved June 22, 2004, from http://www.lotus.com.

Indiana Higher Education Telecommunication System. (2004). *Guiding principles for faculty in distance education.* Retrieved June 21, 2004, from http://www.ihets.org.

Johnson, C. G. (1999). Evaluating preceptorship experiences in a distance nursing program. *Journal of National Black Nurses' Association, 10*(2), 65–78.

Jones, R. (2003) A recommendation for managing the predicted growth in college enrollment at a time of adverse economic conditions. *Online Journal of Distance Learning Administration, VI,* (I). Retrieved June 2, 2004, from http://www.westga.edu.

Kennedy, D. M. (2002). Dimensions of distance: A comparison of classroom education and distance education. *Nurse Education Today, 22*(5), 409–416.

Koeckeritz, J., Malkiewicz, J., & Henderson, A. (2002). The seven principles of good practice: Applications for online education in nursing. *Nurse Educator, 27*(6), 283–287.

Larsen, L. S., Logan, C. A., & Pryor, S. K. (2003). Redesign of clinical nurse specialist role course for distance education. *Clinical Nurse Specialist, 17*(1), 25–33.

Lieb, S. (2004). *Principles of adult learning.* Retrieved June 21, 2004, from http://honolulu.hawaii.edu/intranet/committees/FacDevCom/activity/news0403.htm.

MacIntosh, J. (2001). Learner concerns and teaching strategies for video-conferencing. *Journal of Continuing Education in Nursing, 32*(6), 260–265.

Michigan Virtual University. (2004). *The technology source. The brain, technology, and education. An interview with Robert Sylwester by H. Marcinkiewicz.* Retrieved June 21, 2004, from http://ts.mivu.org.

Ndiwane, A. (2001). Safety net: Student exchange learning and supervision on the World Wide Web. *Journal of Nursing Education, 40*(7), 330–333.

Nesler, M. S., Hanner, M. B., Melburg, V., & McGowan, S. (2001). Professional socialization of baccalaureate nursing students: Can students in distance education nursing programs become socialized? *Journal of Nursing Education, 40*(7), 293–302.

Oehlkers, R. A., & Gibson, C. C. (2001). Learner support experiences by RNs in a collaborative distance RN-to-BSN program. *The Journal of Continuing Education in Nursing, 32*(6), 266–273.

Osciak, S. Y., & Milheim, W. D. (2001). Multiple intelligences and the design of web-based instruction. *International Journal of Instructional Media, 28*(4), 355–361.

Pinch, W. J. E., & Graves, J. K. (2000). Using Web-based discussion as a teaching strategy: Bioethics as an exemplar. *Journal of Advanced Nursing, 32*(3), 704–712.

Pond, W. K. (2004). *Distributed education in the 21st century: Implications for quality assurance.* Retrieved June 21, 2004, from, http://www.westga.edu.

Sackett, K., Dickerson, S. S., McCartney, P., & Erdley, S. (2001). Interactive connections: technologies used in nursing education. *Journal of the New York Nurses Association, 32*(1), 7–10.

Sechrist, K. R., Lewis, E. M., &Rutledge, D. N. (1999). *The California nursing workforce initiative. Planning for California's nursing work force. Phase II final report.* Sacramento: Association of California Nurse Leaders.

Shomaker, D., & Fairbanks, J. (1997). Evaluation of an RN-to-BSN distance education program via satellite for nurses in rural health care. *Journal of Nursing Education, 36*(7), 328–330.

Sobralske, M., & Naegele, L. M. (2001). Worth their weight in gold: The role of clinical coordinator in a family nurse practitioner program. *Journal of the American Academy of Nurse Practitioners, 13*(12), 537–544.

Treistman, J., & Fullerton, J. (1996). Education exchange. Computer-mediated distributed learning: An innovative program design in midwifery education. *Journal of Nurse-Midwifery, 41*(5), 389–392.

Upvall, M. J., Decker, I., & Wilkerson, E. (2000). Essentials of successful distance-learning experience . . . including commentary by Jowett, S. *NT Research, 5*(3), 215–226.

U.S. Department of Education, Institute of Education Sciences. (2004). *Distance Education at Degree-Granting Postsecondary Institutions: 2000-2001. NCES 2003-017.* Tiffany Watts & Laurie Lewis. Project Officer: Bernard Greene. Washington, DC: USDE. Retrieved November 2, 2004, from http://www.ed.gov

Waddell, D. L., Hayes, J. M., Horne, C. D., & Camann, M. A. (2000). Point/counterpoint: Does "online" education short change the RN to BSN student? *Georgia Nursing, 60*(3), 36–39.

Wambach, K., Boyle, D. Hagemaster, J., Teel, C., et al. (1999). Beyond correspondence, videoconferencing, and voice mail: Internet-based master's degree courses in nursing. *Journal of Nursing Education, 38*(6), 267–271.

Watson, J. (2002). Metaphysics of virtual caring communities. *International Journal for Human Caring, 6*(1), 41–45.

Webber, P. B. (2002). A curriculum framework for nursing. *Journal of Nursing Education, 41*(1), 15–24.

WebCT. (2004). Home Page. Retrieved June 22, 2004, from http://www.webct.com.

Wills, C. E., & Stommel, M. (2002). Graduate nursing students' precourse and postcourse perceptions and preferences concerning completely Web-based courses. *Journal of Nursing Education, 41*(5), 193–199.

Yeaworth, R. C. (1996). Consortia arrangements and educational telecommunication. *Journal of Professional Nursing, 12*(3), 147–153.

Zemke, R., & Zemke, S. (1984, March 9). 30 Things we know for sure about adult learning. *Innovation Abstracts, VI*(8). Retrieved June 22, 2004, from http://www.hcc.hawaii.edu/intranet/committees/FacDevCom/guidebk/teachtip/adults-3.htm.

Issues, Trends, and Challenges for the Future

▼

Sarah B. Keating, EdD, RN, FAAN

OBJECTIVES

Upon completion of Chapter 15, the reader will be able to:

1. Analyze the trends in nursing education and the issues and challenges they raise in curriculum development and evaluation.
2. Develop strategies for resolution of the issues raised and ways to meet the challenges with an eye to the future.
3. Critique the proposed parallel career ladder steps and the entry-level doctorate curricula for their application to current and future unified nursing education programs.
4. Evaluate proposed curricula for their responsiveness to future challenges from the health care system and for the health care needs of the populace.

15

▲ OVERVIEW

Chapter 15 discusses trends, issues, and challenges in nursing education as they affect curriculum development. It ends with sample curricula that progress from the lower-division level of higher education to the doctorate and feature step-out points along the way for nurses wishing to enter the workforce at various levels. It integrates some newer prerequisite courses from other disciplines to support the knowledge base for nursing in a complex and ever-changing health care system. It continues the career ladder concept of nursing education so that its practitioners can enter (subsequent levels) of education without repeating previously learned knowledge and skills. At the same time, it promotes a nonstop, progressive curriculum for those who wish to enter the profession at the doctorate level.

Following the sample curriculum that builds on current nursing curricula found in Tables 15.1 and 15.2 is a proposed entry-level doctorate program for the future. It is a blueprint for an 8-year prenursing and nursing curriculum that graduates the student in 8 years with either a Doctor of Nursing Practice (DNP) or a Doctor of Nursing Science (DNSc). A ninth year is added to the program for the student who wishes to pursue a Doctor of Philosophy in Nursing (PhD), which focuses on research and theory building. The author is the first to admit that it is not perfect. Its intent is to raise issues, provoke thought, and generate discussion for future planning.

▲ PERSPECTIVES ON THE INFLUENCE OF HISTORY ON NURSING EDUCATION

There have been few changes to the nursing curriculum in spite of the continuing complaints from nurses in service that new graduates are ill-prepared for practice. To illustrate the lack of change in nursing education, one needs only to peruse the curriculum textbook recommendations of 50 years ago by Bridgman (1953). Within the past 50 years came the end of the Cold War, the Korean War, the Vietnam War, the Gulf War; the war on terrorism in Afghanistan, Iraq, and other places in the world; the rapid growth of technology; the proliferation of knowledge related to the cell, especially in relation to genetics; and the development of health maintenance organizations and health care systems whose services are increasingly taking place in ambulatory care and community settings.

While the Bridgman (1953) curriculum for the 1950s reads much the same as that of 21st century curricula, one can argue that today's hour-to-hour discourse in nursing classrooms and the exchanges of information between students and faculty in the clinical settings are far different from those of the 1950s. Nevertheless, the similarity between yesteryear's curriculum and that of today generates questions for nurse educators. The questions become: What does the future hold, what are the challenges facing nursing education, and how can these challenges best be met in a timely manner?

The history of nursing's responses to shortages in the workforce seemingly repeats itself. The profession scrambles to recruit nurses and succeeds quite well; however, there does not seem to be an equally enthusiastic response to expanding nursing education programs or developing new ones to accommodate increased applications. The number of state-supported programs that expand enrollments is few, except for those that are in partnership with industry, which often prove to be temporary arrangements.

▲ TABLE 15.1 Sample Career Step Ladder and Nonstop Graduate Entry Level Curricula (With Options)

Career Step Ladder Program

Lower-Division Associate Degree

Pre- and Corequisites	Semester Units	Nursing Courses*	Semester Units
Verbal and Written Communications	6	Introduction to Nursing and Health Care	3
Anatomy and Physiology	8	Basic Health Assessment and Skills	2
Microbiology	4	Nursing Process With Skills	2
Pharmacology	3	Geriatric Nursing and Clinical	4
Nutrition	3	Parent–Child Nursing and Clinical	6

Nonstop Graduate Entry-Level Program
(with step-out options)

Lower Division

Pre- and Corequisites	Semester Units	Nursing Courses	Semester Units
Verbal and Written Communications	6	Introduction to Nursing and Health Care	3
Anatomy and Physiology	8	Basic Health Assessment and Skills	2
Microbiology	4	Nursing Process with Skills	2
Pharmacology	3	Geriatric Nursing and Clinical	4
Nutrition	3	Parent–Child Nursing and Clinical	6

(table continues on page 388)

▲ TABLE 15.1 Sample Career Step Ladder and Nonstop Graduate Entry Level Curricula (With Options) (continued)

Career Step Ladder Program

Lower-Division Associate Degree			
Pre- and Corequisites	Semester Units	Nursing Courses*	Semester Units
Human Growth and Development	3	Adult Nursing and Clinical	6
Introduction to Computer Science	3	Psychiatric–Mental Health Nursing and Clinical	6
Competency in a language other than the student's primary language; otherwise, 2 liberal arts electives	6	**12-Week Internship*** (RN licensure eligibility upon completion of ADN degree)	6
Total	**36**	**Total ADN degree units = 65 + Internship**	**29**

Nonstop Graduate Entry-Level Program
(with step-out options)

Lower Division			
Pre- and Corequisites	Semester Units	Nursing Courses	Semester Units
Human Growth and Development	3	Adult Nursing and Clinical	6
Introduction to Computer Science	3	Psychiatric–Mental Health Nursing and Clinical	6
Competency in a language other than the student's primary language; otherwise, 2 liberal arts electives	6		
Total	**36**	**Total lower-division units = 65**	**29**

* Student and faculty choose a mutually agreed upon area of clinical specialty for a 12-week, 35 hours/week internship before taking NCLEX.

▲ TABLE 15.1 Sample Career Step Ladder and Nonstop Graduate Entry Level Curricula (With Options) (continued)

	Career Step Ladder Program			Nonstop Graduate Entry-Level Program (with step-out options)			
	Upper-Division Baccalaureate			Upper-Division Courses Baccalaureate Equivalent			
Pre- and Corequisites	Semester Units	Nursing Courses	Semester Units	Pre- and Corequisites	Semester Units	Nursing Courses	Semester Units
Lower-Division Associate Degree	65 + RN	Introduction to Research	3	Lower Division	65	Introduction to Research	3
Anthropology (Sociology)	3	The Nursing Profession	3	Anthropology (Sociology)	3	The Nursing Profession	3
Chemistry	4	Acute Care With Clinical	6	Chemistry	4	Acute Care with Clinical	6
Economics	3	Nursing Leadership	3	Economics	3	Nursing Leadership	3
Ethics	3	Transcultural Nursing	3	Ethics	3	Transcultural Nursing	3
Genetics	4	Interdisciplinary Health Practice With Clinical	4	Genetics	4	Interdisciplinary Health Practice With Clinical	4
Pathophysiology	4	Community/Public Health Nursing With Clinical	6	Pathophysiology	4	Community/Public Health Nursing With Clinical	6
Statistics	3	Selected Preceptorship**	8	Statistics	3	Selected Preceptorship**	8

(table continues on page 390)

**Student chooses area of clinical specialty with 1-hour seminar and 7 hours clinical preceptorship (total 30 hours/week for 15 weeks or the equivalent).

▲ **TABLE 15.1**   Sample Career Step Ladder and Nonstop Graduate Entry Level Curricula (With Options) (continued)

Career Step Ladder Program				Nonstop Graduate Entry-Level Program (with step-out options)				
Upper-Division Baccalaureate				Upper-Division Courses Baccalaureate Equivalent				
Pre- and Corequisites	Semester Units	Nursing Courses	Semester Units	Pre- and Corequisites	Semester Units	Nursing Courses	Semester Units	Step-out
						Optional 12-week Internship* (RN licensure eligibility upon completion of degree)		Step-out
Total	24	**Total BSN degree:** 36 lower division +24 upper division pre- or corequisites +29 lower-division and 36 upper-division nursing courses =125	36	**Total**	24	**Total baccalaureate units:** 36 lower-division+24 upper-division pre- or corequisites +29 lower-division and 36 upper-division nursing courses = 125	36	

*Student and faculty choose a mutually agreed upon area of a clinical specialty for a 12-week, 35 hours/week internship before taking NCLEX.

▲ TABLE 15.1 Sample Career Step Ladder and Nonstop Graduate Entry Level Curricula (With Options) (continued)

Career Step Ladder Program				Nonstop Entry-Level Graduate Program (with step-out options)			
Graduate Level Master of Science in Nursing				Graduate Level Postbaccalaureate			
Pre- and Corequisites	Semester Units	Nursing Courses	Semester Units	Pre- and Corequisites	Semester Units	Nursing Courses	Semester Units
Baccalaureate with RN and 36 units in upper-division nursing or equivalent	125	Nursing Research	3	Baccalaureate with selected prerequisites and 36 units in upper-division nursing or equivalent	125	Nursing Research	3
Cognate for Specialization or Functional Area	3	Nursing Theories	3	Cognate for Specialization or Functional Area	3	Nursing Theories	3
Advanced Pathophysiology	3	Health Care Policy and Political Action	3	Advanced Pathophysiology	3	Health Care Policy and Political Action	3
Advanced Pharmacology	3	Advanced Health Assessment	3	Advanced Pharmacology	3	Advanced Health Assessment	3
	6	Clinical/Functional* Specialization I With Internship			6	Clinical/Functional* Specialization I With Internship	
	6	Clinical/Functional Specialization II With Internship			6	Clinical/Functional Specialization II With Internship	

(table continues on page 392)

*Clinical specialization examples: Adult, Community Health, Geriatric, Parent–Child, Psychiatric–Mental Health Nursing
Functional specialization examples: Case Management, Supervision, Staff Development/Patient and Family Education, Nurse Educator for Lower Division and Technical Nursing Program

▲ **TABLE 15.1** Sample Career Step Ladder and Nonstop Graduate Entry Level Curricula (With Options) (continued)

Career Step Ladder Program				Nonstop Entry-Level Graduate Program (with step-out options)			
Graduate Level Master of Science in Nursing				Graduate Level Postbaccalaureate			
Pre- and Corequisites	Semester Units	Nursing Courses	Semester Units	Pre- and Corequisites	Semester Units	Nursing Courses	Semester Units
		Research Project	3			Research Project	3
						Optional 12-week Internship (NCLEX eligibility upon degree completion and internship)	Step-out
Total	**9**		**27**	**Total**	**9**	**Total**	**27**
	Total MSN = 36 units					Total Graduate = 36 units	
	Total BSN & MSN = 164					Total BSN & MSN = 164 + Optional Internship if stepping out	

▲ **TABLE 15.1** Sample Career Step Ladder and Nonstop Graduate Entry Level Curricula (With Options) (continued)

Career Step Ladder Program				Nonstop Graduate Entry-Level Program			
Doctorate Level DNP/DNSc/PhD*				Doctorate Level DNP/DNSc/PhD*			
Pre- and Corequisites	Semester Units	Nursing Courses	Semester Units	Pre- and Corequisites	Semester Units	Nursing Courses	Semester Units
BSN & MSN or their equivalent with RN	164	**Core Courses** (DNP, DNSc and PhD*)		Baccalaureate and graduate study with equivalent pre- and corequisites and nursing courses	164	**Core Courses** (DNP, DNSc and PhD*)	
Advanced Statistics and Computer Science (DNP and DNSc)	6	History and Philosophy of Nursing	3	Advanced Statistics and Computer Science (DNP and DNSc)	6	History and Philosophy of Nursing	3
Advanced Statistics and Computer Science (PhD)	9	Nursing Science and Its Domains	3	Advanced Statistics and Computer Science (PhD)	9	Nursing Science and Its Domains	3
		Health Care Issues, Ethics, Policies, and Actions	3			Health Care Issues, Ethics, Policies, and Actions	3
Research Methodologies Qualitative and Quantitative (DNP, DNSc, PhD)	6	**Nursing Research Courses** Nursing Research I, II, III (PhD)	9			**Selected Program and Research**	

(table continues on page 394)

▲ **TABLE 15.1** Sample Career Step Ladder and Nonstop Graduate Entry Level Curricula (With Options) (continued)

Career Step Ladder Program

Doctorate Level DNP/DNSc/PhD*

Pre- and Corequisites	Semester Units	Nursing Courses	Semester Units
	3	Nursing Research I (DNP and DNSc)	
		Nursing and Related Discipline Theories and Application (DNP, DNSc, PhD)	
	3	Theory Analysis (DNP, DNSc, PhD)	

Nonstop Graduate Entry-Level Program

Doctorate Level DNP/DNSc/PhD*

Pre- and Corequisites	Semester Units	Nursing Courses	Semester Units
Two Cognates for Selected Program (DNP, DNSc, PhD)	6	Seminar in Selected Program and Applied Research (DNP, DNSc, PhD)	3
		Seminar in Research for Entry-Level PhD	3
		Clinical Residency in Selected Program (DNP, DNSc, PhD for eligibility for licensure upon completion of degree)	12
		Nursing and Related Discipline Theories and Application (DNP, DNSc, PhD)	
Research Methodologies Qualitative and Quantitative (DNP, DNSc, PhD)	6	Theory Analysis (DNP, DNSc, PhD)	3

▲ TABLE 15.1 Sample Career Step Ladder and Nonstop Graduate Entry Level Curricula (With Options) (continued)

Career Step Ladder Program			Nonstop Graduate Entry-Level Program		
Doctorate Level DNP/DNSc/PhD*			Doctorate Level DNP/DNSc/PhD*		
Pre- and Corequisites	Semester Units	Nursing Courses	Pre- and Corequisites	Semester Units	Nursing Courses
	3	Theory Application (DNP, DNSc, PhD)		3	Theory Application (DNP, DNSc, PhD)
	3	Theory Testing (DNSc and PhD)		3	Theory Testing (DNSc and PhD)
	6	Theory Development (PhD)		6	Theory Development (PhD)
		Selected Program or Research		9	**Nursing Research Courses** Nursing Research I, II, III (PhD)
Two Cognates for Selected Program (DNP, DNSc, PhD)	3	Seminar in Selected Program or Research (DNP, DNSc, PhD)		3	Nursing Research I (DNP, DNSc)
	12	Residency in Selected Program (DNP, DNSc)			
		Clinical Project or Dissertation			**Clinical Project or Dissertation**

(table continues on page 396)

▲ **T A B L E   1 5 . 1**   **Sample Career Step Ladder and Nonstop Graduate Entry Level Curricula (With Options)** (continued)

Career Step Ladder Program

Pre- and Corequisites	Doctorate Level DNP/DNSc/PhD*		
	Semester Units	Nursing Courses	Semester Units
		Proposal (DNP, DNSc, PhD)	3
		Clinical Project (DNP)	6
		Dissertation (Application) (DNSc)	6
		Dissertation (PhD)	6
Total 18 (DNP) 18 (DNSc) 21 (PhD)		**Total Doctorate** DNP = 60 DNSc = 63 PhD = 66	42 (DNP) 45 (DNSc) 45 (PhD)

Nonstop Graduate Entry-Level Program

Pre- and Corequisites	Doctorate Level DNP/DNSc/PhD*		
	Semester Units	Nursing Courses	Semester Units
		Proposal (DNP, DNSc, PhD)	3
		Clinical Project (DNP)	6
		Dissertation (Application) (DNSc)	6
		Dissertation (PhD)	6
Total 18 (DNP) 18 (DNSc) 21 (PhD)		**Total Doctorate** Entry-level DNP = 60 Entry-level DNSc = 63 Entry-level PhD = 81	42(DNP) 45 (DNSc) 60 (PhD)

* DNP = Doctor of Nursing Practice
Examples: Clinical Nurse Specialist, Nurse Anesthetist, Nurse Midwife, Nurse Practitioner
DNSc = Doctor of Nursing Science
Examples: Applied nursing and other disciplines' sciences to administration, advanced practice, education, informatics and technology, public policy
PhD = Doctor of Philosophy
Examples: Research and theory development in administration, education, informatics and technology, nursing science, public policy

▲ TABLE 15.2 Proposed Entry-Level Doctorate Curriculum

Life, Physical, and Social Sciences	# of Courses (Units or Credits)	General Education, Liberal Arts, and Humanities	# of Courses (Units or Credits)	Mathematics and Statistics	# of Courses (Units or Credits)	Nursing and Health Care	# of Courses (Units or Credits)
Prenursing **Freshman Year (9 courses with 31 semester units or credits)**							
Anatomy	1 (4)	Communications-Written	1 (3)	Mathematics	1 (3)		
Physiology	1 (4)	Communications-Oral	1 (3)				
Psychology	1 (3)	History	1 (3)				
Chemistry	2 (8)						
Subtotal	**5 (19)**	**Subtotal**	**3 (9)**	**Subtotal**	**1 (3)**		
Sophomore Year (10 courses with 32 semester units or credits)							
Microbiology	1 (4)	Language (or elective if proficient)	2 (6)	Computer Science	1 (3)	The Health Care System and Professions	1 (3)
Physics	1 (4)	Government and Politics	1 (3)				
Human Growth and Development	1 (3)	Electives or General Education Requirements	1 (3)				
Sociology	1 (3)						
Subtotal	**4 (14)**	**Subtotal**	**4 (12)**	**Subtotal**	**1 (3)**	**Subtotal**	**1 (3)**
Junior Year (10 courses with 32 semester units or credits)							
Genetics	1 (4)	Bioethics	1 (3)	Statistics	1 (3)	History of Nursing	1 (3)
Anthropology (Sociology)	1 (3)	Economics	1 (3)			Transcultural Nursing	1 (3)
Biochemistry	1 (4)	Electives or General Education Requirements	2 (6)				
Subtotal	**3 (11)**	**Subtotal**	**4 (12)**	**Subtotal**	**1 (3)**	**Subtotal**	**2 (6)**

(table continues on page 398)

▲ TABLE 15.2 Proposed Entry Level Doctorate Curriculum (continued)

Life, Physical, and Social Sciences	# of Courses (Units or Credits)	General Education, Liberal Arts, and Humanities	# of Courses (Units or Credits)	Mathematics and Statistics	# of Courses (Units or Credits)	Nursing and Health Care	# of Courses (Units or Credits)
Senior Year (10 courses with 30 semester units or credits: 1 clinical experience course)							
Pharmacology I	1 (3)	Electives or General Education Requirements	1 (3)	Introduction to Research	1 (3)	The Nursing Process and Skills	1 (3)
Nutrition	1 (3)	Introduction to Business Administration	1 (3)			Health Assessment	1 (2)
Gerontology	1 (3)					Care of the Older Adult With Clinical	1 (4)
Pathophysiology	1 (3)						
Subtotal	4 (12)		2 (6)		1 (3)		3 (9)
Grand Total	16 (56)		13 (39)		4 (12)		6 (18)

Graduation at the end of 4 years with baccalaureate and 125 semester units or credits

Nursing Sciences	# of Courses (Units or Credits)	Nursing Practice	# of Courses (Units or Credits)	Cognates	# of Courses (Units or Credits)	Nursing Research	# of Courses (Units or Credits)
4-Year School of Nursing First Year (11 courses with 32 semester units or credits)							
Care of the Adult	1 (3)	Advanced Nursing Skills	1 (2)	Pharmacology II	1 (3)	Introduction to Nursing Research	1 (3)
Parent–Child Nursing	2(6)	Clinical Practice	3 (9)	Advanced Statistics and Computer Science I	1 (3)	Nursing Science and Domains	1 (3)
Subtotal	3 (9)		4 (11)		2 (6)		2 (6)

▲ **TABLE 15.2** Proposed Entry Level Doctorate Curriculum (continued)

Nursing Sciences	# of Courses (Units or Credits)	Nursing Practice	# of Courses (Units or Credits)	Cognates	# of Courses (Units or Credits)	Nursing Research	# of Courses (Units or Credits)
Second Year (11 courses with 32 semester units or credits)							
Mental Health Nursing	1 (3)	Advanced Health Assessment	1 (2)	Advanced Statistics and Computer Science II	1 (3)	Theories Analysis	1 (3)
Acute Care Nursing	1 (3)	Clinical Practice	3 (9)	Advanced Pathophysiology	1 (3)		
Community Health Nursing	1 (3)						
Leadership and Management	1 (3)						
Subtotal	**4 (12)**		**4 (11)**		**2 (6)**		**1 (3)**
Third Year (11 courses with 32 semester units or credits)							
Selected Nursing Specialty I and II	2 (6)	Role Development	1 (2)	Research Methodologies	1 (3)	Nursing Research I	1 (3)
History and Philosophy of Nursing	1 (3)	Clinical Practice	2 (6)			Theory Application	1 (3)
Health Care Issues, Ethics Policies and Actions	1 (3)					Research or Project Proposal	1 (3)
Subtotal	**4 (12)**		**3 (8)**		**1 (3)**		**3 (9)**

(table continues on page 400)

▲ TABLE 15.2　Proposed Entry Level Doctorate Curriculum (continued)

Nursing Sciences	# of Courses (Units or Credits)	Nursing Practice	# of Courses (Units or Credits)	Cognates	# of Courses (Units or Credits)	Nursing Research	# of Courses (Units or Credits)
Fourth Year (7 courses with 30–33 units or credits)							
Theory in Selected Program	1 (3)	Internship in Selected Specialty	1 (12)	Two Cognates to Support Specialty	2 (6)	Theory Testing	1 (3)
Seminar in Selected Program	1 (3)					Research Project or Dissertation	1 (3 to 6)
Subtotal	2 (6)		1 (12)		2 (6)		2 (6–9)
Grand Total	12 (36)		12 (42)		8 (24)		8 (24–27)
Graduation with DNP or DNSc with 126–129 semester units or credits							
Fifth Year (8 courses with 30 semester units or credits)							
Seminar in Selected Function or Practice	1 (3)	Residency in Selected Program	1 (6)	Advanced Statistics III or Computer Science	1 (3)	Nursing Research II	1 (3)
				Research Methodology	1 (3)	Theory Development Seminar in Dissertation	1 (3)
						Dissertation	1 (6)
Grand Total	1 (3)		1 (6)		2 (6)		4 (15)
Graduation with PhD in Nursing							

Brown (2002) states that it is time to overcome past barriers for graduates of diploma and associate degree programs to earn bachelor's degrees. For example, in 2000 the basic educational preparation for the nursing workforce in the United States was 30% at the diploma, 40% at the associate degree and 29% at the baccalaureate levels (U.S. Department of Health and Human Services, Health Resources and Services Administration, Bureau of Health Professions, Division of Nursing, 2001). Thus, there is potential for a large percentage of the nursing workforce to return to school to obtain additional degrees. Brown adds that additional programs are crucial for persons seeking second careers and/or holding non-nursing degrees. Brown urges nurses to unite in preparing for the future and to keep nursing's strong roots in caring because it is still a profession trusted by the public. Fitzpatrick (2002) repeats the need for one voice for nursing and advanced education to keep pace with society's health care needs.

The role of professional nursing organizations in nursing education has implications not only for their impact on curricula, but also for their role in the professional socialization of neophytes. Zungolo (2002) traces the history of nursing organizations, with 1952 a hallmark year when two primary organizations (the American Nurses' Association [ANA] and the National League for Nursing [NLN]) were forged. The ANA was to focus on practice and the NLN to set standards for nursing service and education. In addition to meeting the health care needs of the population, both organizations shared a common goal to involve other health care disciplines and non-nurses in the work of the organizations. As Zungolo reflects on the changes in the nursing profession in the past 50+ years and the fact that there are over 100 existing nursing groups in the early 21st century, one wonders how nursing can effectively speak with one voice.

▲ THE IMPACT OF THE NURSING FACULTY SHORTAGE

It is interesting to see a citation in the literature dated 1995 about a looming nursing faculty shortage, which should have served as a portent for the crisis in the early 21st century (DeYoung & Bliss, 1995). The contributing factors to the shortage listed at that time included aging faculty, burnout, noncompetitive salaries, and fewer nurses entering graduate study for preparation as teachers. These factors continue today, and it is imperative that the profession address them as one measure to ease the shortage. The shortage is not confined to North America; for example, England reported a similar shortage and pointed out the effect it would have on the quality of nursing education programs (Stephen, 1998).

More recently, the American Association of Colleges of Nursing (AACN) (2004a) published a white paper on the faculty shortages in baccalaureate and graduate programs that described the scope of the problem and strategies for expanding the supply. Berlin and Sechrist (2002) describe the problem as especially dire as senior faculty with doctorates plan to retire in the near future, leaving a gap of experienced faculty and leaders in nursing education programs. Of course, these shortages of nursing faculty are but the tip of the iceberg because the aforementioned articles only apply to baccalaureate and graduate programs. Diploma, associate degree, and licensed practical/vocational program are equally short-handed. An example of the faculty shortage for all types of programs in one state can be found at the California Strategic Planning Committee for Nursing Web site: http://www.ucihs.uci. edu/cspcn (California Strategic Planning Committee for Nursing, 2001).

Adversity usually results in innovation. As faculty looks to the future, it must prepare to assume new and, perhaps, different responsibilities for the development and evaluation of curricula. AACN's aforementioned white paper (2004a) recommends many strategies for recruiting faculty and, at the same time, covering teaching loads. The suggested strategies include using non-nurse faculty for subjects such as pharmacology, pathophysiology, nutrition, and statistics; targeting practicing nurses as candidates for continuing their education and entering academe; making graduate courses accessible to working nurses who wish to continue their education; offering accelerated programs for nurses with degrees other than nursing to earn their nursing credentials; and utilizing the experience and wisdom of retired nurse faculty as part-time teachers or administrators.

Tanner (2002) recommends innovation in nursing education regarding faculty responsibilities, such as simulated clinical experiences through the use of technology; re-examining the old formula of one instructor to eight to ten students and its effectiveness; rapid responses to changes in the health care system in place of the long, tedious processes of curricular change in the past; and wide dissemination of innovations in the literature to share new knowledge and techniques with nurse educators. In addition, this author recommends that accreditation and state program approval agencies reconsider regulations that hamper the use of well-qualified nurses with degrees other than nursing (e.g., the Master of Public Health, the Master of Business Administration, PhDs and master's degrees in the sciences, and the LLD (Doctorate of Laws) as nursing faculty).

While there is a need to recruit additional faculty, recruitment does not end with increasing the supply of faculty; it mandates that experienced faculty members act as mentors for new faculty. The majority of nursing faculty members comes to academe with education and experience in their chosen specialties or research. They do not have the education or experience in curriculum development and evaluation, instructional design, student evaluation, and the triplicity of the faculty role—teaching, scholarship, and service. It behooves nursing education to offer courses, workshops, and degree and certificate programs in education to supplement the knowledge base of faculty who lack preparation for the teaching role (Kelly, 2002).

▲ A CULTURALLY DIVERSE FACULTY AND STUDENT BODY

The diversity of the population requires a nursing workforce that is culturally competent and representative of that population. Thus, recruitment of faculty and students who are representative of the multicultural and ethnic population is necessary (Sochalski, 2002). It is critical that minority nursing faculty members act as role models for culturally diverse students and share their knowledge and experience in cultural awareness with other faculty members and students. Braithwaite (2002) describes her experience of mentoring four African-American nursing students in South Africa to provide them with experiences in phenomenological research and immersion in another culture. She describes in detail the many benefits of the mentoring relationship for students, faculty, and host academicians.

While increases in minority students occurred in the mid- and late-1990s and early 21st century, there is a need for continued recruitment to meet the goal of a representative nursing workforce (Sochalski, 2002). In 2003, the Association of Black Nursing Faculty formed a task force to increase the number of minority nurses and minority nursing faculty

(Tucker-Allen, 2003). Other nursing faculty members need to join efforts in recruiting and retaining nursing faculty. It would be remiss not to add the need for recruiting men into nursing, who represent about half the general population and only represent 5.4% of the nursing workforce (U.S. Department of Health and Human Services, Health Resources and Services Administration, Bureau of Health Professions, Division of Nursing, 2001).

Although the representation of men in nursing remains low, some of the stereotypes regarding their role in nursing are being shattered. With the nursing shortage, the changing U.S. economy, deliberate recruitment campaigns for men in nursing, and some positive depictions of male nurses in the popular media, more men are choosing nursing as a career (Cullen, 2003). The profession and nurse educators have the responsibility to champion men in nursing as well and to educate the public about their equal role in such specialties as maternity and family nursing instead of continuing to support notions that certain specialties should not be open to men (Burton, 2003; Morin, Patterson, Kurtz, and Brzowski, 1999).

Boughn (2001) reported on a study that compared men and women nursing students' reasons for choosing nursing. It found that both sexes were quite similar in their commitment to provide care; however, there were differences in their views of empowerment, with women interested in empowering their clients while men were interested in empowering themselves as professionals and the profession. Men indicated a strong motivation for practical reasons to enter the profession, such as salary and working conditions. The author raised the issue of the need for women who continue to dominate the profession in numbers to become socialized into empowerment for the profession and raise issues related to the practical conditions of working.

The racial/ethnic breakdown of minority nurses remains underrepresented, much like the gender representation. According to the 2000 National Sample Survey of Registered Nurses (U.S. Department of Health and Human Services, Health Resources and Services Administration, Bureau of Health Professions, Division of Nursing, 2001), the racial breakdown for the nursing workforce was as follows:

▲ White	86.6%
▲ Black/African American (non-Hispanic)	4.9%
▲ Asian (non-Hispanic)	3.5%
▲ Hawaiian/Pacific Islander	0.2%
▲ American Indian/Alaskan Native	0.5%
▲ Hispanic/Latino (any race)	2.0%
▲ Two or more races	1.2%

While this is an increase in non-white representation, it does not reflect the general U.S. population. The National Advisory Council on Nursing Education and Practice, in its executive summary of an agenda for nursing workforce racial/ethnic diversity, recognizes the need to continue to increase the numbers of underrepresented groups in the nursing workforce with an emphasis on the provision of culturally competent care for clients of nursing. The summary puts forth many recommendations toward reaching the goal of a culturally diverse and competent workforce. Several of those recommendations directly relate to curriculum development and evaluation, for example:

"identify the educational environments and programs that successfully support recruitment, admission, retention, and graduation of minorities and more widely implement successful models; increase the numbers of minority faculty; increase the overall number and percentage of baccalaureate-prepared minority nurses in the basic nurse workforce; and establish cultural competence standards in education and practice" (U.S. Department of Health and Human Services, Health Resources and Services Administration, Bureau of Health Professions, 2003).

Entry-Level Issues and Articulation Challenges

The previous discussion leads into entry-level issues and articulation challenges as they apply to curriculum development and evaluation. The term "entry-level" traces its history back to the American Nurses Association's position paper for the baccalaureate as the credential for entry into professional practice (American Nurses Association, 1965). As discussed in Chapter 1 of this text, the issues raised by this statement continue to haunt nursing and are contributing factors to the hesitancy on the part of nurse educators at both the associate and bachelor's degree levels to collaborate in planning articulation agreements.

Bargagliotti (2003) relabels the term entry into practice to "exit into practice," thereby removing the stigma of the old term and refocusing the thinking of nurse educators toward collaborative educational patterns. At the same time, she pleads the case for reasonable total credit expectations for each degree level of nursing education, for example, 72 credits for the associate degree, 120 to 124 for the bachelor's, 36 for the master's, and 44 for the doctorate. It is time for nursing to provide curricula that encourage young people to enter the profession and that do not require years and years of education and practice at each level of education.

There is recognition on the part of the health care system and nursing leaders in practice and education that nurses for today and tomorrow must have greater knowledge and skills than any previous eras. During a nursing shortage, it is tempting to lower educational standards and to accelerate the preparation of nurses to fill workforce demands. However, health care needs change, and in the current highly evolving society, nurses with advanced knowledge and skills are required. Nursing curricula must be assessed for their relevance to the industry's demands as well as to the needs of the learner and, ultimately, the client. The situation calls for collaboration between industry and education and among the various levels of nursing education. Fitzpatrick (2002) calls for "courageous crusaders" who are willing to take these issues and challenges and bring about change.

It is time to stop the bickering between industry, who claims educators do not know the real world of practice and are not producing the clinicians they need for practice, and educators, who resist change and believe that nurses in the practice setting cannot appreciate the constraints placed upon education for curriculum revisions. Both parties must collaborate in the examination of the practice and education settings and resolve to change them for the benefit of the clients they serve, to utilize nursing services more efficiently, and to define levels of practice based on education and practice, always with the respect to which professionals are entitled.

Nursing and Interdisciplinary Study

Nurses function in most health care settings with other health disciplines; thus, it is necessary to include content and clinical experiences in the curriculum that reflect interdisciplinary practice. Interdisciplinary education is defined by AACN (2002) as "an educational approach in which two or more disciplines collaborate in the learning process with the goal of fostering interprofessional interactions that enhance the practice of each discipline. Such interdisciplinary education is based on mutual understanding and respect for the actual and potential contributions of the disciplines" (p.1). The paper justifies interdisciplinary education in nursing owing to the complexity of the health care system and the multihealth care problems faced by consumers of care. They recommend that interdisciplinary concepts and clinical experiences take place early in the curriculum to professionally socialize nursing students and prepare them for collaborative relationships with other health care professionals.

Leininger (2001) chooses to discuss another discipline for its application to nursing, specifically, anthropology and transcultural nursing. She discusses the role of nurse anthropologists and medical anthropologists in nursing research and in nursing education. She laments the fact the anthropologists interested in health behaviors and issues continue to label themselves as medical anthropologists, though the current health care system and people's health care needs call for "health anthropologists" (p. 795). With the ever-increasing diversity of the general population and the shift from parochial views to a worldview, transcultural nursing and anthropology can serve as examples of interdisciplinary practice, research, and education.

Owing to the nursing faculty shortage, there is no better time to take advantage of the situation and integrate other disciplines' expertise into the teaching and learning process. Planning curricula that mandate other disciplines' participation is a win-win situation. It not only helps to fill in gaps created by the faculty shortage, it also facilitates interdisciplinary education. Cloonan, Davis, and Burnett (1999) describe an example of two health disciplines' collaboration for an interdisciplinary curriculum. The curriculum was developed for Georgetown University's medical and nursing students and focused on ethical decision making. Faculty and students from both disciplines participated in the curriculum that was implemented at the turn of the century. The authors discuss the justification for the program and some of the practical aspects for its implementation. An evaluation plan of the curriculum was in place, and it would be interesting to see a follow-up on the success of the program. It can serve as a model for the development of interdisciplinary curricula that should be inclusive of health disciplines including medicine, nursing, and others.

Zungolo (2003) reviews the advantages of merging academic health sciences into one educational entity. Some of the advantages are shared resources and faculty, integration into the curriculum of interdisciplinary concepts and practice, unified development activities, and consolidation of clinical experiences for all disciplines. However, she points out that the literature is sparse on the successes or failures of these mergers, and she cautions that there is a need for further information related to them to avoid pitfalls that might exist toward success. She observes that while the health disciplines recognize the need for collaboration, in reality they remain isolated from one another in many ways. Examples that she cites are the different foci on prerequisite courses for the professions, learning experiences, and curriculum plans. Interdisciplinary education as it applies to the development of nursing education continues to remain a challenge for the future and, yet, it is a necessity.

▲ CHALLENGES FOR FUTURE NURSING CURRICULA

The fact that the shortage in the nursing workforce will persist means that newer, more efficient methods for the utilization of nurses in the work setting must be developed. According to the U.S. Department of Health and Human Services (2002), the demand for nurses from 2000 to 2020 will increase by 29% nationwide. Yet, the projected growth of the nursing supply will reach only 10% by 2011 and then begin to decline when even more nurses retire. Schools of nursing need to increase enrollments without imperiling quality and work with nurses in the practice setting to redefine the expectations of nurse performance and promote the most efficient use of the nurse. Curricula must be streamlined so that a full-time associate degree program takes no more than 2-1/2 years, a baccalaureate 4, and a master's 1 to 1-1/2.

In 2000, only 59.1% of the nursing workforce was employed in hospitals, with the fastest-growing segment of the workforce (18.9%) in public and community health settings (including occupational and school health settings) (U.S. Department of Health and Human Services, Health Resources and Services Administration, Bureau of Health Professions, Division of Nursing, 2001). Today's hospital settings still employ a majority of the nursing workforce; however, practice has changed radically. Acute care facilities now include 1-day surgeries and emergency care on one end of the continuum and critical care units on the other end. The days of extended in-patient care are long gone, calling for very different approaches to quality nursing care in hospitals. It is no wonder that nurse educators have a difficult time changing curricula when examining the rapid changes in the delivery of care. Current and future hospital settings call for nurses who can provide high-technology care, and at the same time incorporate the patient and family in education for follow-up care owing to the revolving door of acute care. It appears that this trend will continue for the future, and therein lies the challenge to nursing education.

The changes in acute care will continue to result in increases in community health care, owing to demands for continuing care of the acutely ill and health maintenance for those with chronic disease. Both settings call for basic and advanced levels of preparation for nurses. One challenge is to ensure coordination between the two settings so that patients and families are not lost by the wayside, which can result in poor outcomes, readmission to acute care, and higher costs. The other challenge is to prepare nurses who function in both settings and have coordination of care and health education skills. In addition, owing to the shortage of RNs, ancillary personnel will increase in numbers, resulting in the need for nurses who have case management and supervisory skills.

Nursing must examine the practice setting for the more parsimonious use of nurses, so that nurses render professional care and non-nursing tasks are completed by support personnel. This seems such a simple solution; yet, nursing has a poor history of supporting additional assistive personnel for fear it will undermine the role of the professional nurse. It is time to re-examine the use of technical support staff and ensure that nursing has a supervisory role to maintain quality of care. At the same time, nursing is beginning to measure patient outcomes and finding that level of education, nursing care by RNs, overtime, and appropriate staffing ratios make a difference in quality of care (Aiken, Clarke, Cheung, Sloane, & Silber, 2003; Aiken, Clarke, Sloane, Sochalski, & Silber, 2002; Blegen & Vaughn, 1998; Greene, Allan, & Henderson, 2003).

The major breakthrough with the human genome project calls for knowledgeable nurses who provide counseling for clients related to family planning and gene therapies. Public health, with its services of prevention of disease and health promotion, demands nurses who provide case finding, health teaching, coordination of care, preventive services, and care for aggregates and populations. There has been a rejuvenation of public health owing to international concerns related to infectious and communicable diseases and the threats of terrorism, in addition to the goals of Healthy People 2010 (U.S. Department of Health and Human Services, 2002). The majority of nurses for these settings must have advanced education in the care of families, aggregates, and populations, including specific knowledge related to primary, secondary, and tertiary levels of prevention and the major health problems that occur at these levels of prevention.

Ambulatory care settings will continue to need nurses at the staff level as well as the advanced level for primary care roles. In 2000, 9.5% of the nursing workforce was employed in ambulatory care (U.S. Department of Health and Human Services, Health Resources and Services Administration, Bureau of Health Professions, 2001). Advanced-practice nurses are crucial to the care of the acute and critically ill, unserved and underserved people, and those vulnerable populations who suffer disparities in health care. To achieve the highest level of health for all people, nurses must become political activists and leaders to create a health care system responsive to health problems and issues. All of these activities demand nurses with the education and experience in advanced practice and leadership roles, economics, government and politics, and the art of persuasion.

While nurses in nursing homes and extended care facilities accounted for a small percentage of the nursing workforce (6.9%) in 2000, the population of the very old continues to increase. It is expected that:

> "The subgroup 65 years old and older is projected to grow 54 percent between 2000 and 2020, adding 19 million people to the 65-and-over age group . . . . Individuals 65 and over have a high incidence of chronic conditions such as: arthritis (50 percent), hypertension (36 percent), and heart disease (32 percent). Many also have multiple conditions requiring more regular care. The greatest per capita demand for health care, and thus the services of RNs, will quite naturally come from the very old, those 85 and over. This is the fastest growing segment of the population and a major user of long-term care facilities, home health care, and other employers of RNs" (U.S. Department of Health and Human Services, Health Resources and Services Administration, Bureau of Health Professions, 2002, p. 4).

These trends indicate the need for additional advanced-practice nurses, administrators, case managers, and staff nurses for care of the elderly across the healthcare system.

AACN's (2004b) white paper on the role of the clinical nurse leader speaks of many of the challenges mentioned thus far for nursing education to meet the health care demands of the future. The role is described as a nurse who will "provide clinical leadership, implement outcomes-based practice and quality-improvement strategies, will remain in and contribute to the profession . . . and will create and manage systems of care" (p.3). The paper also specifies the education necessary for preparing the clinical nurse leader, including a liberal education, core nursing knowledge, core competencies, and role development. Details and updates on the project can be found at the AACN Web site: http://www.aacn.nche.edu/NewNurse/index.htm.

The implications from these trends are for nursing curricula that prepare professionals to function across all settings with about half in the acute care setting and the remaining in community settings. No one level of nursing education will be confined to a specific setting, and levels of practice must be defined through education and experience. Additionally, it is time for partners from education and service to develop internships for all levels of new graduates to provide them with the experience they need to apply the knowledge gained in the educational program and reinforce critical-thinking and clinical decision-making skills (Keating, Rutledge, Sargent, & Walker, 2003).

Herdrich (2004) reported on a 1-year residency program between a health care system and university. The purpose of the residency program was to promote critical-thinking skills, competence in skills, role transition into professional practice, job satisfaction, institutional commitment, and satisfaction. Based on the pilot program of five participants, the program was very successful. The participants were satisfied with the program, and they reported that goals of the program were met. All passed NCLEX for the first time. Herdrich reported that the residency program is serving as a model for similar statewide programs.

▲ RECOMMENDED CURRICULA FOR THE FUTURE

Evidence-based practice and education contribute to the assurance of quality in the care of clients and the preparation of tomorrow's professionals. The National Council of State Boards of Nursing (NCSB) is in the process of adding this concept to their regulation statements to ensure the protection of the public. According to the NCSBN (2004), the accepted definition of evidence-based practice comes from Sackett, Straus, Richardson, Rosenberg, and Haynes (2000), who describe it as the integration of the best research with clinical expertise and patient values.

The NCSB uses this definition and reports on its Website a study conducted by Smith and Crawford (2003), who surveyed newly graduated associate degree and baccalaureate nurses on their perceptions of the adequacy of their education programs. Included in the list of outcomes were the graduates' competencies to provide caring and respect for patients, commitment to professional development, involvement with errors, or difficulty in their patient assignments. The study raised many concerns regarding the participants' opinions about their education. It is an important document for educators to read, analyze, conduct further study, and think about the application of evidence-based practice and education to the development of curricula.

The Institute of Medicine (2003, p.1), in its summit on education, recommends the following preparation for health care professionals, including nursing for the 21st century:

▲ "delivering patient-centered care,
▲ working as part of interdisciplinary teams,
▲ practicing evidence-based medicine,
▲ focusing on quality improvement and
▲ using information technology."

In addition, it recommends that accreditation agencies, licensing agencies, and certification organizations ensure that the programs include this content in their curricula.

For issues related to graduate curricula, McEwen (2000) reviewed the literature for the content of nursing theory courses and found little change in the content from the mid-1980s to the late 20th century. The author cites the American Association of Colleges of Nursing's (1996) *Essentials of Master's Education for Advanced Practice Nursing's* recommendations for theoretical foundations of nursing as core content for the master's curriculum. McEwen surveyed a randomly selected sample of faculty in master's programs (n = 44) regarding the teaching of theory courses to identify any changes in the content in the past 2 decades. The survey revealed similar core content in the theory courses and the opinion by a majority of the respondents that grand nursing theories are overemphasized and middle-range theories are underemphasized. It was recommended that more middle-range theories and shared theories from other disciplines be integrated into the curriculum content and that more emphasis on the application of nursing and shared theories be applied to practice. McEwen and Sperlac and Goodwin (2003) point out the need for updating theory courses at the graduate level, while AACN's position paper for integrating nursing theory into master's level curricula was published in 1996, the implications remain that nursing and shared discipline theories must continue as part of the graduate curriculum at the master's level for application to practice.

Based on the need to plan for the role of nurses in advanced practice in the future, Mundinger et al. (2000) reviewed current master's and doctoral level programs in nursing for their similarities and differences. Their focus was on nurse practitioners, owing to the increased recognition of their role in primary care by other disciplines and health care payers. They discuss the need to raise the level of education to a doctorate to prepare nurse practitioners for the full scope of practice for managing all aspects of care. The authors propose a Doctor of Nursing Practice (DNP), similar to the Medical Doctor (MD), the Doctor of Dental Surgery (DDS), and the Doctor of Pharmacy (PharmD), all of which are practice-based, versus the research-focused Doctor of Philosophy (PhD). They point out that other advanced levels of nursing practice could be included for a DNP, such as community health and other clinical specialties.

Mundinger et al. (2000) found three major categories of doctoral degrees in nursing: the Nursing Doctorate (ND), which is an entry to professional nursing that usually does not require a dissertation, but rather requires a clinical practice project that applies research; the Doctor of Nursing (DNS, DNSc, DSN), which focuses on research but emphasizes its application to practice; and the Doctor of Philosophy (PhD), which is research based and emphasizes theory development and testing. The authors believe that the current doctorates do not offer preparation for advanced practice that "is independent, sophisticated, analytical, and cross-site" (p. 327).

Standing and Kramer (2003) further explicate the myriad doctoral degrees used by nursing. They urge that the profession place a moratorium on new titles for degrees until the debate about the purpose of each degree is settled, especially in a time when new programs are underway. Their descriptions of the existing degrees include a discussion of the purposes and underlying philosophies for the degrees and provide a basis for differentiating among the degrees. Members of the American Association of Colleges of Nursing endorsed a position statement on the Practice Doctorate in Nursing at its semi-annual meeting in October 2004 (AACN, 2004c). Detailed information on the statement may be found at: http://www. aacn.nche.edu.

Doctoral education preparation in nursing has long been argued as it applies to research, advanced practice, and education. While Mundinger et al. (2000) and the AACN (2004) position statement make persuasive arguments for the advanced-practice doctorate, there is an equal need for an education doctorate. There are only a few doctoral programs that prepare nursing faculty *per se*, except for some that include courses in curriculum development and instructional design. Thus, the argument is the same for the need to prepare nursing faculty at the doctoral level for specific educator roles and for research in education.

McGivern (2003) proposes that nursing education foster the development of nurse researchers through the integration of research experiences from the baccalaureate to the doctoral level. She reiterates traditional nursing curricula plans with baccalaureate level graduates as consumers of research, master's-prepared nurses as participants in research, and doctoral level nurses as testers of theories and generators of research. Furthermore, she advocates research-intensive tracks from the baccalaureate through the doctorate so that bright young scholars are titillated by research opportunities to become researchers prepared at the doctorate level. It is her belief that schools of nursing with strong track records in research funding and which have three levels of degree preparation (BSN, MSN, and doctorate) should be the institutions of preference for these types of tracks. McGivern supports her thesis with the critical need for research at this time of change for the health care system, the role of nursing, and the Healthy People 2010 goals (U.S. Department of Health and Human Services, 2002). McGivern discusses the role of faculty in these tracks for mentoring students in research and the need to reward their research activities.

Based on McGivern's notion of "the scholar's nursery" and the need for developing nursing researchers, the issue is raised for the equally important demand for nurse clinicians and practitioners, educators, case managers, and administrators. As to education, she advocates integration of pedagogy knowledge into the curriculum of master's and doctorate programs, owing to the frequency that students and graduates in these programs assume teaching roles. This author agrees with this idea; however, nursing education and research at the doctorate level should be available to those nurses interested in focusing on nursing education. There are many other topics in education such as history of education, philosophy, curriculum development, program evaluation, student assessment, instructional design, educational research, and so forth that cannot be completed at the master's level.

McGivern proposes that there should be Centers for Nursing Excellence (Research); this author proposes Centers for Nursing Education and that both centers should be open to international nurses as well. Kirschling (2003) served as a moderator for a panel of international educators (though it was not held in person but rather by correspondence). The major themes of the panel revealed common strategies for recruiting additional nurses into the profession, owing to the worldwide shortage, and a trend toward higher education as the entry into practice. Looking into the future, North American schools of nursing have an obligation to provide the most current findings in research, evidence-based nursing practice, and nursing education for their international colleagues. As the world becomes smaller and health problems become global, North American nurses have the expertise to share their nursing knowledge and practice with nurses from other countries. In so doing, they must avoid the temptation that occurred so often in the past to retain these nurses in the United States instead of ensuring that they return to their home nation to provide nursing services for their people.

Lindeman (2003), in her *Thoughts about the Future and Nursing Education,* suggests two major considerations related to nursing practice in the future. The first is a change from nurses providing direct care to a practice "based on prevention and education" (p.12). The second is that institutions within the health care system will disappear, owing to the portability of technology that allows quality care to be rendered in most any location. Thus, nursing care in hospitals will continue to decrease and nurses will render more care in community settings. Lindeman points out that such practice requires different knowledge sets and skills from those in the hospital and should be taken into account when planning curricula.

Lindeman identified five trends affecting nursing education in the next 5 years: an emphasis on learning and outcomes, competition of traditional schools with virtual universities, seamless education (there should be no barriers between segments of higher education), benchmarking, and findings based on productivity.

▲ NURSING RESEARCH AND ITS INFLUENCE ON NURSING CURRICULA

The National Institute of Nursing Research (NINR) (2004) posted its nursing research themes for the future that reflect much of the discussion thus far. The themes were developed through a series of meetings with experts and at advisory board meetings and roundtable discussions. Each of the themes has implications for content in nursing curricula, research projects for faculty and students, and opportunities for research in the practice setting. The five themes are:

1. Changing Lifestyle Behaviors for Better Health
2. Managing the Effects of Chronic Illness to Improve Quality of Life
3. Identifying Effective Strategies to Reduce Health Disparities
4. Harnessing Advanced Technologies to Serve Human Needs
5. Enhancing the End-of-Life Experience for Patients and Their Families

▲ INDIVIDUAL NURSE RESPONSIBILITIES FOR THE FUTURE

Carpenito (2001) talks about the future and the individual responsibilities of nurses in meeting the challenges of the future. She charges individual nurses to nourish each other and includes specific responsibilities for faculty, students, administrators, managers, and clinical nurses. She lists the behaviors to thrive in nursing as "intellectual honesty and curiosity, assertiveness, compassion, realistic optimism, comfort with imperfection and messes, ability to prioritize, takes work seriously but has fun, hopeful" (p. 3). This places the responsibility on every nurse to become an advocate for the profession by publicizing its vital role in the health care delivery system, providing high-quality nursing care services in collaboration with other disciplines, shaping public policy as it applies to health disparities and services for the unserved and underserved, and advocating for compensation that is appropriate to the professional services rendered.

These words of advice not only apply to individuals, but also provide topics that should be included in nursing curricula. With these in mind and the issues and challenges nursing education faces for the future, the following are curricula offered to readers for discussion, debate, refinement, and perhaps consideration as plans for the future.

▲ SAMPLE FUTURE CURRICULA

Sterubert Speziale (2000) studied Mid-Atlantic schools of nursing in regard to their RN-to-MSN programs. In the process of collecting data, she discovered that these curricula held on to traditional prerequisites for nursing, not taking into account some of the changes in the health care system such as the breakthroughs in genetics research and the need for business administration and economics knowledge. Speziale found that the respondent schools had a wide range of credit awarded for transfer and experiential learning as well as credits required for graduation. This is but one example of the need for uniformity of credits, courses, and requirements across all schools of nursing, if not for the logic of it, at least for the marketability of schools to potential students wishing to continue their education.

Until professional nursing education transforms into doctoral education, the career step ladder curriculum is essential for the majority of nurses who are educated at the diploma, associate degree, and baccalaureate levels to continue their education and, at the same time, increase the number of entry-level doctorates in nursing that model nursing education by the mid-21st century. Table 15.1 provides parallel career step ladder and entry-level graduate curricula that propose a unified approach to nursing education, allowing for entry into practice at several points, maintaining the career ladder option for persons wishing to enter the workforce in a short time with re-entry later, and offering a nonstop option to facilitate persons completing a doctorate in nursing much like other professions.

The proposed curriculum is not revolutionary; there are no new concepts that have not been discussed in the past. Instead, traditional courses in nursing are included and the pre- and corequisites are much the same as current curricula, except for the addition of proficiency in a language other than the student's primary one, genetics, economics, and computer science. These latter additions should be self-explanatory for their relevance to the nursing curriculum, that is, the multicultural and ethnic population for whom nursing cares, the breakthroughs in genetic research, the major role of health care economics in the delivery systems, and the ever-expanding world of technology-driven communications.

The two parallel curricula in Table 15.1 are much the same, although the order may be varied according to the student's place in the respective programs, (i.e., undergraduate or graduate levels). As much as possible, generic labels are assigned to courses to indicate the core content and concepts in courses, recognizing that each institution has different titles for courses that contain the same or similar content. The lower- and upper-division level courses are prescriptive; however, the choices at the graduate levels are flexible, allowing for each institution to determine the pre- and co-requisites and nursing courses for the functional roles or practice specialties at the master's level and for the selected program of practice, education, or research at the doctorate level.

The major argument for or against professional education becomes apparent in the undergraduate programs. If the curriculum is maintained at 65 units for completion of the lower division and a total of 125 units for the lower and upper divisions, and the necessary pre- and co-requisite knowledge for nursing are retained, there is no room for electives. Adding electives or prerequisites to nursing pre-or corequisites adds to the length of the program and, thereby, the time for students to enter the workforce and to meet health care demands. An analysis of the prescribed curriculum reveals that the nursing major has a total of 65 nursing units (a little over half of the total 125) with the remaining in the arts and sciences. There also isn't room for the institutions' general education requirements that might or might not allow for double counting from the requirements prescribed in the nursing major.

For too long, nursing has been dominated by other disciplines in academe that have a major influence on the length, composition, and type of degree nursing will have. This is especially true in academic health science institutions and state-supported systems of higher education. Diers' (1976) article describing the combined basic-graduate program for college graduates at Yale University discusses this very issue in a school that can claim itself as the first to offer nursing in an institution of higher learning. Convincing other disciplines in higher-education institutions of the need to educate nurses with a strong foundation in the arts and sciences, and at the same time prescribing the nursing curriculum that remains within the usual number of units for associate degrees (65 to 70) and the baccalaureate (120 to 125) is difficult. There are numerous courses that nurses value as foundations for practice such as history, the arts, political science, and even business as it applies to health care. Yet, there is no room for courses in these disciplines in the 125-unit nursing degree program.

The proposed unified curriculum in Table 15.1 is ideal but unrealistic, owing to the aforementioned issues. Yet, nurse educators should strive to revise or build curricula that are close to the unit requirements rather than continuing to require excess units in undergraduate degrees. At the same time, uniform curricula for both levels that allow seamless entry into the next level are necessary to provide the existing nurse workforce with career ladder opportunities and options for the current applicants to nursing programs.

These issues related to undergraduate education elucidate the need for nursing to move into graduate education. If nurse educators try to integrate the missing arts and sciences components into the curriculum, they add units far exceeding the usual 120 to 125 for the baccalaureate. One needs only to interview nurses who are 40+ years old with baccalaureates to discover the excess number of credits in their degree work and realize the enormity of the problem and the injustices nurses suffered in gaining education beyond the diploma and associate degree with no academic recognition of their additional work. Going one step further, nurses in that age group or older who hold master's and/or doctorates suffer the same overabundance of credits, earning far more than their colleagues in medicine, pharmacology, education, engineering, religion, and law. Table 15.1 summarizes current requirements for nursing degrees and can serve in the interim while schools of nursing with bravado develop doctoral programs that accommodate the foundations of a liberal, scientific, and professional education that can serve as a model for the future.

Based on the curricula in Table 15.1, the argument for "entry into practice" ends with the idea that a candidate is eligible for licensure at various points of the education track, such as after completing the associate degree (lower division) and 3-month internship, the bachelor of science with an internship, the master's with an internship, or, finally, the doctorate with completion of a clinical residency. Thus, students have a choice for entering practice through licensure at the associate's, bachelor's, master's, or doctorate degree levels. At the same time, the curricula contain the same courses or content, thus allowing nurses to enter at the next step of their education to continue their career opportunities. If these generic curricula were adapted by schools of nursing, there would be no need for challenge examinations and repetition of knowledge and skills already assimilated.

Schools of nursing bear the responsibility for evaluating the credentials of applicants with prior education or degrees not in nursing. There is a need for flexibility in granting credit for courses equivalent to those pre- and corequisites in nursing and nursing courses (for registered nurses [RNs] with degrees not in nursing) to enter into the curricula and to complete the next academic level. Examples are RNs with baccalaureates in other disciplines and non-nurses with baccalaureates or higher degrees who matriculate directly into master's programs rather than repeating the baccalaureate. Of course, RNs need upper-division level nursing courses or their equivalent and non-nurses need nursing courses equivalent to the baccalaureate but offered at the graduate level before entering master's or doctorate level nursing courses.

Another divergence from the traditional curriculum occurs in the graduate program proposed in Table 15.1. It moves advanced-practice roles such as nurse practitioners, midwives, anesthetists, and clinical specialists to the doctoral level. It is time to make this move, because these programs far exceed the usual 30 to 36 units expected for master's degrees. While changing the undergraduate programs to entry-level graduate programs will take time, these advanced-practice programs should be relatively easy to convert in the near future. If they do not initiate this change, the unfairness of adding more units, time, money spent by students to an overloaded curriculum with no credential except a master's will continue. Mundinger et al.'s (2000) arguments for a Doctor of Nursing Practice apply in this instance.

It is apparent that nursing needs to expand entry-level doctorate programs to accommodate the vast body of knowledge and skills expected of the professional nurse today and in the future. It has been more than 50 years since baccalaureate and associate degree programs began to flourish. In that time, major revolutions in technology and health-related sciences have taken place. It is no wonder that the undergraduate programs can no longer accommodate all of the new knowledge and skills that must be included in a nursing curriculum. Table 15.2 introduces an 8-year entry-level doctorate curriculum with a ninth year for a PhD option. The program is divided into a 4-year prenursing program ending with a baccalaureate and continuing into a 4-year school of nursing. See Table 15.2 for an outline of the program.

The development of entry-level doctoral programs should not disenfranchise education programs that prepare nurses at the undergraduate and master's levels. In fact, increasing numbers of programs will become graduate programs and the need for foundation courses will still exist at the lower- and upper-division levels of undergraduate education. A prenursing curriculum in the undergraduate program should contain introductory courses to nursing and health care and require faculty at that level. Nursing courses in graduate level programs require nursing faculty members who are expert in the specialties to facilitate students' assimilation of the knowledge and skills required for the specialties.

Table 15.2 outlines a prenursing and nursing school curriculum plan that should be considered for the future. It is dangerous to set a deadline but, ideally, the mid-21st century is a desirable target. To accomplish the task, existing and new programs could begin to initiate these programs and eventually phase out the old. While it is difficult to predict the development of a nationwide licensing program that could help to define a unified code of requirements for licensure eligibility, these new programs would continue to meet licensing requirements. The entry-level doctorate programs could be of two types: the research-focused PhD and the practice-focused DNSc or DNP.

The advantages to the entry-level doctorate program are numerous. It would facilitate high school graduates' entry into a nursing program with graduation 8 years away, thus producing expert clinicians, researchers, and educators who are relatively young in age. If these candidates choose not to pursue nursing in the first 4 years, their options are many for changing majors. The prenursing curriculum provides a strong scientific and liberal arts background for the increasingly complex professional world of nursing. Graduates of the programs will be on equal footing with other health care professionals. The 4-year nursing school would be open to applicants with baccalaureates who seek major or career changes. The 8-year total curriculum plan provides the time for in-depth education and the production of quality graduates prepared for practice, teaching, and research roles.

If the profession embraces this transformation of nursing education, then it must come to grips with the reality that there are roles for personnel such as the licensed practical/vocational nurses. The proposed model calls for an expansion of that technical model comparable to the expansion of technical and support services within the health care system. It is logical that these programs fall into the community college genre, thus raising the specter of the "Civil War" in nursing yet again. This author leaves that debate to the nurse educators reading this text and the nursing profession over the next few decades.

▲ SUMMARY

Though the world order, the national society, and the health care system change so rapidly and it is difficult to predict the future, there are prevailing trends that should have an impact on the development and evaluation of nursing curricula over the next decade. If nursing chooses not to respond to these changes, the danger is that education will not transform and instead will maintain a status quo existence much as it has in the past 50 years. This could mean that the profession will continue to be splintered with less opportunity for it to help in shaping public policy toward optimal health care for the populace. Nurse educators have a responsibility to work with their colleagues in practice and research to develop curricula that prepare nurses who are competent and caring and who are scholars and researchers. A nursing education system for the future will have the following characteristics:

1. Clearly defined levels of education and differentiated practice based on education and experience
2. At least a 3-month internship in a selected arena of practice following graduation from all levels of professional nursing education
3. Quality institutions of higher education that specialize in the preparation of staff nurses for entry into practice in a timely fashion
4. Quality institutions that focus on the faculty role of excellence in teaching, community service, and the application of knowledge from nursing science and related disciplines
5. Quality institutions of higher education that specialize in the preparation of nurses to provide evidence-based advanced-practice nursing services for families and aggregates
6. Students and faculty who are active participants in nursing and related disciplines' research activities
7. Quality institutions of higher education that specialize in the preparation of staff nurses for entry into practice and for providing advanced-practice nursing services for families and aggregates
8. Academic and health science centers for nursing research and development for the advancement of nursing science through evidence-based practice; testing of theories; the development of new theories, concepts, and models; and educational innovations on the national and international levels

DISCUSSION QUESTIONS

1. What major changes in the health care system are occurring that call for an immediate response from nursing education for curriculum revision? Do these changes take into account the future? How would you go about revising the curriculum in a timely fashion?

2. What actions do faculty need to take to integrate interdisciplinary theories, concepts, and clinical practice into the curriculum plan? Which of the disciplines would have the highest priority for placement in the curriculum? Do you believe that faculty other than nursing could teach nursing courses? Explain your answer.

3. What teaching and learning strategies should be integrated into the curriculum plan for meeting the needs of an increasingly diverse student body? Describe how nursing can recruit and retain racially/ethnically diverse faculty and what effect they can have on the education of a diverse student body.

4. Given the rapid changes in the health care and education systems and the ongoing shortage of nurses, what changes in nursing education do you envision within the next 5 to 10 years?

5. What strategies for changing nursing education worked in the past, and how can these success stories apply to needed changes in nursing education today? What are the lessons from the past that prohibited nursing from moving its educational agenda forward? How can today's nurse educators use these lessons to bring about change?

LEARNING ACTIVITIES

Student Learning Activities

1. Synthesize the information in this text into a "Dream School of Nursing." Develop a curriculum that prepares nurses for practice 10 years from now, keeping in mind that practice and the setting in which it is delivered will be different. Let your imagination run wild!

Faculty Development Activities

1. Hold a faculty meeting focused on brainstorming and let creative thoughts flow freely. List the characteristics of the ideal nurse prepared to practice 5 to 10 years from now. Examine these characteristics and decide how a curriculum can be developed that provides the kind of education necessary to prepare this kind of nurse. Focus on creativity and newer theories of learning. Compare these ideas to your existing curriculum. How can it be transformed into the one you envision?

REFERENCES

Aiken, L. H., Clarke, S. P., Cheung, R. B., Sloane, D. M., & Silber, J. H. (2003). Educational levels of hospital nurses and surgical patient mortality. *The Journal of the American Medical Association, 290*(12), 1617–1623.

Aiken, L. H., Clarke, S. P., Sloane, D. M., Sochalski, M. J., & Silber, J. H. (2002). Hospital nurse staffing and patient mortality, nurse burnout, and job dissatisfaction. *The Journal of the American Medical Association, 288*(16), 1987–1993.

American Association of Colleges of Nursing. (1996). *The essentials of master's education for advanced practice nursing.* Washington, DC: Author.

American Association of Colleges of Nursing. (2002). *Interdisciplinary education and practice.* Position Paper. Washington, DC: Author. Retrieved May 31, 2003, from http://www.aacn.nche.edu/Publications/postions/interdis.htm

American Association of Colleges of Nursing. (2004a). *White paper on faculty shortages in baccalaureate and graduate programs: Scope of the problem and strategies for enhancing the supply.* Washington DC: Author. Retrieved June 24, 2004, from http://www.aacnb.nche/Publications/WhitePapers/FacultyShortages.htm

American Association of Colleges of Nursing. (2004b). *White paper on the role of the clinical nurse leader.* Retrieved June 24, 2004, from http://www.aacn.nche.edu/NewNurse/index.htm

American Association of Colleges of Nursing (2004c). AACN position statement on the practice doctorate in nursing. Retrived November 3, 2004 from: http://www.aacn.nche.edu.

American Nurses Association. (1965). *Educational preparation for nurse practitioners and assistants to nurses: A position paper.* New York: Author.

Bargagliotti, L. A. (2003). Reframing nursing education to renew the profession. *Nursing Education Perspectives, 24*(1), 12–16.

Berlin, L. E., & Sechrist, K. R. (2002). The shortage of doctorally prepared nursing faculty: A dire situation. *Nursing Outlook, 50*(2), 50–56.

Blegen, M. A., & Vaughn, T. (1998). A multisite study of nurse staffing and patient occurrences. *Nursing Economics, 16*(4),196–203.

Boughn, S. (2001). Why women and men choose nursing. *Nursing and Health Care Perspectives, 22*(1), 14–19.

Braithwaite, D. (2002). Mentoring relationships with conducting international research. *Journal of Multicultural Nursing & Health, 8*(1), 36–41.

Bridgman, M. (1953). *Collegiate education for nursing.* New York: Russell Sage Foundation.

Brown, B. J. (2002). From the editor. *Nursing Administration Quarterly,* 26, 5, VI-VIII.

Burton, D. A., (2003). Are you man enough...to be a nurse? *Nursing Education Perspectives, 24*(1), 6–7.

California Strategic Planning Committee for Nursing. (2001). *Anticipated need for faculty in California schools of nursing for school years 2001-2002 and 2002-2003.* Irvine, CA: Author. Retrieved June 25, 2004, from http://www.ucihs.uci.edu/cspcn

Carpenito, L. J. (2001). The future of nursing. *Nursing Forum, 36*(2), 3–4.

Cloonan, P. A., Davis, F. D., & Burnett, C. B. (1999). Interdisciplinary education in clinical ethics: A work in progress. *Holistic Nursing Practice, 13*(2), 12–19.

Cullen, L. T. (2003, May 12). I want your job. *Time,* 52–56.

DeYoung, S., & Bliss, J. B. (1995). Nursing faculty – An endangered species? *Journal of Professional Nursing, 11*(2), 84–88.

Diers, D. (1976). A combined basic-graduate program for college graduates. *Nursing Outlook, 24*(2), 92–98.

Fitzpatrick, M. A. (2002). Wanted: Courageous crusaders. *Nursing Management, 33*(7),4.

Greene, D. L., Allan, J. D., & Henderson, T. (2003). The role of states in financing nursing education. National conference of state legislatures. The nursing workforce. Institute for primary care and workforce analysis. Washington DC: National Conference of State Legislature.

Herdrich, R. (2004). Creating new avenues for learning: Covenant's nurse residency program. *NURSINGMATTERS, 15*(2), 1,3.

Keating, S. B., Rutledge, D., Sargent, A., & Walker, P. (2003). A demonstration model of the California competency-based role differentiation model. *Managed Care Quarterly, 11*(1), 40–46.

Institute of Medicine. (2003). *Health professions education: A bridge to quality.* Retrieved June 25, 2004, from http://www.iom.edu/report.asp?id=5914

Kelly, C. M. (2002). Investing in the future of nursing education: A cry for action. *Nursing Education Perspective, 23*(1), 24–29.

Kirschling, J. M. (2003). Nursing education: Global perspectives. *Reflections on Nursing LEADERSHIP,* fourth quarter, 21–24.

Lindeman, C. (2003). *Thoughts about the future and nursing education.* Paper Presented at the Annual Meeting of the California Deans and Directors of Nursing, Sacramento, CA.

Leininger, M. M. (2001). Current issues in nursing anthropology in nursing education and services. *Western Journal of Nursing Research, 23*(8), 795–806.

McEwen, M. (2000). Teaching theory at the master's level: Report of a national survey of theory instructors. *Journal of Professional Nursing, 16*(6), 354–361.

McGivern, D. O. (2003). The scholars' nursery. *Nursing Outlook, 51*(2), 59–64.

Morin, K. H., Patterson, B. J., Kurtz, B., & Brzowski, B. (1999). Clinical scholarship.

Mothers' responses to care given by male nursing students during and after birth. *Journal of Nursing Scholarship, 31*(1), 83–87.

Mundinger, M. O., Cook, S. S., Lenz, E. R., Piacentini, K., Auerhahn, C., & Smith, J. (2000). Assuring quality and access in advanced practice nursing: challenge to nurse educators. *Journal of Professional Nursing, 16*(6), 322–329.

National Institute of Nursing Research. (2004). *Research themes for the future.* Retrieved June 24, 2004, from http://www.nih.gov/ninr/research/themes.doc

National Council of State Boards of Nursing. (2004). *Evidence-based nursing education.* Retrieved June 24, 2004, from http://www.ncsbn.org/regulation/nursingeducation_nursing_education_evidence_based.asp

Sackett, D. L., Straus, S., Richardson, S., Rosenberg, W., Haynes, R. B. (2000) *Evidence-based medicine: How to practice and teach EBM* (2nd ed.). London: Churchill Livingstone.

Smith, J., & Crawford, L. (2003). The link between perceived adequacy of preparation to practice, nursing error, and perceived difficulty of entry-level practice. *JONA'S Healthcare, Law, Ethics, and Regulations, 5*(4), 100–103.

Sochalski, J. (2002). Nursing shortage redux: Turning the corner on an enduring problem. *Health Affairs, 21*(5), 157–164.

Sperhac, A. M., & Goodwin, L. D. (2003). Using multiple data sources for curriculum revision. *Journal of Pediatric Health Care, 17*(4), 169–175.

Standing, T. S., & Kramer, F. M. (2003). Preparing nurses for clinical and educational leadership. *Reflections on Nursing LEADERSHIP,* fourth quarter, 35–37.

Stephen, H. (1998). Nurse teacher shortages threaten training quality. *Nursing Standard, 13*(7), 7.

Sterubert Speziale, H. J. (2002). RN-MSN admission practices and curricula in the Mid-Atlantic region. *Nursing Education, 23*(6), 294–299.

Tanner, C. A. (2002). Education's response to the nursing shortage: Leadership, innovation, and publication. *Journal of Nursing Education, 41*(11), 467–468.

Tucker-Allen, S. (2003). Increasing minority nurses means increasing minority nursing faculty members. *The American Black Nursing Faculty Journal, 14*(1), 3.

U.S. Department of Health and Human Services. (2002). *Healthy people 2010: Understanding and improving health* (vol. I and II). Boston: Jones and Bartlett.

U.S. Department of Health and Human Services, Health Resources and Services Administration, Bureau of Health Professions. (2003). *Nursing. National Advisory Council on Nursing Education and Practice: A National Agenda for Nursing Workforce Racial/Ethnic Diversity. Executive Summary.* Retrieved May 30, 2003, from, http://bhpr.hrsa.gov/nurswing.nacnep/divrepex.htm

U.S. Department of Health and Human Services, Health Resources and Services Administration, Bureau of Health Professions, Division of Nursing. (2001). *The registered nurse population. National survey of registered nurses– March 2000. Preliminary findings.* Retrieved May 25, 2003, from   http://bhpr.hrsa.gov/healthworkforce/reports/rnsurvey/default.htm

U.S. Department of Health and Human Services, Health Resources and Services Administration, Bureau of Health Professions, National Center for Health Workforce Analysis. (2002). *The projected supply, demand, and shortages of registered nurses: 2000-2020.* Retrieved June 24, 2004, from http://bhpr.hrsa.gov/healthworkforce/reports/rnproject/report.htm#supplytrends

Zungolo, E. (2002). Nursing organizations: Visiting the past/envisioning the future. *Nursing Education Perspectives, 23*(5), 106–107.

Zungolo, E. (2003). Nursing and academic mergers of the health sciences: A critique. *Nursing Outlook, 51*(2), 52–58.

GLOSSARY

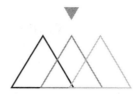

A

Accreditation: A process that education programs undergo to receive recognition for meeting basic standards or criteria set by national, regional, or state organizations.

Affective Domain: A domain of knowledge that deals with individual feelings or emotions that are reflected in values and interests.

Andragogy: The science of adult learning.

Articulation: The process by which students can transfer credits from one educational institution to another for previously completed courses or degrees. Institutions usually have formal articulation agreements for facilitating transfer between specific programs such as nursing (e.g., associate degree to baccalaureate).

Asynchronous Learning: Learning that takes place between the teacher and learners through web-based education and occurs at varying times.

Axiology: "Seeks to describe that which is ethical, logical, and of value" (Csokasy, 2002, p. 32).

B

Behavioral Domain: "The domain of knowledge involved with developing knowledgeable, acculturated and competent individuals" (Hauenstein, 1998, p. 3). The behavioral domain consists of acquisition, assimilation, performance, and aspiration (a holistic approach to learning).

Behaviorism: The belief that "instruction is achieved by observable, measurable and controllable objectives set by the instructor and met by students" (Leonard, 2002, p. 16).

Benchmarking: The setting of specific standards or criteria by which an educational program can measure its success and/or compare itself to other like institutions.

Body Politic: The people power(s) behind the official government within a community. It is composed of the major political forces and the people who exert influence within the community.

C

Career Ladder Concept: In nursing practice and education, the concept that one can enter nursing practice at a certain basic level of education and continue along certain intervals— for example, from a nursing aide to licensed practical/vocational nurse to registered nurse through an associate degree or baccalaureate, master's, or doctoral education. Depending on the educational program, experience may be credited toward degree work as well as previously completed course work.

Cocurriculum: See *Informal curriculum*.

Continuous Quality Improvement (CQI): The implementation of a system designed for ongoing evaluation, analysis of findings, and implementation of plans for improvement within an organization.

Cognitive Domain: The domain of knowledge that addresses intellectual skills and types of knowledge.

Cognitivism: "The belief that human thinking and learning are similar to that of computer information processing" (Leonard, 2002, p. 29).

Community: "People and the relationships that emerge among them as they develop and use in common some agencies and institutions and a physical environment; a locality-based entity composed of systems of formal organizations reflecting society's institutions, information groups, and aggregates" (Stanhope & Lancaster, 2000, p. G-5).

Community-Based Nursing: The provision of nursing care that takes place in the community setting and focuses on the care of individuals, families, aggregates, and communities.

Component Display Theory (CDT): A learning theory by Merrill (1983) that puts the learner in control of the sequencing of learning based on the instructional components in a lesson plan. The cognitive bases of the theory include associative memory (a hierarchical network structure) and algorithmic memory (using schema).

Concept-Mapping: The graphic demonstration of the learners' thinking processes to illustrate the interconnectedness of concepts and data.

Conceptual Framework: "A logical grouping of related concepts or theories, usually created to draw together several different aspects that are relevant to a complex situation such as a practice setting or an educational program. Term used synonymously with theoretic framework. A knowledge from within the empirics pattern" (Chinn & Kramer, 1999, p. 252).

Constructivism: "The belief that learners, having had some prior knowledge and experience as a basis from which to test their hypotheses, build upon their own set of content to solve a particular problem posed by the instructor. Constructivism is a learner-centric educational paradigm, in which content is constructed by the learners in a team-based, collaborative learning, constructivist learning environment rather than by the instructor" (Leonard, 2002, pp. 37-39).

Core Curricula: Courses within a curriculum that are common to and required for all majors (or tracks) and that meet a portion of graduation requirements.

Creative Thinking: A global or holistic pattern of thinking. It is emotive, intuitive, and creative and is a visual, tactile, or kinesthetic model of the thinking process.

Criterion-Referenced Instruction (CRI): Focuses on the job activities of learners and seeks to determine the specific competencies (knowledge and skills) needed to perform the job successfully.

Critical Thinking: "...The intellectually disciplined process of actively and skillfully conceptualizing, applying, analyzing, synthesizing, and/or evaluating information gathered from, or generated by, observation, experience, reflection, reasoning, or communication, as a guide to belief and action" (Scriven & Paul, 2002, p. 1).

Cultural Competence: "A set of academic and interpersonal skills that allow an individual to increase their understanding and appreciation of cultural differences and similarities within, among and between groups. This requires a willingness and ability to draw on community-based values, traditions, and customs and to work with knowledgeable persons of both and from the community in developing targeted interventions, communications and other supports" (Health Resources and Services Administration, Bureau of Health Professions, Division of Nursing, 2004, p. 1).

Curriculum: The formal plan of study that provides the philosophical underpinnings, goals, and guidelines for the delivery of a specific educational program.

Curriculum Evaluation: "The process of delineating, obtaining, and providing information useful for making decisions and judgments about a program of learning" (Applegate, 1998, p. 179).

D

Demographics: Data that describe the characteristics of a population (e.g., age, gender, socioeconomic status, ethnicity, education levels).

Distance Education: Any learning experience that takes place a distance away from the parent institution's home campus or central headquarters.

Discovery Learning Theory: A theory that believes "learners are more likely to remember concepts if they discover them on their own, apply them to their knowledge base, and structure them to fit their own backgrounds and life experiences" (Leonard, 2002, p. 38).

E

Educational Taxonomy: A form of classifying, categorizing, clarifying, and defining the features of elements found on a continuum, from simple to complex.

Empirical: An epistemological way of knowing that reflects observation and experimentation.

Entry-level Programs: Programs that prepare students for eligibility to take the licensure examination (NCLEX) for registered nurses (RNs). The programs include associate degree, baccalaureate, master's, and doctorate levels.

Epistemology: "Is the study of nature, the validity of knowledge, and how the truth differs from opinion" (Csokasy, 2002, p. 32).

Evaluation: The determination of the worth of a thing. It includes obtaining information for use in judging the worth of a program, product, procedure, or objective or the potential for utility of alternative approaches to attain specific objectives" (Worthen & Sanders, 1974, p. 19).

Evidence-Based Practice: The integration of the best research with clinical expertise and patient values (Sackett, Straus, Richardson, Rosenberg, & Haynes, 2000).

External Frame Factors: Those factors that influence curriculum development in the environment and outside the parent institution.

Extracurricular Activities: See *Informal curriculum.*

F

Formative Evaluation: Assessment that takes place during the implementation of the program or curriculum. It can also be viewed as process evaluation. In education, this type of evaluation is often linked to course or level objectives.

Frame Factors: The external and internal factors that influence, impinge upon, and/or enhance educational programs and curricula. As a conceptual model, they serve to collect, organize, and analyze information that is useful for the development and evaluation of curricula. There are two major categories of frame factors: external and internal.

G

Generic Programs: See *Entry-level programs.*

Goal-based Evaluation: Based on the stated goals of the entity undergoing evaluation. It is frequently used in education and tied to the stated goals, purpose, and end-of-program objectives of the program or curriculum.

Goal-free Evaluation: A method for evaluators to assess and judge some thing or entity. That person has no prior knowledge of the entity (program or curriculum) that he or she is evaluating. The person must be an expert in the field of evaluation and in the type of entity under evaluation. The value of this type of evaluation is that it is relatively bias-free.

I

Interdisciplinary Education: "An educational approach in which two or more disciplines collaborate in the learning process with the goal of fostering interprofessional interactions that enhance the practice of each discipline. Such interdisciplinary education is based on mutual understanding and respect for the actual and potential contributions of the disciplines" (AACN, 2002, p.1).

Informal Curriculum: The activities that take place outside of the formal or planned curriculum-for example, convocations, ceremonies, athletic activities and events, and student organization meetings (see also *Co-curriculum* and *Extracurricular activities*).

Instructional Transaction Theory: A learning theory that focuses on individual learners who interact with a set of knowledge objects to perform a specific job and progressively build competence (Merrill, 1996).

Internal Frame Factors: Those factors that influence curriculum development and are within the environment of the parent institution and the program itself.

L

Learning Domain: A class or category of knowledge and the learning processes involved in which abilities or types of knowledge are defined based on the relative complexity or difficulty.

M

Mentor: An experienced clinician who is either assigned formally or selected informally by mutual agreement between the mentor and the person being mentored and acts as counselor, teacher, and advocate for that person.

Metaparadigm: The discipline of nursing's four major concepts around which theory and models are organized. The four domains are nursing (the profession), person (client or consumer of care), health, and environment.

Metaphysics: "Seeks to answer the basic questions of reality and what is real and true" (Csokasy, 2002, p. 32).

Multiple Intelligences: According to Gardner (2000), there are eight intelligences: musical, linguistic, logical-mathematical, spatial, bodily-kinesthetic, interpersonal, intrapersonal, and naturalist.

N

Needs Assessment: The process for collecting and analyzing information that can influence decisions to initiate a new program or revise an existing one.

Noetic: An epistemological way of knowing that reflects an intellectual understanding.

Nonsectarian: Not associated with a religious organization.

O

Operant Conditioning: A part of behaviorism learning theory that centers on the reinforcement of a response to a stimulus.

Outcome Evaluation: Similar to goal-based evaluation; however, it may include other items to measure outcomes (e.g., graduation rates, NCLEX results, career success for its graduates).

P

Pedagogy: "The art, science, or profession of teaching" (Merriam-Webster, 2004).

Philosophy: The critical examination of the grounds for fundamental beliefs and an analysis of the basic concepts employed in the expression of such beliefs (Encyclopedia Britannica, 2003).

Preceptor: A clinician assigned to a new employee or student who provides knowledge regarding nursing science, clinical skills, agency policies and procedures, and professional behaviors for the employee or student in the provision of nursing care.

Process Evaluation: See *Formative evaluation.*

Program Approval: A process whereby regulating bodies review programs to ensure consumer safety. Nursing education programs are subject to state regulations that are usually administered by the State Board of Nursing.

Psychomotor Domain: The development of physical abilities and skills that result from the input of information and content.

Q

Quality Assurance: "Consistently meeting product specifications or getting things right the first time, every time" (Sallis, 2002, p.17).

Quality Control: "The detection and elimination of components or final products that are not up to standard" (Sallis, 2002, p.17).

R

Rational: An epistemological way of knowing that reflects understanding by the process of reasoning.

Regulatory: A form of approval, recognition, or accreditation required by a federal, state, or provincial government agency.

Research: "The activity aimed at obtaining generalizable knowledge by contriving and testing claims about relationships among variables or describing generalizable phenomena. This knowledge, which may result in theoretical models, functional relationships, or descriptions, may be obtained by empirical or other systematic methods, and may or may not have immediate application" (Worthen & Sanders, 1974, p. 19).

S

Satellite Campuses: Programs that offer the curriculum in whole or in part in off-campus sites from the parent institution.

Sectarian: Associated with or supported by a religious organization.

Social Learning Theory: The belief that learning occurs through imitation of others.

Standardized Patient (SP): A person who is trained to portray an actual patient by simulating an illness.

State-Regulatory Agencies: Agencies that recognize or approve colleges, universities, or programs for operation with the state as governed by state statutes.

Stimulus-Response Theory: A theory of learning that proposes that learning occurs through close associations between stimuli and responses to them. It is believed that these associations guide all behavior, including learning.

Subsumption Theory of Learning: New material learned in a school setting that is related to previously presented ideas and concepts and that is processed and extant to the cognitive structures of the learner's brain.

Summative Evaluation: Takes place at the end of the program and measures the final outcome. In education, summative evaluation is often linked to the goal(s) or purpose of the program.

Synchronous Learning: Learning that takes place simultaneously with live interactions between the teacher and learners through web-based education.

T

Theoretic Framework: See *Conceptual framework.*

Threaded discussion: a form of asynchronous, web-based discussion that tracks the entries of students and the teacher according to selected topics.

Total Quality Management (TQM): Continually assessing an educational program, correcting errors as they occur, and continually improving the quality of the program.

Transformative Learning Theory: Assumes that individual learners have their own perspectives and expectations about the world that influence the meaning derived from personal experiences. Learning, therefore, takes place when the individual changes his or her perspectives concerning the meaning of certain phenomena.

V

Videoconferencing/Teleconferencing: An interactive delivery system of education that transmits learning materials through cable or closed circuit television.

W

Web-Based Education: An educational system that utilizes computer technology to deliver learning materials through synchronous or asynchronous activities.

REFERENCES

American Association of Colleges of Nursing. (2002). *Interdisciplinary education and practice.* Position Paper. Washington, D.C. Author. Retrieved May 31, 2003 from: http://www.aacn.nche.edu/Publications/postions/interdis.htm.

Applegate, M.H. (1998). Curriculum evaluation. In D. Billings & J. Halstead (Eds.). *Teaching in nursing: A guide for faculty.* Philadelphia: WB Saunders.

Chinn, P.L. and Kramer, M.K. (1999). *Theory and nursing. Integrated knowledge development. Fifth edition.* St. Louis: Mosby.

Csokasy, J.C. (Jan. 2002). A congruent curriculum: Philosophical integrity from philosophy to outcomes. *Journal of Nursing Education.* 41 (1), 32–33.

Encyclopaedia Britannica. "Philosophy." Encyclopædia Britannica Retrieved February 7, 2003, from Encyclopædia Britannica Online.

Gardner, H. (2000). *Intelligence reframed: Multiple intelligences for the 21st century.* Boulder, CO: Basic Books: Perseus.

Hauenstein, A.D. (1998). A Conceptual Framework for Educational Objectives: A Holistic Approach to Traditional Taxonomies. New York: University Press of America.

Health Resources and Services Administration, Bureau of Health Professions, Division of Nursing. *Other definitions of cultural competence: Division of Nursing.* Retrieved November 4, 2004 from: http://bhpr.hrsa.gov/diversity/cultcomp.htm.

Leonard, D.C. (2002). *Learning theories A to Z.* Westport, CT: Greenwood Press.

Merriam-Webster (2004) Collegiate Dictionary. *Pedagogy.* Retrieved November 3, 2004, from: http://www.m-w.com.

Merrill, M.D. (1983). *Component display theory.* In C. Reigeluth (ed.). *Instructional design theories and models.* Mahwah, NJ: Lawrence Erlbaum Associates.

Merrill, M.D. (1996). Instructional transaction theory: Instructional design based on knowledge objects. *Educational Psychology* 33, 30–37.

Sackett, D.L., Straus, S., Richardson, S., Rosenberg, W., Haynes, R.B. (2000) *Evidence-based medicine: how to practice and teach EBM.* 2d ed. London, U.K.: Churchill Livingstone.

Sallis, E. (2002). *Total Quality Management in Education. Third Edition.* London: Kogan Page Ltd.

Scriven, M. and Paul, R. (2004). Defining critical thinking. Retrieved from the World Wide Web, November 3, 2004.: http://www.criticalthinking.org/University/univclass/Defining.html).

Stanhope, M. and Lancaster, J. (2000). *Community and Public Health Nursing. Fifth Edition.* St. Louis: Mosby.

Worthen, B.R. & Sanders, J.R. (1974). *Educational Evaluation: Theory and Practice.* Belmont, CA: Wadsworth Publishing Company.

INDEX

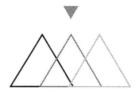

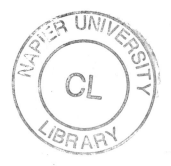